SPORTS TRAINING PRINCIPLES

6th Edition

WITHDRAWN

8 MAR 2024

D0322978

3 8025 00608963 8

SPORTS TRAINING PRINCIPLES

6th Edition

FRANK W. DICK

YORK ST. JOHN
LIBRARY & INFORMATION
SERVICES

BLOOMSBURY

LONDON · BERLIN · NEW YORK · SYDNEY

Note: While every effort has been made to ensure that the content of this book is as technically accurate and as sound as possible, neither the author nor the publishers can accept responsibility for any injury or loss sustained as a result of the use of this material.

Published by Bloomsbury Publishing Plc
50 Bedford Square
London WC1B 3DP
www.bloomsbury.com

Bloomsbury is a trademark of Bloomsbury Publishing Plc

Sixth edition 2014, Fifth edition 2007, Fourth edition 2002, Third edition 1997,
Second edition 1989, First edition published in 1980 by Lepus Books,
an imprint of Henry Kimpton (Publishers) Ltd

Copyright © 1980, 1989, 1997, 2002, 2007, 2014 Frank W. Dick

ISBN (print): 9781472905277
ISBN (epub): 9781472905284
ISBN (epdf): 9781472905291

All rights reserved. No part of this publication may be reproduced in any form or by any means – graphic, electronic or mechanical, including photocopying, recording, taping or information storage and retrieval systems – without the prior permission in writing of the publishers.

Frank W. Dick has asserted his rights under the Copyright, Design and Patents Act, 1988, to be identified as the author of this work.

A CIP catalogue record for this book is available from the British Library.

Acknowledgements
Cover photograph © Shutterstock
Inside photographs © All inside images © Shutterstock.com with the exception of the following: p.102 © Daniel Goodings / Shutterstock.com; p.116 © Steve Yager / Shutterstock.com; p.156 © Ike Li / Shutterstock.com; p.270 © Radu Razvan / Shutterstock.com; p. 284 © Sergey Golotvin / Shutterstock.com
Illustrations by Dave Saunders and Dave Gardner
Commissioning Editor: Kirsty Schaper
Editor: Sarah Cole

This book is produced using paper that is made from wood grown in managed, sustainable forests. It is natural, renewable and recyclable. The logging and manufacturing processes conform to the environmental regulations of the country of origin.

Typeset in Minion by Seagull Design
Printed and bound in Great Britain by CPI Group (UK) Ltd, Croydon CRO 4YY

10 9 8 7 6 5 4 3 2 1

CONTENTS

Part 5 Planning the Programme

PREFACE

It has always fascinated me that athletes are able to produce almost identical times over their racing distance, yet their training plans seem extremely diverse. This fascination naturally led me to enquiry, and I began with a study of the relevant aspects of anatomy, physiology and psychology.

In presenting my interpretation of these aspects, I wish to acknowledge, with both respect and gratitude, the counsel of several authorities. Dr H. Robson (Loughborough University) and Dr Siggerseth (University of Oregon), who were my lecturers in anatomy and kinesiology. Tom Craig (formerly physiotherapist to Glasgow Rangers Football Club), who wrapped much 'meat around the bones' of part 1. Dr Soderwall (University of Oregon), Dr Clyde Williams (Loughborough University), and Dr Craig Sharp (West London Institute of Higher Education), guided me through the complexities of physiology, which I present as part 2. Professor Miroslav Vanek (Charles University, Prague), Peter Hill and Jean Carroll (both formerly of Dunfermline College of Physical Education), and Dr Pamela F. Murray (Royal Air Force, Cosford) provided new insight into the world of psychology, as set out in part 3. Bridging anatomy, physiology and psychology is the theme of applying each science to the growing child, a concept made much clearer for me by Dr Ivan Szmodis (Central School of Sports, Budapest).

The sciences of anatomy, physiology and psychology are essential basics in pursuing this enquiry, but are as far from being an explanation as bricks are to being a house. Part 4 might then be thought of as the 'cement', giving these bricks context. So many associates have helped me in this area of study that it would be impossible for me to list them all here. However, I would like to record my deep indebtedness to them and to mention especially: Dr Geoff Gowan, Basil Stamatakis, Tony Chapman, Ron Pickering, Wilf Paish, Friedhelm Endemann, Stewart Togher, Vladimir Kuznyetsov, Peter Radford, Sandy Ewen, Gerard Mach, Carlo Vittori, Wilson Young, Gordon Forster, Denis Watts, Harry Wilson, Alex Naylor, Bill Bowerman, Dr Elio Locatelli, Seppo Nutilla, Peter Coe, Max Jones, Carlton Johnson, John Issacs, Erkki Oikarinen, Rita Englebrecht, Dr Ekkart Arbeit, and Norman Brooke for their thoughts and comments on strength, speed, mobility and endurance.

It would be very difficult to say exactly when I first began to draw together the detail of the final part of this book – whenever it was will coincide with the origins of that fascination referred to earlier. I see part 5 as the design or blueprint, and it is my opinion that every coach I have ever met (from several sports) is responsible for its content.

It has also become very clear to me that central to the education and development of any coach is what he can learn from the athletes themselves. I owe each one of the athletes I have coached an immense debt in this respect.

Although the book began to grow several years before pen was put to paper in the autumn of 1975 for the first edition, the nature of its contents means the subject matter requires regular review. The second edition did, in fact, consider again certain aspects of strength, speed and endurance training, and, in particular, focused more tightly on the area of regeneration in the 'Training v straining' chapter.

In the third edition, three colleagues contributed their specialist knowledge to take the components of training theory, as set out here, to a new level. Dr Craig Sharp (West London Institute) reviewed and edited part 2, while Professor Miroslav Vanek (Charles Institute, Prague) and Dr Pamela F. Murray (researcher, Royal Air Force, Cosford) wrote and introduced new material for part 3. I am very grateful for their continued professional and authoritative input.

In the fourth and fifth editions I enhanced the content relating to process in parts 4 and 5, with the help of Andy Roxborough (UEFA Technical Director), Josef Vengelos (UEFA), Ian McGeechan (former Chief Coach Scotland RU), Dr Ekkart Arbeit, Dr Elio Locatelli (IAAF Technical Director), Dr Peter Bonov, Dr Dane Korica, Dr Ron Maughan, Peter Kesne and Dr Wolfgang Ritzdorf. I have also received personal communications from Erkki Oikarrinen (Finland), Peter Tschiene (Germany), Helmar Hommel (Germany), Dr Ekkart Arbeit (Germany), and Elio Locatelli (Italy), and am grateful for their exchange of views.

In the sixth edition I have adopted the same principle as used in the 'partnership system' in coaching. Developments in the performance sciences and in training theory suggest that in these areas, I involve internationally acknowledged experts as co-authors. All have worked with athletes or teams to Olympic and world level while being leaders in their chosen fields of expertise. *Sports Training Principles* 6th edition is significantly and substantially improved as a consequence and I am deeply grateful to them. Their brief biographies are appended and underline how privileged I am to enjoy their outstanding contributions.

As a student, it was put to me that each one of us is exposed to thousands of facts and opinions and that any ideas we think of as our own are, in fact, simply an interpretation of these facts and opinions. My objective here has been to present my understanding of the principles which may help you establish your presentation of training theory to the advantage of the athletes in your charge. I hope you discover this to be the case.

Throughout this book athletes and coaches are, in the main, referred to individually as 'he' rather than 'he or she'. This has been agreed with the publisher as an expedient only.

Finally, I would like to acknowledge with sincere gratitude, the excellent work of five assistants in typing this text from really bad handwriting! Janet Leyland (1980), Jackie Brown (1989, 1997, 2002), Anna Stanforth (2002), Elvie-Jo Shergold (2007) and Donna Fischetto (2014).

CONTRIBUTORS TO THE SIXTH EDITION

Professor John Brewer, chapters 4–9

Professor of Applied Sport Science and Head of the School of Sport, Health and Applied Science at St Mary's University, Twickenham, having previously been Professor of Sport at the University of Bedfordshire and Director of Sports Science at GlaxoSmithKline. He also managed the Lilleshall Human Performance Centre for 18 years, where he worked with many of the UK's top sportsmen and women, and was a member of the England backroom staff at two World Cups, 1990 (soccer), and 1992 (cricket). Currently a board member of UK Anti-Doping, and Chair of British Ski and Snowboard, and previously Chair of British Handball during the London 2012 Olympics. He has published papers in peer reviewed journals, and the popular press, and appeared regularly on various media channels providing opinions on sport and exercise science. Married with two daughters, he is a keen skier and has run the London Marathon 15 times.

Professor Timothy Noakes, chapter 4

Timothy Noakes is the Discovery Health Professor of Exercise and Sports Science at the University of Cape Town, director of the UCT/MRC Research Unit for Exercise Science and Sports Medicine and co-founder of the Sports Science Institute of South Africa (SSISA). He is an A1-rated scientist with the National Research Foundation and has received the Order of Mapungubwe, Silver from the State President for 'excellent contribution in the field of sports and the science of physical exercise'. He has authored many books and papers over the years. His books include *Lore of Running, The Art and Science of Cricket, Challenging Beliefs: Memoirs of a Career* and *Waterlogged: The Serious Problem of Overhydration in Endurance Sports*. He has just co-authored *The Real Meal Revolution* with David Grier, Jonno Proudfoot and Sally-Ann Creed. This book covers the science of good nutrition, the dos and don'ts of healthy eating and fabulous recipes.

Dr Penny Werthner, chapter 10

Penny Werthner, PhD is a Professor and Dean of the Faculty of Kinesiology, University of Calgary, Alberta, Canada. Her areas of research include coaching and learning, women and coaching, and the use of bioneuro-feedback for Olympic coaches and athletes (the latter research funded by Own the Podium, the agency responsible for high-performance sport in Canada). Dr Werthner has been published in *The Sport Psychologist, The International Journal of Sports Science and Coaching,* and the *International Journal of Coaching Science*. She currently serves as an editorial board member of the *International Sport Coaching Journal* and is a member of the *International Council for Coaching Excellence* (ICCE). Dr Werthner was also one of the founding members and Chair (2009–2013) of the Canadian Sport Psychology Association (CSPA). She was an Olympic athlete in athletics, medalist in the Pan American Games and Commonwealth Games, and continues to work as a sport psychology consultant to Olympic coaches, athletes, and teams.

Vern Gambetta, chapter 14

Vern is considered the father of 'Functional Sports Training'. Currently Director of Gambetta Sports Training Systems, Vern's coaching experience spans 44 years at all levels of competition in a variety of sports. He has authored over 100 articles and nine books on various aspects of training. He received his BA from Fresno State University; his teaching credential with a coaching minor from University of California Santa Barbara; and his MA in Education from Stanford University.

Vern's decades of coaching saw him take on such roles as: track and field coach at all levels, including Division I head coach for the women's cross country and track and field team at University of California in Berkeley; director of conditioning and director of athletic development to two major baseball league teams; basketball conditioning coach to Canadian national teams (men's and women's); soccer conditioning coach to US men's World Cup team; and dry land training consultant for swim teams/clubs including Harvard Women's team.

Dr Cliff Mallett, chapter 15

Dr Cliff Mallett is an Associate Professor of Sport Psychology and Coaching in the School of Human Movement Studies at The University of Queensland. He was previously a National High Performance Coach in track and field (sprints and relays) with Athletics Australia and the Australian Institute of Sport. Cliff has coached extensively at the elite level – coaching 15 international athletes and national relay teams many of whom were medallists in major international competitions. He has been a national team coach on several Australian teams, including two Olympics and five World Championships. He teaches undergraduate and graduate students and actively researches in the area of high performance sport. Cliff has published extensively in sport coaching and sport psychology peer reviewed journals and presented at numerous international sport conferences. He regularly consults with elite coaches and athletes, as well as national and professional sporting organisations.

Professor David Jenkins, chapter 16

Professor David Jenkins is an Associate Professor in Exercise Physiology at the University of Queensland. He has had a long-standing involvement in Rugby Union and was the editor of the first and second editions of the Australian Rugby Union's Level II Sports Science manual. He edited *Training for Speed and Endurance* (published by Allen and Unwin in 1996), has published 130 scientific papers and maintains a strong interest in the physiology of high intensity intermittent exercise.

Dr Scott Drawer, chapter 18

Dr Scott Drawer is currently the Athletic Performance Manager at the Rugby Football Union. He is responsible for all performance services (science, medicine and technology) across all age group teams, women's and 7s. The department is tasked with working in partnership with England's leading rugby clubs to support the development of an over supply of talent for future success.

Prior to this role Dr Drawer headed up the research and innovation (R&I) programmes at UK Sport and EIS working across multiple Olympic and Paralympic sports. The R&I programme was tasked with supporting GB's leading sports with key innovates to impact directly on medal winning performances, covering everything from custom equipment design to sensor and software technologies and training science and injury / illness management solutions. Dr Drawer was educated at Brunel (BSC Hons), Loughborough (MSC, PhD) and Nottingham Trent (PGCE).

INTRODUCTION

'Those who are enamoured of practice without science are like a pilot who goes into a ship without rudder or compass and never has any certainty of where he is going.'

(Leonardo da Vinci)

Coaching is mainly an art and, like the artist, the coach must have two attributes. The first is creative flair, that marriage of aptitude and passion which enables him to draw an athlete's dream towards realisation. The athlete, moved to express himself within a social mosaic, chooses to do so in pursuit of competitive excellence in sport. The coach creates order and direction for that expression.

The second attribute is technical mastery of the instruments and materials used. The athlete is the instrument and the material with which the coach works. Structurally, he is a system of levers, given movement by the pull of muscle, and obedient to the laws of physics. Functionally, he is a dynamic integration of adaptive systems. But more than that, he is a reasoning being.

A gardener who works to create ever greater beauty in a plant, does so on the basis of his knowledge of the plant's behaviour in certain conditions. His art lies in the adjustment of these conditions. The coach may have the advantage over the gardener in that the athlete, unlike the plant, can perceive his total environment, rationalise situations, compare present with past, predict the consequences of actions and rapidly adapt his behaviour within his personal framework of attitude, values and motivation. At first sight, the active involvement of the athlete makes the coach's task seem simpler than that of the gardener. After all, 'two heads are better than one'! Yet the infinitely variable behaviour, which might result from even one simple adjustment to the athlete's environment, confirms the extra-ordinary complexity of the coach's art. The coach must clearly understand the purpose of each practice and its relevance to the total scheme of preparation, yet comprehend fully the role of sport as but one part of the life of a growing and changing person. So the coach is not only in the technical business; he is in the people business.

To accept the full weight of this responsibility, the coach, in this first quarter of the twenty-first century, must move towards a deeper appreciation of those sciences which relate to the athlete. This is not to say that pragmatism is dead; there will continue to be situations where the coach 'knows' a practice is correct, according to his 'feel' for coaching athletes. This is, of course, part of the coach's art and it should stimulate rather than inhibit pursuit of explanation. Many established practices may work (and for good reason) but, until underlying principles are defined, what basis do we have for developing further practices or for communicating experience in coaching to *all* sports?

And there are at least two reasons why we should feel confident that coaches will continue to increase their effectiveness in delivering their art. First, there is the certain knowledge that the sciences which influence performance are accelerating the intelligence resource coaches need to ensure athletes fulfil their performance potential. Next, there is irrefutability to the words of Arie de Geus:

'Probably the only sustainable competitive advantage we have is the ability to learn faster than the competition.'

So we enjoy an advantage in a world where the performance-related database is expanding exponentially. That world is one of constant change where, on the one hand, we are exposed to change and learn to adapt to it, and on the other we learn to introduce change and are creative in this.

In drawing together the substance of the following pages it has not, then, been my intention to create an apotheosis of sports science. The various changes will, I hope, contribute to the coach's sources of reference, form part of a basis for understanding current coaching research, and offer a framework of training principles for an ever-expanding source of practices designed to help the athlete in preparation for excellence in his sport. *Sports Training Principles* has been written to provide a launching platform for your lifelong learning as a coach.

The coach is most certainly not 'enamoured of practice without science', but I would not wish to make him a bookworm, equipped only with sports science jargon. His art is to weave his understanding of related sciences into the fabric of coaching an athlete. It is a practical art, based on careful appraisal of all relevant knowledge. I hope this book will contribute to your interpretation of this fine art.

PART 1
RODS TO LEVERS

An athlete may be thought of, structurally, as a series of connected rods. The design of each connection will determine the nature and range of movement between adjacent rods and, consequently, their potential function. These connections are the joints; the rods are the bones. Combined, they form the skeletal system. The movement at any given joint is made possible by the pull of muscle on bone across the joint. The total arrangement of muscle and its attachment to bones forms the muscular system. Part 1 looks at these two systems, and the mechanical laws which they must obey, to effect an appreciation of the athlete's aggregate movement potential for the expression of energy.

So, part 1 serves as an introduction to the sciences of anatomy, kinesiology and biomechanics. These sciences are fundamental to the coach in the design and selection of exercise on the one hand, and technique development and analysis on the other.

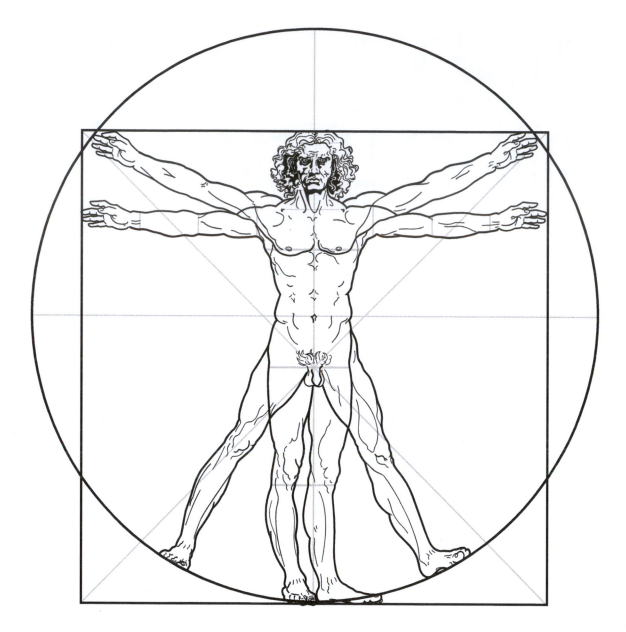

1 THE WORKING PARTS

AXES

It is easy to understand how a wheel spins about an axle, and at right angles to that axle. If the athlete had wheels instead of arms and legs, the axles being located at the shoulders and at the hips, it would again be easy to understand why the wheels would rotate or spin at right angles to the body and on the same plane as the direction in which the athlete was moving. If the axles are now faded out in the mind's eye and the arms and legs are considered as rotating like wheels – not round and round, but forwards and backwards like pendulums – it appears that the body is equipped with invisible axles, or axes, and that the movement at the joints is rotation. However, whereas the wheel may rotate on one plane only, the body's joints permit greater freedom of movement.

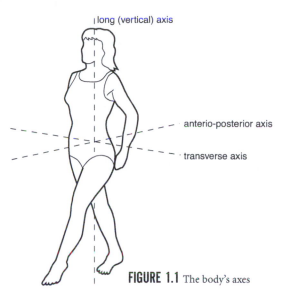

FIGURE 1.1 The body's axes

Our bodies are three-dimensional. There are three axes of rotation – vertical, transverse and anterior-posterior – for the body as a whole and, in principle, at each joint. We will now look at the axes and consider them in the light of the whole body movement and the movement at various joints (figure 1.1).

Vertical axis

The vertical axis is the long axis of the body and is that about which the figure skater spins, or the ballet dancer pirouettes.

If the body is tilted to lie parallel with the ground (i.e. horizontal) rotation is still possible about the long axis (e.g. the child rolling sideways downhill). Although horizontal, the rotation is described as about the body's vertical axis. In describing rotations, it is important to identify clearly the axes under consideration as if the person is standing. Very little confusion arises when discussing the whole body in flight, but occasionally problems arise with a particular joint action. For example, just as the long axis of the body is referred to as the vertical axis, so also is the long axis through a joint. Hence the actions of turning out one's feet like Charlie Chaplin, twisting one's head and shoulders to the rear, and turning off a tap (with elbow extended) are all examples of rotation about the long/vertical axis. Taking the last example, however, consider the arm held out to the side (abducted) and swung forwards, as in a discus throw. This rotation is about the vertical axis through the shoulder, while long axis rotation of the arm which will influence the attitude of the discus, will, in this case, be about the transverse axis through the shoulder. The moral of the story is to *be precise in defining axes.*

Transverse axis

The transverse axis is that described in the 'wheels for limbs' reference above. These particular axes would apply to shoulder and hip. Examples of rotation about these axes in the athlete are: kicking a ball, the pulling action of the arms in swimming, and the piking to extension movements of the gymnast. Returning to the vertical axis situation mentioned above, rotations about the transverse axis become rotations about the vertical axis when the arm is abducted. For example, the actions of underarm bowling and the forehand in tennis are similar in terms of movement at the shoulder joint, although different muscles may be involved due to changing angles of pull on levers. Consequently, when considering transverse axis rotations, one must also consider rotations with an abducted limb. These include the pull-through of the hurdler's trail leg into the line of running, and the golfer's swing.

The transverse axis of the body as a whole is that about which the trampolinist or springboard diver rotates in a front or back somersault. The high jumper who uses the flop technique rotates about the vertical axis at take-off and about the transverse axis in bar clearance.

Anterio-posterior axis

The cartwheel somersault of an acrobat is a useful visual image of an athlete rotating about the body's anterio-posterior (A–P) axis. This axis is from front to back and is seen in joint actions where, for example, a rider presses her knees against the flanks of her mount. A soldier standing at ease, then responding to a command to stand to attention, would be rotating the leg on the hip about the A–P axis. Similarly, arms raised sideways or returned to the side are rotating on the shoulder about the A–P axis. Other examples are the hip/spine movements of the side-step or body swerve in football, the tilting of the pelvis in recovering the hurdler's trail leg, and certain expressions of lateral movement in dance.

JOINT ACTIONS

Related to the axes of rotation outlined, there are the specific actions of flexion, extension, adduction, abduction and rotation. An understanding of these actions affords fuller appreciation of movement and technique.

Flexion

Flexion is the rotating of one lever about another in such a way that the angle between these levers is reduced. Bringing hand to shoulder is an example of flexion at the elbow. The soccer player who can keep the ball in the air by using his knee is doing so by flexing his thigh on his hip and, simultaneously, flexing his lower leg on his thigh. The spine too may be considered as a lever or a series of levers. As a guide, any movement which curls the athlete into a tucked shape or round, like a ball, is flexion of the spine.

Two more types of flexion are described, at the shoulder and the ankle. Flexion at the shoulder is the raising forward of the arm above the head, as in swimming backstroke arm recovery. Plantar flexion is pointing the toe, standing on tiptoe. Dorsiflexion at the ankle is turning the toes up towards the knee (as in Aladdin's shoes!). Horizontal flexion at the shoulder is in such actions as bench press, discus arm, forehand in tennis, and shot-put arm.

Extension

Extension might be thought of as the opposite of flexion and is the rotating of one lever away from another. Thus the angle between the levers increases towards 180°. If greater than 180°, the action is referred to as hyperextension. At the moment of delivery in shot-put, the arm is completely extended (straightened) at the elbow. As the basketball player leaves the floor for a jump shot, extension takes place at the hip, knee and ankle. As the volleyball player jumps to block an opposition spike, the elbows, wrists and fingers are extended. In a hollow-back somersault, the extreme arching of the spine is hyperextension.

Extension of the arm on the shoulder is the opposite action to that described for flexion and is demonstrated in the overhead smash shots in tennis, squash and badminton, also in javelin arm and in the powerful pull phases of the arm action when swimming butterfly, freestyle or breaststroke. Extension at the ankle is the action of plantar flexion, making the line of the lower leg/foot straight, or even convex. Ballet dancers and gymnasts are capable of the latter. Horizontal extension at the shoulder is seen when the athlete, standing in the crucifix position, presses the arms backwards, or when in reverse flies in weight training.

The actions of flexion and extension are considered as rotations about the transverse axis of a given joint, and the body's tendency to a total flexion or extension is also about this axis.

Adduction

Adduction is the drawing of a lever towards the midline of the body, for example moving the legs from standing astride to standing with the legs together, or in returning the arms from a position in which they are out from the side back to the side. Thus the action of bringing the legs towards each other in breaststroke leg action is one of adduction, as is gripping the body of a horse with one's knees when riding.

The action of adduction may take a lever past the midline, for example in crossing one's legs or in sweeping a soccer ball across the body from one side to the other. Obviously, to perform such an action, the leg would have to be either slightly extended or flexed on the hip to permit passage of one leg beyond the obstruction of the other.

Abduction

Abduction is the opposite movement to adduction and is therefore the movement of a lever *away* from the midline. Raising an arm to the side and moving the legs from being together to legs astride are examples of abduction. The shot-putter emphasises the abduction of his putting arm and the hurdler abducts the trailing leg to ensure clearance of the barrier.

The actions of adduction and abduction are normally considered to take place about the A–P axis.

Rotation

All movements of levers are rotations, but the expression 'rotation', when considered with the anatomical actions of flexion, adduction, abduction and extension, is taken to mean long-axis rotation. When Charlie Chaplin turned his feet outwards, the action was outward or lateral rotation. When he turned them inwards, so that he was pigeon-toed, the action was inward or medial rotation. Lateral means 'to the outside or outwards', medial means 'to the inside or inwards'. Abduction, then, could be described as a lateral movement and adduction as a medial movement.

The action of rotation is normally understood to take place about the vertical axis, but, again, care must be taken to define the axes precisely.

BASIC STRUCTURE
Bone

The rods are the athlete's bones and they become levers via the joints. The structure of each joint will dictate its function potential, hence the contrast between the mobility of the shoulder complex of joints and the stability of the hip joint; the difference between cervical intervertebral movement and the lumbar intervertebral movement; and the functional variable available to the elbow as opposed to the knee. For the serious student of movement, whether in general or specific to sport, a working knowledge of the skeleton (figure 1.2) and how bones relate to each other as skeletal components of join actions is fundamental.

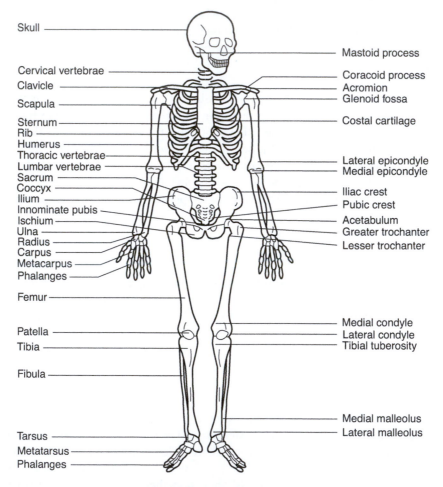

FIGURE 1.2 The skeleton

Muscle

Muscles, by converting chemical energy into mechanical energy, pull on the bones via tendinous attachment and bring about the actions already described. The specific action of a muscle will be defined by the bony lever systems it connects and the position and angle of attachment.

Muscles have two attachments; the origin (proximal) and insertion (distal). In anatomy the term proximal means nearer the centre of the body (spine); distal means farther from it.

In several instances, a muscle may cross two joints (e.g. gastrocnemius, biceps femoris) and is therefore responsible for two separate actions. The efficiency of each action is critically affected by the stability status of each joint; the position of the bones connected at each joint; and the consequent relationship of relevant muscle origin and insertion. The major muscles are illustrated in figure 1.3. Once again, for the serious student of movement, it is fundamental to have a strong working knowledge of the muscular system and muscle actions in order to select exercises and design exercise programmes.

It is essential to understand that in any movement, it is not one or two but several muscles working in harmony that are brought into play. The 'harmony' involves *agonists*, *antagonists*, *fixators* or *stabilisers* and *neutralisers*. An agonist is a muscle that actively contracts to produce a desired movement. So in extending the knee in kicking a ball, the quadriceps are agonists. An antagonist is a muscle that opposes the movement produced by the agonist. So in extending the knee, the hamstrings (biceps femoris, semimembranosus and semitendinosus) are antagonists. A fixator or stabiliser is a muscle that anchors or supports a bone or body part in order that the agonist can do its job. So the fixators in kicking the ball will include gluteus medius and minimus, obturator externus and internus. A neutraliser is a muscle that contracts in order to counteract an undesired action of another contracting muscle. The collective function of fixators and neutralisers renders them synergists.

There are two kinds of synergy: helping synergy and true synergy. The former occurs during the action of two muscles that primarily share a joint action yet their secondary action is antagonistic to that of the other. True synergy occurs when one muscle contracts statically to prevent any action in one of the joints traversed by a contracting two-joint or multi-joint muscle.

Tendon

Tendon attaches muscle to bone. The Achilles tendon, for example, attaches the calf muscles responsible for ankle extension to the large bone at the rear of the heel (the calcaneus). Gripping this tendon between forefinger and thumb, gives an idea of the extreme toughness of this tissue. Due to this strength, the tendon itself is seldom injured. However, the connections of tendon to muscle or tendon to bone are more vulnerable to injury.

Ligaments

The ligaments are bands of white fibrous tissue connecting bones about a joint. They may be considered as guardians of the joint's stability as they are extremely resistant to distortion and stretching. Certain types of mobility work are geared to passive stretching of ligaments to permit a greater freedom or range of movement. However, it must be borne in mind that such work restricts their role as stabilisers. Once stretched, the ligament will maintain its new length, having plastic rather than elastic properties (figure 1.4).

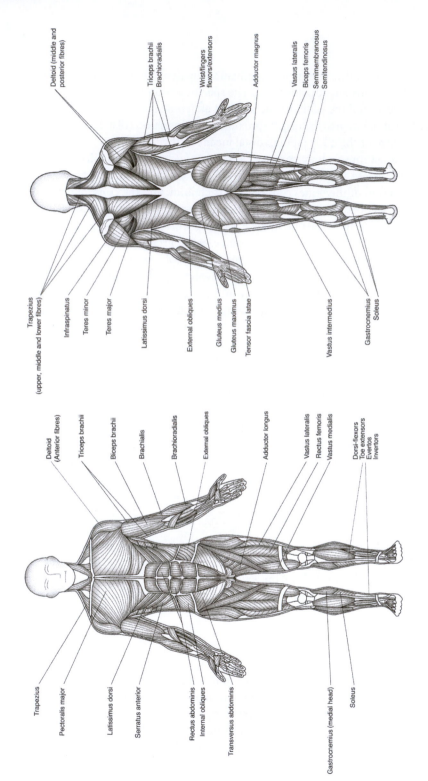

Deltoid (middle and posterior fibres)
Triceps brachii
Brachioradialis
Wrist/fingers flexors/extensors
Adductor magnus
Vastus lateralis
Biceps femoris
Semimembranosus
Semitendinosus

Trapezius (upper, middle and lower fibres)
Infraspinatus
Teres minor
Teres major
Latissimus dorsi
External obliques
Gluteus medius
Gluteus maximus
Tensor fascia latae
Vastus intermedius
Gastrocnemius
Soleus

Deltoid (Anterior fibres)
Triceps brachii
Biceps brachii
Brachialis
Brachioradialis
External obliques
Adductor longus
Vastus lateralis
Rectus femoris
Vastus medialis
Dorsi-flexors
Toe extensors
Evertors
Invertors

Trapezius
Pectoralis major
Latissimus dorsi
Serratus anterior
Rectus abdominis
Internal obliques
Transversus abdominis
Gastrocnemius (medial head)
Soleus

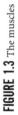

FIGURE 1.3 The muscles

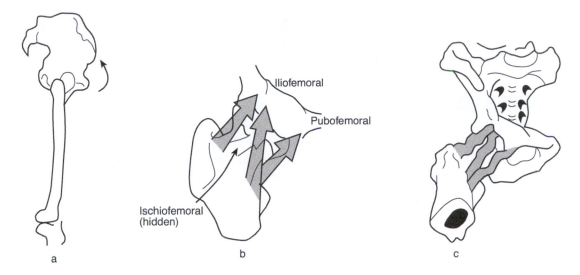

FIGURE 1.4 The ligaments of the hip (from Kapandji, 2010). As the child develops from the quadruped posture to the erect posture, and the pelvis tilts upwards and backwards (a), all ligaments become coiled round the neck of the femur, in the same direction. Extension winds these ligaments tighter (b); flexion unwinds, and slackens them (c). The stretching of these ligaments in the quadruped to upright posture demonstrates plastic, rather than elastic, properties of ligaments.

Periosteum

The connective tissue surrounding the bone is periosteum. In the grown organism it has a supporting function and when strong tendon, ligaments or muscle are attached to a bone, the periosteum is incorporated with them. This is the final connection of muscle to bone. While it is obviously a strong connection, it is nevertheless vulnerable to injury when strained. Stress may accumulate or occur as a result of fatigue and strong muscle contraction, or in maximal contraction when imbalance has caused an unnatural alignment of the joint. In the growing organism, periosteum protects a layer of tissue containing the 'bone-growing' cells. It is an unstable material, which is why extremes of muscular fatigue or force of contraction may cause damage.

Synovia

Most joints of the body are completely surrounded by a capsule lined with a synovial membrane. This membrane lines the whole of the interior of the joint except the actual ends of the bones which meet in that particular joint. The membrane releases a constant small flow of a lubricant called synovia or synovial fluid. Exercise maintains a healthy supply of released fluid, while inactivity reduces it and joint injury causes an extremely rapid flow. The latter causes swelling in the joint concerned.

Cartilage

Cartilage may be thought of as a shock-absorbing or reducing agent. In the knee, cartilage discs not only cushion the impact of movement between the two bones, but also serve to ensure perfect contact between them. Fibrocartilage discs act as cushions between the various bones or vertebrae which are stacked one upon the other in the spine. Finally, the ends of each bone meeting at a joint are protected by *articular* cartilage.

It should be remembered that cartilage has no blood supply and consequently cannot repair itself once damaged. However, it would appear that synovia provides cartilage with nutrients and it has been shown that with exercise the amount of available fluid increases. This flow increases the efficiency of joint movement.

THE UPPER LIMBS

Reflection on the number of movements and actions performed by the upper limb complex will point to its primary characteristic – mobility. Mobility depends on combinations and permutations of actions at four joints. These joints will be considered in order from the proximal to the distal.

Shoulder

The skeletal components involved in the shoulder girdle actions are:

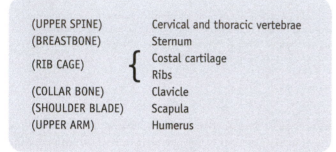

(UPPER SPINE)	Cervical and thoracic vertebrae
(BREASTBONE)	Sternum
(RIB CAGE)	Costal cartilage
	Ribs
(COLLAR BONE)	Clavicle
(SHOULDER BLADE)	Scapula
(UPPER ARM)	Humerus

They variously afford origin and/or insertion attachments for those muscles which produce the following actions about the axes indicated. For each action two muscles involved in producing the action are given as examples.

Transverse axis: *flexion* – arm raised forwards; *extension* – arm pulled downwards or backwards. These opposing actions can be seen clearly in the arm movements in running. The plane in which these movements take place is the *sagittal* plane (figure 1.5a).

E.g.   Flexion: pectoralis major (clavicular)
                              coracobrachialis
       Extension: latissimus dorsi
                              pectoralis major (sternocostal)

Anterioposterior axis: *abduction* – raising the arm out from the side; *adduction* – returning the arm from a position of abduction to the side. These actions are in the *frontal* plane (figure 1.5b).

E.g.   Abduction: middle deltoid
                              supraspinatus
       Adduction: teres major
                              infraspinatus

Vertical axis (arm parallel with spine): *rotation outward* (*lateral*) – clockwise movement of the straight right arm, for example turning a tap off; *rotation inward* (*medial*) – anticlockwise movement of the straight right arm, for example turning a tap on.

E.g.   Medial rotation: subscapularis
                                   teres major
         Lateral rotation: teres minor
                                   infraspinatus

Vertical axis (arm abducted): *horizontal flexion* – starting from a position with arm held out from the side (abducted), the arm is brought forward towards the midline. This is seen in the discus arm action, in bench press, or in wrapping the arms about the body to keep warm; *horizontal extension* – the reverse to horizontal flexion. These actions are in the *horizontal* plane (figure 1.5c). Circumduction through combinations of these actions permit immense adaptability, for example slipping an arm into a coat sleeve, combing the hair at the back of the head, scratching the opposite shoulder blade from above or below, throwing in a ball at soccer, and even dislocations on the gymnastic rings.

E.g.   Horizontal flexion: pectoralis major
                                       anterior deltoid
        Horizontal extension: posterior deltoid
                                       latissimus dorsi

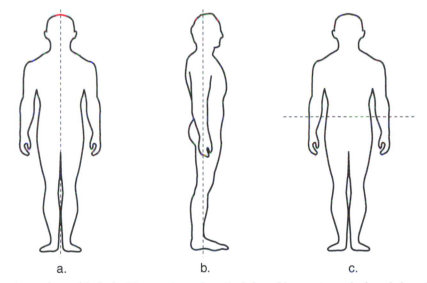

a.   b.   c.

FIGURE 1.5 The primary planes of the body: (a) separation at the sagittal plane; (b) separation at the frontal plane; (c) separation at the horizontal plane

Application examples of shoulder mobility

Arm action in high jump: a coaching point often quoted for high jump arm action is 'thumbs in, elbows out'. By turning in the thumbs, the arms are medially rotated and this in turn slides the wing-like scapulae (shoulder blades) laterally round the rear wall of the rib (thoracic) cage. As this happens, the joint between the humerus and the part of the scapula which receives it (glenoid fossa), is brought forward allowing greater range of extension.

Discus arm: in discus, the abducted arm must be supported by the powerful abductor muscles and the discus aligned by controlled inward rotation of the arm, yet the action which applies force to the discus is one of fast horizontal flexion over as great a range as possible. The limited degree of inward rotation must cause the scapula to be a restricting agent to a great range of horizontal extension, but this is preferable to the outward rotation employed by the beginner who struggles to keep the discus securely gripped by the distal phalanges of his throwing hand at the limit of extension. If the athlete continued this outward rotation, his arm would assume the starting position for javelin throw. Many top discus throwers hang the discus low and behind the hip as if they were attempting to place the throwing hand in their hip pocket. Here the arm is kept inwardly rotated until the athlete moves into his throwing position, when the discus is then allowed to swing the arm out to an increased range of movement. Tennis strokes at below shoulder level involve similar principles.

Javelin arm: the arm in the javelin throw is withdrawn prior to the actual throw, as in the outward rotation of the arm, the horizontal extension of the shoulder (arm abducted), the backward movement of the shoulder girdle, and rotation about the long axis of the spine. A fundamental adjustment must then be made to allow the thrower to pull along the length of the javelin and forcefully project it. This involves even greater rotation and a consequent sliding of the entire shoulder under the javelin. In fact, what is involved is a rapid positional change from extreme horizontal extension to extreme flexion. There is a clear relationship between this action and that of the tennis serve, the forehand smash in racket sports, the volleyball spike, the soccer throw-in, and the arm action in butterfly and freestyle swimming.

Elbow

The skeletal components involved in elbow actions are:

(UPPER ARM)	Humerus
(FOREARM)	Radius
	Ulna

At the elbow joint, two axes of rotation are evident.

Transverse axis: *flexion* – hand brought to the same shoulder; *extension* – elbow straightened. These opposing actions can be seen clearly in activities such as chinning the bar (flexion) and push-ups (extension).

    E.g. Flexion: biceps brachii
                               brachialis
           Extension: triceps brachii
                               anconeus

Vertical axis: *pronation* – forearm is rotated medially to a palm down or overgrasp position; *supination* – forearm is rotated laterally to a palm-up or undergrasp position. These actions are applied when using a screwdriver to screw or unscrew with the right hand. The clockwise action of screwing on a nut is supination, while the anticlockwise action of unscrewing a nut is pronation. The right-handed pole-vaulter supinates the right forearm and pronates the left in gripping the pole. The tennis player serves with pronation but supinates for backhand shots.

E.g. Pronation: pronator teres
                      pronator quadratus
      Supination: supinator
                      biceps brachii

Elbow mechanics

Flexion efficiency depends on the position of the forearm (i.e. pronation or supination) and the position of the arm relative to the shoulder. Extension efficiency depends on the position of the arm relative to the shoulder. The relative efficiency is illustrated in strength measurements listed in table 1.1.

Position	Etension force	Flexion force
Arm stretched above shoulder	43 kg	83 kg
Arm flexed at 90°	37 kg	66 kg
Arm hanging at side of the body	52 kg	51 kg

TABLE 1.1 Elbow extension and flexion force compared in three different positions (Kapandji, 2007)

From this we can deduce man's suitability to climbing and certain implications of limb alignment for vaulters and apparatus gymnasts. Considerable difference can be measured at 90° of flexion when the forearm assumes varying points of rotation between supination and pronation (table 1.2). The difference has been explained by Provins and Salter (1955) as (1) biceps are stretched but poor leverage, (2) brachioradialis is the same, (3) brachialis is the same, and (4) pronator teres is at greatest length and leverage.

Position	Strength force	Standard deviation
Supination	19.64 kg	3.82
Mid-position	21.60 kg	4.05
Pronation	13.41 kg	2.00

TABLE 1.2 Isometric flexion strength relative to elbow joint position (adapted from Rasch, 1968)

This will obviously make a difference in how chinning the bar and biceps curls are performed, and how high bars, poles, etc., are gripped. It should also be pointed out that in gripping a bar in pronation, with the object of performing biceps curls, the weight of the bar will place considerable stress on the extensor muscles of the wrist as the bar is raised. As the stress increases, the wrist will be pulled to a position of flexion, thus stretching the extensors of the fingers and forcing the flexors to release their grip on the bar. The total effect is similar to the action performed in unarmed combat when attempting to disarm an opponent who holds a weapon. The hand containing the weapon is seized, the wrist forced into flexion, and the weapon is dropped.

Returning to extension of the elbow, the triceps are at their greatest mechanical advantage and are stretched when the arm is abducted. However, it must be realised that there is a problem since the action at the elbow and the shoulder are really opposing each other. Immediate connection should be clear, keeping the elbow high in shot. There is another little muscle involved in extension and that is the anconeus. Its main function is to pronate as the elbow extends, for example in javelin long axis spin and in imparting spin to tennis shots.

Wrist

The skeletal components involved in wrist action are:

(FOREARM)	Radius
	Ulna
(WRIST)	8 carpals (scaphoid, lunate, triquetrum, pisiform, hamate, capitate, trapezoid, trapezium)
(HAND)	5 metacarpals
(FINGERS)	14 phalanges (fingers 3 each; thumb 2)

The wrist is a very adaptable complex of joints, offering rotation about three axes.

Transverse axis: *flexion* – palm of hand is moved towards the forearm; *extension* – back of hand is moved towards the forearm. These actions are immediately recognisable in the final wrist flick in shot-put (flexion), or the whip cracking action of a badminton backhand (extension).

E.g. Flexion: flexor carpi ulnaris
palmaris longus
Extension: extensor carpi radialis
extensor digitorum

Anteriorposterior axis: *adduction* – small finger side of the hand is moved towards the forearm; *abduction* – thumb side of the hand is moved towards the forearm. The former is seen when chopping wood with a hand axe, the latter in the final flicking action of the wrist when imparting spin to the discus.

E.g. Adduction: extensor carpi ulnaris
flexor carpi ulnaris
Abduction: extensor carpi radialis longus
extensor carpi radialis brevis

Vertical axis: rotation about the vertical axis is circumduction rather than rotation as described earlier. It is the combination of the abduction, adduction, flexion and extension function, plus supination and pronation function of radius and ulna. This contributes to the total manipulative capacity of the fingers. Little wonder then the spinners' and pitchers' magic in cricket and baseball; the subtleties in slice, spin and racket face angle in tennis and squash; the delicate touch in moving the blade of the foil in fencing; or in high velocity steering adjustment in Formula 1. On the other hand it must be borne in mind that the force efficiency of this joint is limited, but must be developed if an accumulated force from leg, hip, trunk, shoulder and elbow are to be transferred to an implement held in the hand. This is particularly the case with a heavy implement such as shot, where wrist or finger injury can terminate an athlete's ambitions for an entire season. It is also pertinent for lighter implements such as javelin, racket or golf club.

Fingers

The skeletal components involved in finger actions are:

(UPPER ARM)	Humerus
(FOREARM)	Radius
	Ulna
(WRIST)	8 Carpals (scaphoid, lunate, triquetrum, pisiform, hamate, capitate, trapezoid, trapezium)
(HAND)	5 Metacarpals
(FINGERS)	14 Phalanges (fingers 3 each; thumb 2)

Although these are the bones which host muscle origins and insertions, in one way or another it is the whole upper body complex from shoulder girdle to fingertips that combine to allow the discrete manipulation capacity of the fingers to function efficiently and effectively. The grab of a mechanical digger cannot perform its tasks efficiently if the arm has not been driven to the most efficient functioning site. Similarly, the control of shoulder, elbow and wrist are basic to the working of the fingers. These small joint complexes make fine movement possible by rotation about two axes for the four fingers and thumb.

Transverse axis: *flexion* – the beckoning action of curling the finger towards the palm; *extension* – the straightening of the finger to point or indicate. The fingers are flexed in all gripping activities like holding a bar, bat or a throwing implement. Actions of extension are mainly seen as a return from flexion, but static extension may be held as, for example, in karate.

E.g. Flexion: flexor digitorum superficialis
flexor digitorum profundus
Extension: extensor digitorum
extensor pollicis longus

Anterioposterior axis: *abduction* – spreading the fingers; *adduction* – bringing the fingers and thumb together as in the characteristic 'karate chop' position. The fingers are abducted to grip a discus or give maximum area to present to a basketball or water (in swimming). Adduction is used when the talon grip is used in javelin. The upper limb joint complexes afford immense movement potential, from the foundation of mobility. This is demonstrated from subtleties of finger and wrist actions in the pianist and strings musicians; to the touch of the racket player or bowler in cricket; to the power of throwers, gymnasts and weightlifters. Conditioning enhances that potential by building on mobility and motor coordination programmes.

E.g. Abduction: dorsal interossei
abductor pollicis brevis

Adduction: palmar interossei
                  adductor pollicis

In addition, the thumb and little finger are capable of *opposition*. This action is where the thumb can be brought across the palm towards the little finger, which for its part, is drawn forward and rotates to meet the thumb.
    E.g. Opposition: opponens pollicis
                            opponens digiti minimi

One final reflection on the truly remarkable functional adaptability of the hand in terms of grip: the same joint complex can adjust with ease to hold a needle in completing a delicate surgical movement; hold bodyweight with fingertips on a rock face; finger at speed the strings on a violin; pull weight on the oar in rowing; hold fork and knife; pluck the strings of a harp; raise a heavy barbell; or flight a dart to one hundred and eighty!

SPINE

The spine is the pillar on which all skeletal function is founded. Its own movement potential, however, is made possible by the involvement of a number of other skeletal components.

(SPINE)	Vertebral column: 7 cervical vertebrae (1st atlas, 2nd axis), 12 thoracic vertebrae, 5 lumbar vertebrae, sacrum (5 sacral vertebrae – fused), coccyx (4 coccygeal vertebrae – fused)
(COLLARBONE)	Clavicle
(SHOULDER BLADE)	Scapula
(UPPER ARM)	Humerus
(RIB CAGE)	Ribs and costal cartilage
(HIPS)	Pelvis (iliacus, ischium, pubis) (sacrum inserts into iliacus and is connected by ligaments to the iliacus and ischium)
(THIGH)	Femur

The spine, spinal column or trunk is at once a single rigid lever and a series of levers. As a single lever it can sustain great burdens, or accept the powerful extension of the lower limbs, in connection with the upper limbs, to propel an object or the body itself. As a series of levers it is capable of immense mobility and can absorb the shock of impact from above or below. Thus the spine offers the body an extremely wide range of movement by virtue of its adaptability. The spine may be likened to a series of cotton reels joined end to end with a piece of string passing along the central tunnel. Each cotton reel represents a *vertebra*: man is a vertebrate because he has a backbone, a worm is invertebrate because it has none.

Vertebrae and discs

The vertebrae gradually increase in size from neck to tail. This is because each vertebra must bear the weight of all parts of the body above it. The farther down the spine, the greater the weight, hence its solid structure.

In the hole in the middle, the spinal cord passes through, like a vast bundle of wires in a telephone cable. This is the communications system linking brain and body. Damaging this cable will cut off communications to parts of the body below the level of the damage, hence the terrible consequences of spinal injury and the classification system according to the level of injury in paralympic sport.

The discs are the cushions between vertebrae and damaging them brings considerable pain and discomfort. This is caused not so much by the pressure of bone on bone, but by pressure on the cord, or branches of the cord. These would normally leave the main cable via the gap between the two vertebrae kept free by the disc in question.

Shape of the spine

Of course, the picture of a column of cotton reels is not too accurate, because the spine is not straight whether viewed from the side or from behind. The spine has a characteristic series of curves, the evolution of which is interesting.

Babies at birth have only one curve, that which gives the body the appearance of a comma (figure 1.6a). The cervical (neck) curve is formed by the strong intermittent pull of the infant's muscles on the spine as

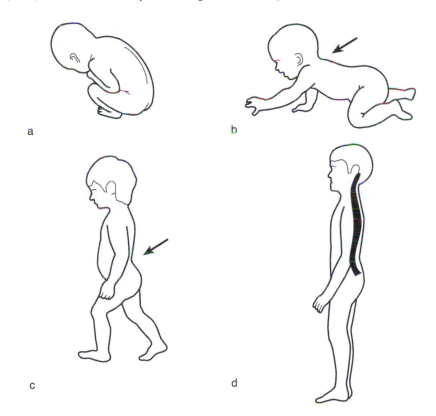

a

b

c

d

FIGURE 1.6 The developing spine: (a) the newborn baby has one spinal curve – making the basic shape something similar to a comma. This curve will remain in the thoracic region. (b) The young child has already introduced a second curve in the cervical region; (c) once upright, the third curve is developed in the lumbar region as early as three years, becoming obvious by eight years and assuming characteristic adult shape around 10 years (d).

he begins to sit up and hold up his head. It is emphasised further in the tilting back of the head to see where he is crawling to, or in looking for his next meal (figure 1.6b). Once he is on his feet, the pelvis (hip bone) is pulled forwards and downwards by ligaments attached to the bone of the thigh (figure 1.4). This action, combined with the body's weight bearing down on the lower spine as he pulls himself erect, pulls the lower spine forwards, completing the final curve of the spine (figure 1.6c).

The curvature perfectly aligns the holes (vertebral foramen) in the vertebrae to ensure a clear channel for the spinal cord. It is clear then, that the integrity of the spine's shape must be robust and is maintained by appropriate strength and mobility exercise. Core strength work should be considered as fundamental for all exercise programmes, and has specific import for those in sports or activities where there is a one-sided or dominant-sided action, for example golf, tennis; occupational posture stressors, for example lifting; or uneven lateral stressors on the pelvis, for example leg length variation. In such cases, exercise programmes and/or orthotics to compensate for strength imbalances/leg length variation must be introduced early and continued to avoid persistent structural compromise to the spine.

Movements in the spine

The tension of ligaments joining vertebrae, and the shape of vertebrae at different levels of the spine, dictate the movements of which the spine is capable. (Exceptions are the two vertebrae upon which the head rests; the atlas and axis vertebrae.) Rotation is possible about three axes in the spine, rendering it a most mobile complex of joints.

Transverse axis: *flexion* – the curling forwards of the head towards the hips. It takes place in all regions of the spine, but is most free at the cervical and lumbar regions. The contribution of head and hip movement to the overall picture of spine flexion is worth noting. Tension of extensor muscles and solid restrictions, such as the ribs or excess weight about the middle, are the main limiting factors to spine flexion. Flexion is seen in front somersault or in the rock-back position in pole-vault. The shoulders may readily become rounded, encouraging flexion of the spine at its upper third. This shows in a stoop and can be brought about by tiring or weakening of the extensors, occupational postures, or over conditioning of flexors. The ease with which this may happen creates a problem in weight bearing on the shoulders, where instability is introduced and injury may result due to exceptional pressure for which this part of the lever system is ill-prepared.

Extension – the straightening of the spine. It takes place most freely at the cervical and lumbar spine, but is restricted in the thoracic spine. The expression of hyperextension is used to describe a degree of extension which moves far beyond normal postural extension. This movement is very evident in arching positions in gymnastics, such as the hollowback somersault, and so on. The total maximum range of flexion of the spine from sacrum to skull as a whole is approximately 110° and extension 140° (Kapandji, 2008). These values will, of course, vary considerably with age and ability levels.

E.g. Flexion: sternocleidomastoid
                       rectus abdominis
      Extension: interspinales
                       iliocostalis cervicis

Anterioposterior axis: *lateral flexion* – the curving of the spine to either side, as in reaching the right fingers towards the right ankle while looking straight ahead. It is possible at all levels, but is greatest at the junction between thoracic and lumbar spine. The tilting of the pelvis to recover the trail leg in hurdles involves a degree of lateral flexion, as do twisting movements involved in the complex patterns of agility displayed in diving, or in body swerve in field games, slalom skiing, etc. The total maximum range of lateral flexion from sacrum to skull is approximately 75–85° (Kapandji, 2008). Again, there are variations related to age and ability.

E.g.   Lateral Flexion: quadratus lumborum
                                 longissimus thoracis

Vertical axis: rotation/twisting along the length of the spine is most free in the cervical region and through the thoracic region, but is negligible in the lumbar spine. This particular property of the spine is very important and both strength and mobility must be worked at. The athlete attempts to take the spine to extremes of rotation in order to 'compress the spring' in throws, hence the 'wound-up' position in discus and javelin, or in the preparation phases of tennis strokes, golf swing, etc. The total maximum rotation from sacrum to skull is approximately 90° (Kapandji, 2008), with variation according to age and ability levels.

The spine is the critical conduit of structure and function in movement potential. Its musculature development is focused on as the pillar on which all posture depends, so core strength protection holds priority in coordinating programmes. There must be sensitivity to even the smallest imbalances. The capacity to respond rapidly to compensate and the strength to counter threat to integrity of structure in this complicated joint complex is critical. Developing movement potential through mobility work and complex motor skills cannot be progressed at the expense of maintaining core strength.

E.g.   Rotation: multifidus
                         semispinalis thoracis

THE LOWER LIMBS

Although the complex of lower limb joints offers a limited movement potential compared with the upper limbs, they are extremely stable. Indeed, this stability is fundamental to the two basic functions of the lower limbs: support of the body's weight, and locomotion.

Hip

The skeletal components involved in hip actions are:

(SPINE)	Lower thoracic vertebrae; lumbar, sacral and coccygeal vertebrae
(HIPS)	Pelvis (iliacus, ischium, pubis)
(THIGH)	Femur
(LOWER LEG)	Tibia, Fibula

It is very important to remember two details when considering hip joint movement. First, some of the muscles which are involved in joint actions at the hip are also involved in joint actions at the knee (figure 1.7). Second, the pelvis (hip) is jointed not only with the femur (thigh) but also with the spine. This means that there must be very careful analysis of movement in any technical sport. For example, tilting the pelvis so that the lumbar spine flattens alters the relationship of the pelvis to the femur. So appropriate alignment of pelvis and spine is critical if maximum advantage is to be gained from the contribution of muscle actions at the hip joint (with femur), knee, ankle and foot. The following actions are possible about the axes indicated.

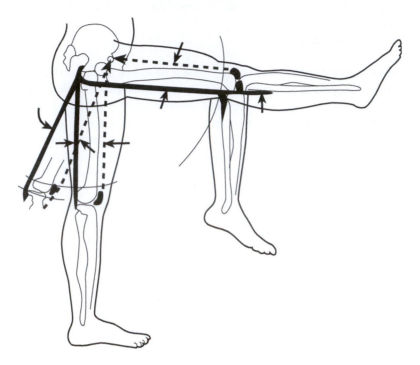

FIGURE 1.7 Effect of two-joint actions on two-joint muscles: rectus femoris (dotted line) and hamstring group (solid line) (Kapandji, 2010)

Transverse axis: *flexion* – the thigh is raised forward towards the chest. A limiting factor in this action is the state of flexion or extension at the knee. This is due to the 'hamstrings' group of muscles bridging two joints. When both hips are flexed, there is a tilting upwards and backwards of the pelvis, flattening the lumbar curve. Tilting the pelvis in this way aids hip flexion; *extension* – the thigh is pulled backwards. A limiting factor again is the state of flexion or extension at the knee. This is due to the rectus femoris bridging two joints. The forwards and downwards tilting of the pelvis helps extension. Hyperextension is brought about by exaggerating the lumbar curve. In effect, then, this does not alter the degree of extension between femur and pelvis but does considerably influence the angle between femur and the erect or extended spine above the lumbar region.

    E.g.   Flexion: iliopsoas
                                rectus femoris
         Extension: gluteus maximus
                                semimembranosus

It should be noted here that the position of flexion is a position of instability due to slackness of ligaments connecting femur and pelvis. Adduction and flexion together as in sitting with legs crossed increases the instability.

Anterio-posterior axis: *abduction* – the drawing apart of the thighs as in moving to stand with legs astride. The movement is limited by the adductor muscles, the iliofemoral and pubofemoral ligaments, and the bony structures themselves. The active maximum is 90°, while passive gives a greater angle only when combined with flexion and the forward tilt of the pelvis; *adduction* – the drawing together of the thighs as in gripping the flanks of a horse. This obviously must be combined with flexion or extension if a thigh is to be adducted past the midline of the body. The maximum degree of adduction beyond the midline is approximately 30°. The position of greatest instability of this joint is when the hip is well flexed and adducted, for example when sitting with the legs crossed.

> E.g.   Abduction: gluteus medius
>   sartorius
>   Adduction: adductor longus
>   gracilis

Vertical axis: *rotation outward (lateral)* – the action of moving towards splayed feet (ballet dancer) is limited by the iliofemoral and pubofemoral ligaments and, consequently, by the state of flexion or extension of femur on pelvis; *rotation inward (medial)* – the action of moving to stand pigeon-toed. This is limited by the ischiofemoral ligament and therefore by flexion or extension at the hip. Inward rotation is the easier, due to the slackness of the ischiofemoral ligament in movements combining flexion/abduction/inward rotation. This particular situation is the root of a problem for the beginner hurdler, who habitually drops the trailing knee to give an abbreviated first stride away from the hurdle.

> E.g.   Lateral rotation: piriformis
>   quadratus femoris
>   Medial rotation: tensor fascia lata
>   gluteus minimus

Outward rotation	Hip	Inward rotation
60°	Flexed	35°–45°
30°	Extended	30°–40°

Combinations of these actions allow circumduction as in hurdlers' trail leg recovery.

Knee

The skeletal components involved in knee actions are:

(HIPS)	Pelvis (iliacus, ischium, pubis)
(THIGH)	Femur
(LOWER LEG)	Tibia, Fibula

This joint must effect a mechanical compromise to reconcile two mutually exclusive requirements: great stability in extension when bodyweight and lever lengths impose stress, and great mobility in flexion when the joint must adapt to irregularities of terrain, changes of locomotive speed and direction, and in control of foot movements as in soccer, dancing, etc.

Satisfying these two requirements completely is almost impossible. Despite the ingenious mechanical devices incorporated in the joint, the poor degree of interlocking of surfaces (an essential for mobility) exposes the joint to immense risk of strain and injury. The following actions are possible about the transverse and vertical axes.

Transverse axis: *extension* – straightening the knee. The knee is considered extended when the thigh and lower leg form what is virtually a straight line. Only a very slight increase (5–10°) is possible beyond this point and may be produced by passive extension, i.e. when standing on a decline. Extension beyond this is abnormal. Extension of the hip aids extension of the knee by stretching the rectus femoris; *flexion* – the action of bringing the heel towards the buttock. The possible range depends on the state of flexion/extension at the hip joint and also whether the knee flexion is active or passive.

Active	Hip action	Passive
140°	Flexed	160°
120°*	extended	110–140°†

* Due to weakened hamstring and stretched rectus femoris, but follow through can bring heel to buttock
† Due to stretch of rectus femoris

E.g.	Extension:	vastus medialis
		rectus femoris
	Flexion:	biceps femoris
		semitendinosus

Vertical axis (leg in natural alignment with body): *rotation* – this is only possible when the knee is flexed, and the degree of rotation varies with the degree of knee flexion until the knee is flexed at 90°; *outward* – the foot is turned outwards, with knees bent as in commencement of the breaststroke leg kick; *inward* – the foot is turned inwards with knees bent, as in the initiation of rotation in javelin and discus.

Outward rotation	Knee flexion	Inward rotation
32°	30°	20°
42°	90°	30°

There is also a phenomenon known as automatic rotation. At the completion of knee extension the lower leg rotates outwards on the femur. Conversely, if the knee is extended while the foot is anchored on the floor (as in standing) then the first action described is seen as the femur rotating inwards on the lower leg. The injury potential in field games such as football and rugby is clear, for example, when there is forced outward rotation of femur on the lower leg, while it is naturally rotating inward in extension.

E.g.   Lateral: biceps femoris – long head
                     biceps femoris – short head
      Medial: gracilis
                popliteus

Ankle

The skeletal components involved in ankle actions are;

(LOWER LEG)	Tibia, fibula
(FOOT)	7 tarsals (talus, calcaneus, navicular, medial, intermediate and lateral cuneiforms, cuboid)
	5 metatarsals
(TOES)	Big toe – 2 phalanges; other 4 toes – 3 phalanges each (14 bones)

Several expressions are used uniquely in describing ankle joint actions. These actions are possible about the transverse, anterio-posterior and vertical axes when the joint is not weight bearing (e.g. when the foot is not in contact with any surface).

Transverse axis: *plantar flexion (flexion)* – this is the action of pointing the toes. To complicate matters, this action is referred to as ankle extension when rising up on the toes (i.e. when the ankle is weight bearing). The main muscles responsible for plantar flexion have greatest efficiency when the knee is extended and the ankle is in dorsiflexion; *dorsiflexion (extension)* – the action of turning the toes up towards the knee. There is less rotation possible in dorsiflexion than there is in plantar flexion.

E.g.   Plantar flexion: gastrocnemius
                            soleus
      Dorsiflexion: tibialis anterior
                            extensor digitorum longus

Anterio-posterior axis: *inversion (supination)* – the action of turning the medial (big toe) side of the foot upwards towards the inside of the knee. Inversion injuries (i.e. where the trauma is sustained on the lateral side) account for 80 per cent of all ankle injuries; *eversion (pronation)* – the action of turning the lateral (small toe) side of the foot upwards towards the outside of the knee.

Due to the demands for directional change in the majority of games, the latter two actions are extremely important. Lateral changes of direction will ultimately require departure from the running surface via inversion or eversion. Moreover, these actions facilitate adaptation to a terrain.

E.g.   Inversion: tibialis posterior
                      extensor hallucis longus
      Eversion: fibularis tertius
                    fibularis longus

Vertical axis: as indicated above, rotation is more free in plantar flexion than in dorsiflexion; *outward (abduction)* – the turning of the foot outwards; *inward (adduction)* – the turning of the foot inwards. Once again, these actions are critical in changing direction and in adjusting balance in variable terrain.

E.g. Lateral rotation: peroneus longus
peroneus brevis
Medial rotation: tibialis posterior
tibialis anterior

Combinations of these actions permit circumduction – critical to footwork with the ball in football.

Foot

The skeletal components involved in the foot and toe actions are:

(LOWER LEG)	Tibia, fibula
(FOOT)	7 tarsals (talus, calcaneus, navicular, medial, intermediate and lateral cuneiforms, cuboid)
	5 Metatarsals
(TOES)	Big toe – 2 phalanges; other 4 toes – 3 phalanges (14 bones)

In discussing the ankle joint actions, especially those of inversion and eversion, the actions of the foot have already been introduced. Man's foot has been the unfortunate victim of the progress of civilisation, and its properties are gradually being lost. Our ancestors may well have been able to oppose their big toes in the same way that we can oppose our thumbs. However, the toes may be flexed, extended, adducted and abducted in much the same way as fingers.

Due to the complex of 26 bones, the foot is well equipped both in strength and mobility to adapt to any type of terrain. This adaptability is obviously fundamental to efficient locomotion. The foot is the first and final contact with the surface of the ground, and a lack of ability to accept loadings of momentum on any given surface will result in dissipation of effort or possible injury.

Kapandji's observations (2010) are worth noting: 'The town dweller always walks on even and firm ground with his feet protected by shoes. There is therefore little need for the arches of his feet to adapt to new terrains and the supporting muscles eventually atrophy: the flat foot is the price paid for progress and some anthropologists go so far as to forecast that man's feet will be reduced to mere stumps. This thesis is borne out by the fact that in man in contrast to the ape the toes are atrophied and the big toe can no longer be opposed.'

This stage is still a long way off and even civilised man can still walk barefoot on a beach or on the rocks and grip with his toes. There can be little doubt that the small muscles of the foot can and should be developed to maintain the integrity of the plantar vault (figure 1.8) and, as a consequence, retrieve its adaptive capabilities. The toes, like the fingers, make movements possible about two axes.

Transverse axis
E.g. Flexion: flexor digitorum longus
flexor hallucis brevis (big toe)

| Extension: | extensor digitorum brevis |
| | extensor hallucis longus (big toe) |

Anterio-posterior axis

E.g.	Abduction:	dorsal interossei
		flexor digiti minimi brevis
	Adduction:	plantar interossei
		adductor hallucis

The function of the toes and foot muscles are critical to maintaining and adjusting balance when weight bearing.

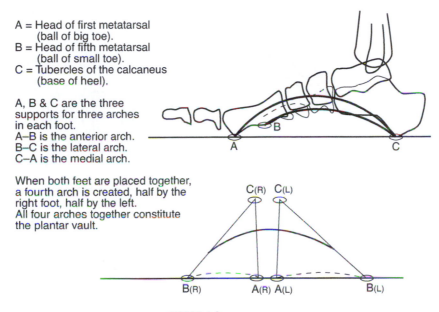

A = Head of first metatarsal (ball of big toe).
B = Head of fifth metatarsal (ball of small toe).
C = Tubercles of the calcaneus (base of heel).

A, B & C are the three supports for three arches in each foot.
A–B is the anterior arch.
B–C is the lateral arch.
C–A is the medial arch.

When both feet are placed together, a fourth arch is created, half by the right foot, half by the left.
All four arches together constitute the plantar vault.

FIGURE 1.8 Plantar vault

The lower limbs joint complexes afford immense potential from the foundation of strength. We are a long way from exhausting that potential. Control of the toes to hold brushes in painting; of the feet and ankles in flamenco and the modern variants of Celtic dancing; and of total lower limb complexes in soccer, skiing, and ice skating, demonstrate this in the area of motor coordination. Gymnasts, acrobats and limbo dancers demonstrate this in the area of mobility. Weightlifters, ski jumpers, throwers and ballet dancers demonstrate this in the area of strength. Mobility and motor coordination embrace lower limb joint complex movement potential by building on strength.

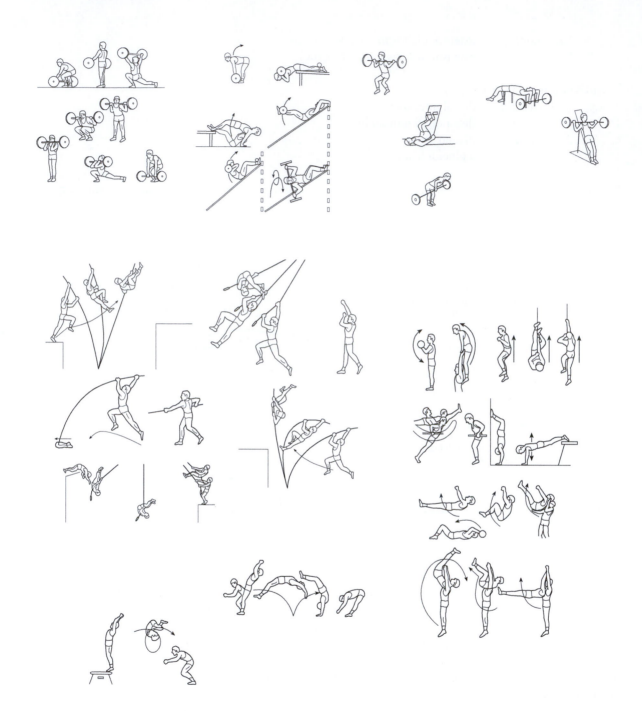

FIGURE 1.9 Examples of exercises demonstrating the total movement potential of the body's system of levers: circuit training; active mobility; passive mobility; basic weight training; related strength exercises and specific strength exercises

MALE/FEMALE BODY VARIATIONS

Before leaving this section, male/female variations are worth noting. Due to the greater width of the female pelvis compared with the male pelvis, the angle between femur and tibia is generally greater for women than for men. This causes a more lateral force as the quadriceps extend the knee which may pull the patella outwards. This is clearly a disadvantage when force of knee and hip extension is required and highlights the high injury potential not only at knee and hip, but at the junction of sacrum and ilium, and pubic symphysis which are less stable in women than in men, particularly in the two or three days premenstruation. Although the head of the female femur is approximately 30 per cent smaller than in the male, affording some degree of extra mobility, stability in the joint is not compromised; nor is there greater stress in the female hip joint due to the support of the fibrocartilaginous rim (acetabular laborum) that lines the socket (acetabulum) into which the head of the femur fits, plus the strength of the transverse acetabular ligaments.

The female shoulders are also narrower than in men and the lateral angle of radius/ulna on humerus is greater, providing a weaker force application potential in 'pulling' and 'pushing' activities. The length of the female spine is approximately 86 per cent that of the male spine and this, combined with a greater distribution of weight towards hips/thighs, gives women a relatively lower centre of gravity and therefore an advantage where potential stability and/or balance is required.

SUMMARY

Whole body movement, and the movement at each joint, can be described in terms of rotations about axes. These movements are classified as actions in specific anatomical terms. In any given activity, several combinations of joint actions, made possible by a specific programme of muscle contractions, will take place. The interplay of these actions will dictate the final efficiency as an expression of energy.

In the first instance, the range of a joint action will be a function of that joint's structure. Secondary limiting factors are imposed by the soft tissue structures bridging and surrounding the joint. A working knowledge of all the body's structures must then be seen as basic to an appreciation of the body's total movement potential and to analysis of technical models. It is convenient to study body movement with reference to three areas.

1. The upper limb complex is designed for mobility and is the final link in a force sequence for many activities. By its nature, it is the fastest link in the force sequence and training is aimed at ensuring that the contribution of this link is synchronised in its application of speed, force, range, and final technical 'touch' after other joint complexes have provided their contributions.

2. The spine is variously a complex of joints providing a remarkable range of movement in some activities and a powerful pillar linking lower and upper limb complexes in others. Both strength and mobility must be developed to ensure that demands of stability and mobility can be met.

3. The lower limb complex is the initiator of a force sequence in many activities. Great force must be generated by the complex, frequently with only instantaneous ground contact. Moreover, it must offer

sufficient mobility to permit rapid adjustment to any given terrain. Consequently the lower limb must provide mobility, stability and the capacity to express force at speed.

It must be stressed that although the coach considers each joint action in analysis of a given movement, no action should be thought of in isolation, but as part of the total movement, in terms of both force contribution and timing. To summarise chapter 1, an understanding of the extraordinary movement potential of the lever system is fundamental to the design of the technical models demanded of sports disciplines, and to the selection of exercises for effective technical development and technical performance. Chapters 3, 6 and 11 build on this understanding, which is then translated through parts 4 and 5 into practice.

REFLECTIVE QUESTIONS

1. In performing a half squat without added weight:
   a. What are the actions at hip, knee, spine, ankle?
   b. What are the principle agonists, antagonists, stabilisers and neutralisers for each joint action named?

2. On the images below of the following bones, indicate in red the origins of relevant muscles and, in green, insertions.
   a. Right pelvis: (ilium, ischium, pubis) lateral and medial surfaces
   b. Left scapula: costal/anterior and dorsal/posterior surfaces

3. Why would someone accustomed to high heeled shoes experience discomfort when in low heeled shoes? Where might such discomfort be felt and what are possible anatomical and mechanical reasons?

4. Reflecting on the importance of synergic function (stabilisers and neutralisers) of muscles, describe some exercises and activities to develop their effectiveness in each of the following:
   a. Foot, ankle, knee
   b. Spine
   c. Hips
   d. Shoulder girdle
   e. Hand, wrist, elbow

5. Weightlifters may use a supportive broad belt around their waist. Some other people, for cosmetic or other reasons wear similar supportive girdles. Discuss the role of these devices mechanically and anatomically in terms of what and how they may contribute to support of the spine and any possible negative effect of persistent use. How would you develop relevant musculature to reduce or eliminate reliance on such devices?

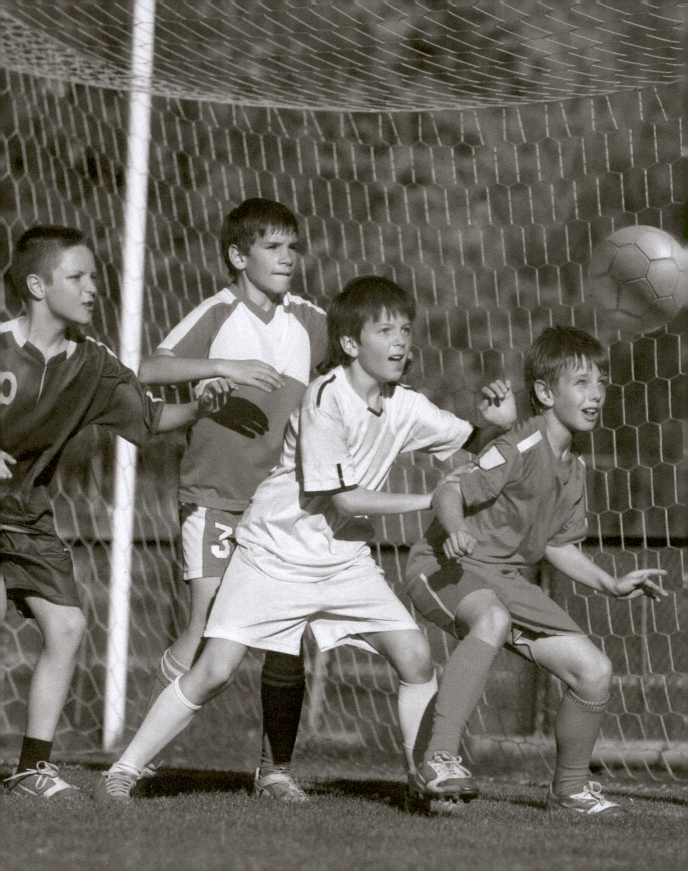

2 STRUCTURAL CHANGES IN THE GROWING CHILD

STAGES OF GROWTH

It takes approximately 20 years for all the morphological, physiological and psychological processes of development to bring the newly born child to maturity. The unfolding of his development is a long but necessary period, during which time growth cannot simply be seen as an increase in height and weight, but as a gentle ebb and flow of differentiating and integrating forms and functions.

The child, in his or her various stages of growth, is not a mini-adult. It must be clearly understood that from stage to stage in his growth, the child varies in the proportion of individual body parts in terms of

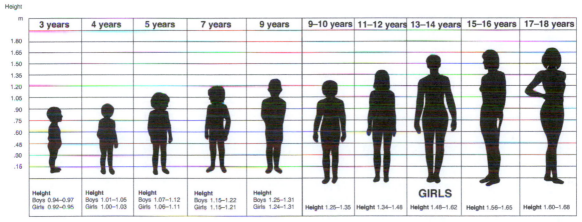

FIGURE 2.1 Growth of the child. Average height progression, showing the 'parting of the ways' after approximately nine years, in terms of relative height increase, and absolute height. Modified from *Family Health Guide* (Reader's Digest, 1972).

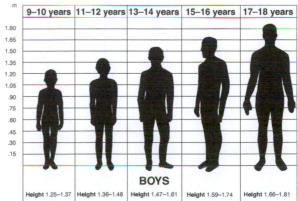

length, volume and weight. Each part grows at a different rate, ranging from twofold expansion (head) to fivefold expansion (legs), between birth and maturity (figures 2.1 and 2.2). Implicit in this is that certain skills may require considerable adjustment of the neuromuscular processes from year to year, according to shifting emphasis of growth. Consequently, as the athlete grows, it seems advisable to maintain principal elements of technique training throughout the year, relating the solutions of short-term technical challenges to long-term technical models.

Several authorities have attempted to classify the stages of development (see table 2.1).

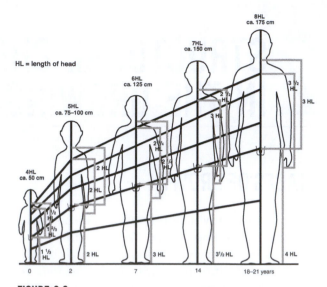

FIGURE 2.2 Alterations in body proportions during growth (from Bammes, 2011)

Stage	Characteristic growth landmarks	Age: male	Age: female
Newly born	Healing of the umbilicus		
Infant	Up to appearance of first milk teeth	0.5	0.5
Crawling age	Up to learning to walk	1–1.5	1–1.5
Small child	Up to appearance of the first permanent tooth	6	6
Early school age (pre-puberty)	Up to first signs of maturity (beginning of growth spurt, rapid genital development, first breast development)	11	9
Puberty	Period between appearance of pubic hair and first menarche or development of male sperms	14	14–15
Adolescence	Puberty and end of physical growth	22	18
Age of achievement	Period of optimal capacity	variations in these stages cover a great range but are normal	

TABLE 2.1 Stages of growth against age and gender (adapted from Grimm, 1966)

Skeletal development

With the exception of the skull and clavicle, all the bones in the body are formed from cartilage. The process starts from before birth and concludes with final ossification of the skeleton between 18 and 22 years of age. Bone lengthens by growing at the junction between the main shaft and the growing end which is known as the epiphysis. In the long bones (i.e. the arms and legs), most growth takes place at one end only. This is extremely significant when one considers that the femur and tibia, for example, grows mostly at the knee end, which is exposed to considerable training loads. Ossification is the destruction and breakdown of cartilage and its replacement with bone tissue. This process is accompanied by the setting down of an increasingly thick layer of bone around the cartilage (perichondral ossification) and from within the cartilage (endochondral ossification).

The growing bone has a greater proportion of softer material in the basic substance, which is essential for compressive and tensile strength. This, and the sponge-like nature of immature bone material, which is still in the process of developing adaptability to loading, means that the growing bone is more elastic but has less bending strength. This is a major cause of the reduced load-bearing capacity of the child's skeleton.

Hormones affect the process and rate of skeletal development, but functional loading may also influence the process. Most research has considered the role of hormones, but a considerable volume of research would indicate that controlled loadings will favourably influence skeletal growth. Research in this area has suggested that: (1) intermittent submaximal loading (80–90 per cent maximum) stimulates height growth (Tittel, 1963); (2) excessive loading in quality or quantity inhibits height growth; and (3) muscle pull, above all, is the functional stimulus for the growth in thickness of the bone (Harre, 1973).

It is an unfortunate fact of modern life that there is a general decline in physical activity of children and young people in their growing years. This will be discussed more fully in chapter 13, but it is appropriate here to point out that physical activity is essential to healthy musculoskeletal development and function. For example, without physical activity, the lateral angel of radius/ulna on humerus (pubertal valgus) remains greater for females than males. However, girls exposed to training programmes in early (pre-pubertal) involvement sport such as gymnastics and swimming have relatively straight arms (Craig Sharp). This is clearly an advantage in further upper body strength development.

A multi-sport approach to activity programme design, in addition to providing a wide range of challenges in coordination/motor skills, joint action and physical demand must also ensure that a balance of strengths is maintained. So, for example, in the growing athlete, it should not be assumed that because a lot of knee extension exercise is evident in training and competition, all four parts of the quadriceps are being developed in parallel. For a number of reasons the strength of muscles which afford lateral pull (e.g. vastus lateralis) may develop disproportionately to the medial side (vastus medialis). This can cause medium and long term problems in the knee.

A thoughtfully balanced yet challenging physical activity programme through an athlete's growing years is the platform on which all further development and performance can be built. This, on the one hand, is preparation for an active life, and on the other, for high performance in sport.

It is my opinion that, in the early growth stages, working the child to a point where loading cannot be repeated due to fatigue and/or insufficient strength is fundamentally working against the most favourable conditions for healthy growth. Although insufficient motivation on the part of the child may terminate activity long before this point is reached, parents, teachers or coaches must exercise responsible judgement in when and when not to push towards limits arrived at through strong external motivation.

Tendencies of growth

We can see from figures 2.3a and 2.3b that, over time, there is a pattern to the increase in weight and height. By plotting this we can identify anomalies in growth and development, and select athletes on the basis of specific anthropometric criteria for a sport or discipline.

There is reference in several papers to phases of extension (growing up) and phases of abundance (growing out) as factors of some importance in the training of athletes. Such changes, then, are not a matter of continuous increase. Several attempts have been made to relate these phases to athletic events and performances (table 2.2).

The changes in relative body dimensions have been mentioned earlier in connection with the possible variations in the development of athletic skill and ability. The amazing complexity of this shift in relative dimension is probably best illustrated in a piece of work conducted on elite swimmers between 8 and 14 years of age in the former German Democratic Republic (GDR), as figure 2.4 shows. Looking to the future, tables may be constructed to show indices of age-specific, strength-weight ratios as this might give a clear guide as to which physical characteristics (age-dependent, or specific growth rate dependent) are temporarily regressive (table 2.2).

Against this background it is important to avoid the temptation to ignore the less proficient in favour of the superior athlete in his early teens. Superiority may well be due to early physical development which frequently leaves an athlete's peers unable to meet him on equal terms. The spread of growth in these years is considerable. Attention must therefore be given to those youngsters who are able to perform skills efficiently,

Feature	Value	Norm value	Value age	Mean value	Value age	Spread	Mean of top 5 athletes by performance
Class 7 x	Height cm	151.6	13	159.2	14.5	150.9–167.3	160.3
+12.8 yrs	Weight kg	40.7	13	43.0	13.5	34.4–51.6	44.5
	Thigh length mm			429		409–447	444
	Lower leg length mm			358		336–378	380
Class 8 x	Height	157.8	14	167.1	15.5	160.9–173.2	169.3
+13.8 yrs	Weight	45.7	14	50.0			52.2
	Thigh length			448		430–466	460
	Lower leg length			376		352–397	386
Class 9 x	Height	163.6	15	173.0	16	168.1–177.9	175.3
+ 15 yrs	Weight	50.7	15	56.6	16	50.9–62.3	60.1
	Thigh length					450–478	469
	Lower leg length					374–408	400

TABLE 2.2 Comparison of body measurements of young middle distance athletes with the average values for the former German Democratic Republic (adapted by Harre 1986 from Marcusson 1961).

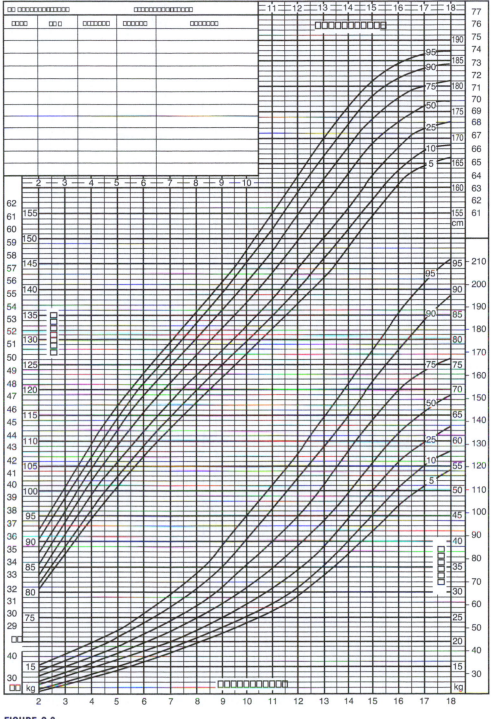

FIGURE 2.3a Boys' physical growth percentiles

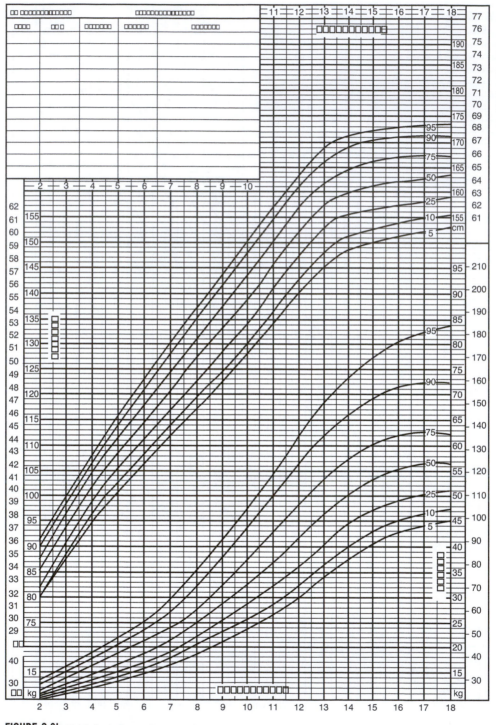

FIGURE 2.3b Girls' physical growth percentiles

and compete with considerable success, but have yet to develop. In short, a judgement of body size based solely on age is unreliable, but can be made reliable if it is seen against the individual's stage of maturity. Early, late and normal developers must be seen in 'performance perspective'.

The total time of pubescent growth lasts longer for boys, although girls start earlier by 1½–2 years. The 14-year-old girl is already approximately 97 per cent final height, and at 18 years of age is 96 per cent final leg length. On the other hand, the 14-year-old boy is approximately 85 per cent final height, and 80 per cent final leg length between 18–22 years of age.

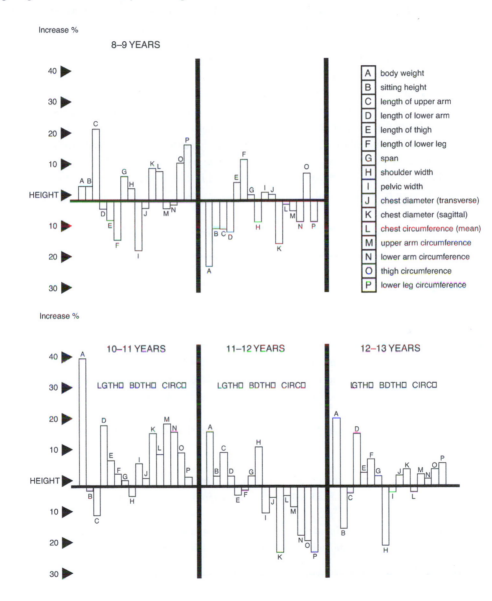

FIGURE 2.4 Relative rate of growth of body parts (from Harre, 1986)

SUMMARY

The period up to and through the adolescence years of rapid growth is not only one of preparation for serious competition in the later peak performance years of their twenties and thirties, it is also a period of preparation for high pressure competition in the growing years. Clearly this is the case in sports such as gymnastics and, to a variable extent, swimming, but it is also true where an early and exceptional level of talent takes an athlete beyond his peers and finds him competitive in top level sport. As a consequence, the coach must understand the athlete's patterns of growth. From these patterns it seems logical to establish the fundamentals of techniques before the pubertal growth spurt, as pubescence and adolescence create disproportionate relationships between body parts. In some instances, a technical model is established to meet the short-term objectives of junior arenas, then changed later. In others, the model will be progressively modified in stages to suit the demands of short-, medium- and long-term performance objectives. Training loads should be progressed via numbers of repetitions and/or speed rather than by increasing resistance, which should not go beyond an estimated 80–90 per cent maximum. Epiphyses are almost certainly damaged if this advice is ignored. Loading which compresses the spine, as in several orthodox weightlifting exercises, must not be employed until the spine has stopped growing and/or has been protected by developed spinal musculature. Prediction of height growth patterns is possible and is used in several countries to select athletes according to anthropometric trends in given disciplines.

REFLECTIVE QUESTIONS

1. Discuss the statement: 'You should fit the activity to the child before trying to fit the child to the activity.'

2. Your group of 12–16 year old athletes have been working over some months on an all-weather surface on activities and exercises for a sport which requires multiple accelerations and decelerations over distances from 5–20m. A number of them are mentioning pain in their shins and knees. Discuss possible anatomical and mechanical reasons and what changes you may make to the programme.

3. Discuss advantages and disadvantages of athletes developing extreme ranges of joint mobility in spine and pelvis in pre-pubertal years.

4. Young children appear to develop skill on skis more readily than adults learning such. Discuss why this may be the case and what advantage or disadvantage this might represent as the young skier grows.

5. Discuss the pros and cons of providing a programme of multiple motor skills/sports and ensuring a foundation of balanced strength and mobility versus early specialisation.

3 BASIC MECHANICS

A detailed knowledge of 'laminae and particles' is not required by the student of training theory, but he should attempt to achieve some working knowledge of those terms which are most frequently used in analyses. To this end, the following is presented.

DEFINITIONS
Motion

Motion is simply a change of position, but should be defined as a change relative to another body, a fixed point, etc. For example, the femur flexes on the pelvis; the basketball player breaks past his opposite number, and so on. Some types of motion are not easily observed because they are too slow (for example the opening of a flower) or because they are too fast (for example the beating of a fly's wing). Video analysis is often used to study motion in sport. Such study may range from an analysis of team play to the analysis of an athlete's technical efficiency.

Rest is the status of an object when its position, with respect to some point, line, surface, etc., remains unchanged. It is important to know that in any given activity there is no movement at some joints while there is at others. Where there is no movement the muscle activity is referred to as *static* and where there is movement the muscle activity is *dynamic*.

A study of motion and rest, relative to limbs or bodies, etc., forms the basis of mechanical analysis. *Linear motion* is motion in a straight line; this is also referred to as translatory motion (e.g. running 60m). *Angular motion* is the motion of rotation; this is also referred to as rotary motion (e.g. a front somersault). *Curvilinear motion* is motion which involves linear and angular motion (e.g. a cartwheel or a hammer thrower advancing and turning across the circle).

Centre of gravity

The centre of gravity is a body's centre of weight. In other words, it is that point about which the body is balanced relative to all three axes. When a body is in flight, any rotation takes place about the centre of gravity. When describing rotation in flight, direction of rotation about an axis is defined as clockwise or anticlockwise.

Vertical axis (long axis of the body): the athlete is standing on the clock face, i.e. a pirouette to the right is a clockwise rotation (figure 3.1b).

Transverse axis (axis through the hips, left to right): the athlete has the clock face on his left, i.e. a front somersault is a clockwise rotation (figure 3.1a).

Anterio-posterior axis (axis from front to back through hips): the athlete faces the clock, i.e. a cartwheel to the right is clockwise rotation (figure 3.1c).

The centre of gravity represents the intersection of these axes, which in the athlete's body is roughly half way between umbilicus and pubic crest and 3cm in front of the spine. This of course, is an approximation and will find slight difference in females compared with males; short and broad athletes compared with tall and thin; the same person as a child and as an adult. Provided the imaginary perpendicular from this point to the ground falls within the athlete's 'base' (e.g. feet), he will not fall over. The relationship of this perpendicular to the body's point(s) of support is critical in the study of sports technique.

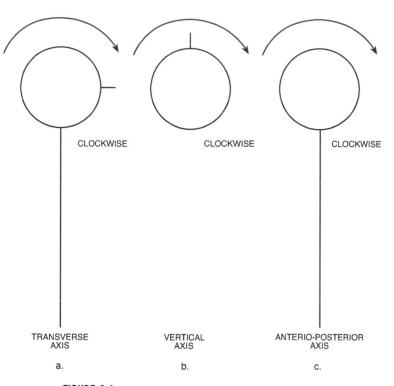

FIGURE 3.1 Basis for defining rotation about the body's axes

Force

Force is anything which produces motion or changes of motion. It could also be seen as a push or pull, a tendency to distort, and so on. As applied to work or movement analysis, three factors must be considered: (1) magnitude of force, i.e. its size (e.g. 400 joules); (2) direction of the force, i.e. in which direction the force is applied (e.g. vertically); and (3) point of application of force, i.e. where the force is being applied (e.g. at the athlete's foot) as in figure 3.2.

Work is the overcoming of a load or resistance and is measured as the product of force × distance moved. In most cases, the force producing work in moving the athlete's limbs is the contraction of muscle. This usually results in a shortening and thickening of the muscle without a change in volume. The product of the force with which it contracts, and the range through which the force is applied, is the measure of the mechanical work performed by the muscle. Some confusion must arise when the muscle contraction is static (isometric). The force provided by the contracting muscle is applied through 0 range – producing mechanical work of force × 0 = 0. In this case there appears to be no mechanical work performed, but energy has certainly been expressed as physiological work which might be measured in terms of heat energy. It becomes convenient, then, to measure mechanical work according to its energy cost.

Energy cost

One joule of work is that performed in raising 1 newton, 1m. One newton is the force acting on the mass of 1kg at normal acceleration of gravity. One joule may also be expressed as 0.239 calories. One calorie is the amount of heat required to raise 1g water, 1°C. The basic unit for most purposes is a kilocalorie (kcal) which is 1000 calories (4186 joules). The energy costs of various activities can be calculated and stand-

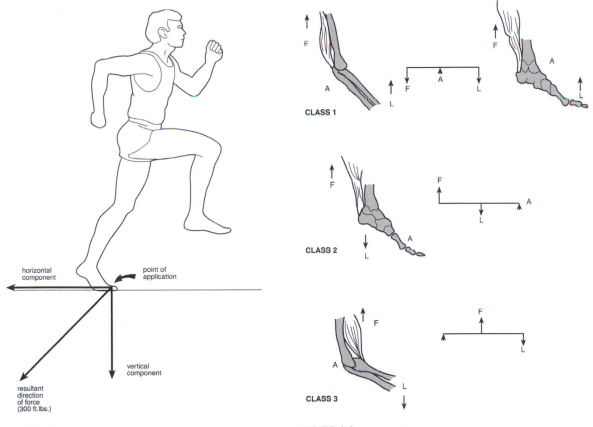

FIGURE 3.2 Force application in long jump

FIGURE 3.3 Classes of lever

ardised as an aid to studying the balance of energy input (nutrition) against energy output (work). For example, sitting at ease = 1.6kcals/minute, while walking at 8.8km/h on flat ground = 5.6kcals/minute (see also table 4.1, p. 55).

The athlete's bodyweight should remain constant if the calorie input (diet) equals the calorie output (activity).

Machines

A machine is a device for performing work. Among the simplest machines are the pulley, the lever, the wheel and axle, the inclined plane, the wedge and the screw. All complex machines comprise simple machines which, in the case of the athlete are almost always levers. Machines are concerned with two forces – that put into the machine (effort, or internal force, or force) and that which the machine attempts to overcome (resistance, or external force, or load).

A lever is a rod turning about a fixed point (axis). In the athlete, the levers are bones. The forces are expressed by the contracting muscles pulling on the bones, and the loads vary from other bones or the athlete's own bodyweight, to external loads such as barbells, , discuses,oars, water, kinetic energies, etc.

The efficiency of the lever depends on certain mechanical factors. Of primary importance are the exact position on the lever of the application of force (F), the location of the load (L), and the axis in question (A).

The relative positions of these points dictate the 'class' of lever. An understanding of how these levers work may help in technical analysis (figure 3.3). Broadly speaking, class 1 is built for equilibrium, class 2 for saving force, and class 3 for speed and range of movement. The distance from F to A is known as the force arm, and the distance from L to A as the load arm. Any lever system will balance when:

force × force arm = load × load arm

What force is required to make each system balance in a class 1 lever system? From the figures in table 3.1, the following can be seen:

- The force required to move the lever is indirectly proportional to the length of the force arm.
- Only when the two arms are equal in length will the force equal the load.
- By adding to the length of the force arm, the force may be reduced to almost nothing.
- The effect of the load follows the same rules as those which determine the effect of the force.
- The force necessary to operate the class 1 lever depends upon the relative length of the lever arms.

With small adjustments these observations also apply to class 2 and class 3 levers.

force	x	force arm	=	resistance	x	load arm	answer
F	x	2	=	10	x	18	F = 90
F	x	8	=	10	x	12	F = 15
F	x	16	=	10	x	4	F = 2.5
F	x	8	=	10	x	2	F = 2.5

TABLE 3.1 Equilibrium exists where force × force arm = load (resistance) × load arm

This brief expansion on the 'mathematics of levers' is not advanced purely for academic interest. It may help, for example, in creating new possibilities for strength training where the total available resistance is relatively low. By thoughtful use of levers, or pulleys, the effect of this low resistance can be increased.

Before moving on from levers, the value should be noted of bony devices which provide greater mechanical advantage of muscle pull. They achieve this by increasing the length of the lever arm, changing the direction of force application, and so on. There are several examples, but few illustrate this better than the patella (kneecap). The force of muscle pull may be thought of as having two components. One provides rotation of one lever on another and the other pulls along the length of the levers, and by so doing provides joint stability. If the direction of muscle pull is almost parallel with the levers concerned, the stabilising component is very great and the rotational component small. The converse is true if the direction of muscle pull is more angular. The patella changes the direction of application of force of the knee extensors by providing a greater angle of insertion of the patellar ligament into the tibial tuberosity. This change of direction raises the effective force of the knee extension by increasing the component of rotation and decreasing the stabilising component.

LAWS OF MOTION

There are three laws of motion – inertia, acceleration and reaction (Newton's three laws).

The law of inertia

A resting or moving body will remain in that state until a force alters this situation. By this law, both motion and rest are states of resistance or loading. The amount of resistance to change of state (inertia) is dependent upon the mass of the body concerned and its velocity. Velocity is the relationship of the distance covered to the time taken – *and it has a direction* (e.g. 45km/h south). It is inertia that must be overcome in making something move from rest (e.g. weightlifting, sprint, rowing, swimming, kayak, cycling, etc. starts); or in arresting movement (e.g. tackling in soccer, rugby, Australian Rules, NFL, etc.); or in changing direction of movement (e.g. changing tack in sailing; slalom in canoe, ski, etc.; sidestepping or swerving in field games, etc).

The law of acceleration

Acceleration is directly proportional to the force causing it and inversely proportional to the mass of the body involved. Acceleration is the rate of change of velocity. This implies increase or decrease in the distance covered in a given period of time but, in addition, since velocity has direction, acceleration must also be implied in a rate of change of direction. Thus centripetal acceleration is that continuous change of direction which permits an athlete or cyclist to move round a curve.

The law of reaction

For every action there is an equal and opposite reaction. When stepping on to a chair or box, one is supported by the counterforce offered by the chair or box. If the counterforce is less, one will fall through! When flight is considered, as in jumping, and a body part moves in one direction, then some other part or equivalence of force must act in the opposite direction.

Gravity

One force which will act on the body at all times is that of gravity. When an athlete launches himself or an object into flight, as soon as flight is commenced, there is a force which causes a reduction in upward velocity at a speed of 981.274 cm/sec^2. The centre of gravity of the object or athlete will be seen to trace a course – a parabola (figure 3.4). It should be noted that whether or not the athlete rotates or moves parts of his body while in flight, the parabola of the athlete's centre of gravity is dictated by the angle and speed of take-off. Should the implement have aerodynamic properties then, of course, the flight path will not be a parabola as it will glide for at least part of its journey.

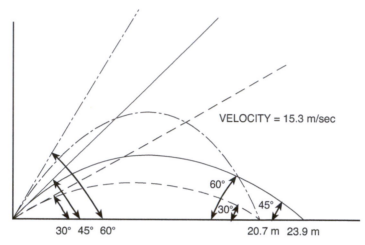

FIGURE 3.4 Once launched, the centre of gravity of an athlete or implement must follow a parabolic path in flight. Here, this is seen in the path of the object projected at various angles at 15.3m/sec.

Momentum

Momentum is the quantity of motion and is therefore the product of mass × velocity. The body is frequently put in motion, or assisted in motion, by transfer of momentum from a part of the body to the whole body, as in the free leg and arms in the high jump. Momentum may be linear or angular.

Mass

Mass is the quantity of matter. It is given dimension from weight/gravity.

Moment of inertia

Moment of inertia is the distribution of a body's mass, i.e. its size. If a gymnast tucks himself into a ball, his moment of inertia is small about the transverse axis. If he extends into a star shape, his moment of inertia is large about the transverse axis. Moment of inertia might well be thought of as the rotating body's radius.

Angular momentum

Angular momentum is the product of the moment of inertia × angular velocity, i.e. revolutions per minute. The importance of understanding angular momentum should not be underestimated because it has a considerable number of applications in sport. This concept may be illustrated by assuming that an imaginary gymnast is rotating at 5 revs/minute with a radius of three units. His angular momentum is $(3 \times 5) = 15$ units. Now, assuming there is no deceleration due to friction, air resistance, and so on, the momentum will remain at 15 units. If the athlete now reduces the radius to one unit, the momentum remaining the same, his angular velocity is now 15 revs/minute. An understanding of this may enable sophisticated control of rotation in flight.

Related in part to this is the fact that the reaction of the body to a long lever will be greater than to a short one. In throwing movements involving rotation of the body, the longer the lever, the less will be the force but the greater will be the instantaneous linear speed at the end of the lever. This is also relevant in all striking activities, ranging from golf to soccer.

Understanding angular momentum is fundamental in learning and applying certain aspects of technique. For example, an ice skater may alter and control the speed of spin by moving arms away from the body (slower) or bringing them tight to the body (faster). The same principles apply in tumbling, trampoline, gymnastics and acrobatics. In discus throw, by commencing rotation from the back of the circle with a wide long sweep of the non-weight bearing leg, then snapping it in tight to the vertical axis on entering the throwing position, the plane of the hips moves from being parallel with the shoulders to being in advance – creating torque and consequent force/speed advantage on release.

When considering rotation, it is worth bearing in mind that it is seldom about one axis only. Also, in several sports, there can be the sudden intervention of an outside force when a body is already rotating. When this happens, the principle of precession applies. When a body is rotating clockwise about one axis, and a force intervenes to make it rotate clockwise about a second axis, the reaction is for the body to rotate clockwise about the third. If the intervening force in this situation makes it rotate anticlockwise about the second, the reaction is anticlockwise about the third (figure 3.1).

Friction

It is important to understand those factors which retard or interfere with motion as it is to understand what creates motion. 'Friction' is the force resisting the relative motion of solid surfaces, fluid layers and material elements sliding against each other. Broadly speaking, there is static friction (between non-moving surfaces) and kinetic friction (between moving surfaces). The positive side of friction, for example, is that it permits intended movement such as locomotion, so we have spiked shoes, boots with studs. Or again, it affords security of grip (e.g. resin/chalk on hands in gymnastics, pole vault, weightlifting) or of balance (e.g. studs and abrasives on shoes and boots). The negative side, on the one hand, can retard progress (e.g. air resistance, heavy underfoot conditions); and on the other, cause damage through uneven or non-free flowing movement (e.g. joint damage, skin chafing, blisters, etc).

Sports like sailing leverage the plusses and minuses of the 'friction' of wind movement, while designing the hull to leverage the plusses and minuses of the 'friction' of water and currents. Alpine skiing seeks an optimal balance between engaging friction and reducing it.

This has implications for the design of clothing, footwear, equipment, surfaces, etc. to maximise factors which support performance, while reducing factors which interfere with performance.

Torque

At its simplest, torque is a force. Normally, a force is a push or a pull. Torque is a twist. It is, then, a turning force producing rotation.

It has an important place in sport techniques where it is applied to create a rotational force which in turn produces change in angular momentum – either as acceleration or deceleration.

For example, in throwing events in athletics, torque is created in the vertical axis by twisting (rotating) the plane of the hips in advance of the plane of the shoulders on entry into the delivery phase, producing an acceleration in angular momentum of the shoulders and consequently implement release speed.

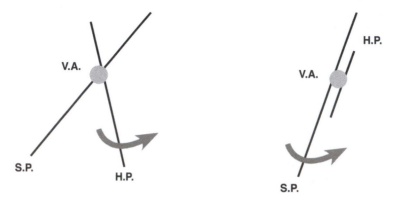

FIGURE 3.5 Hips plane (HP) rotates ahead of shoulders plane (SP) – creating torque about the vertical axis (VA). SP rotation (angular momentum) is then accelerated.

SUMMARY

There has been no intention here to present an exhaustive review of mechanics, but more realistically to establish some understanding of the basic terminology used in mechanical analysis. It must be remembered that in dealing with mechanical laws, the athlete is biomechanical and flexible; he is not a machine, but a living, thinking, self-regulating being. The excellent and more detailed mechanical information available to coaches and students of physical education in specific texts must always be interpreted with this in mind.

Because the neuromusculoskeletal complex is a self-regulating system operating within a framework of mechanical laws, even a well-established technical model may be compromised. Muscular imbalances, poorly monitored practice and fatigue, for example, may produce compensatory biomechanical adjustments which, over a period of time, create less effective technique and, as a consequence, underperformance. Ideally, technical performance should be regularly monitored via biomechanical analysis using digital video. There is a growing resource of software programmes specifically designed for this purpose.

Throughout his career, Jack Nicklaus, the legendary golfer, annually worked with a professional over a two-week period to 'realign my swing'. No matter how expert and experienced the athlete, the rough and tumble of competition through a season or year normally finds introduction of compensatory movements. Compensations must be determined to reestablish technical models which are stable and robust.

REFLECTIVE QUESTIONS

1. Select a technique in a sport of your choice and explain how an understanding of Newton's three laws of motion influences the effectiveness of that technique.

2. From the moment an athlete takes off in long jump, there is forward rotation about the transverse axis. Applying understanding of centre of gravity; Newton's three laws; and of angular momentum, how can the athlete counter his rotation to land with heels ahead of the centre of gravity flight path?

3. Discuss the similarities and differences in technique for a track athlete sprinter and sprinting in field sports. What are the mechanical reasons for the differences? Use two sports to illustrate: one with a ball only and one with an additional piece of equipment such as hockey or lacrosse stick.

4. You are communicating with the International Space Station from Houston. What you see on your screen is an astronaut floating horizontally, facing upwards, his head to your left. You need to have him vertical and facing you as if standing to attention. He cannot reach any fixed object to do so. Explain each instruction in terms of mechanical principles.

5. At Acapulco in Mexico, the divers (clavadistas) dive from a cliff (La Quebara), 41.5m above the water. They need to enter the water 4m out from the cliff base to miss the rocks. What distance must they travel? How long are they in flight from take-off to entry? What will their velocity be on entry?

SUMMARY OF PART 1

When analysing movement or investigating new possibilities of technique, it is tempting to focus attention on a single joint action or on one mechanical principle. However, it is basic to all study of movement that it is the most efficient compromise which must be sought. Moreover, one must be constantly aware of a joint action relative to other joint actions, a joint action relative to whole body movement, and all actions relative to mechanical laws. Consequently, it is suggested that the student of techniques in sport should establish a technical model for a given discipline or sport and athlete. This technical model will represent the most efficient compromise. It will embrace broad principles of movement, such as upward tilting of the pelvis for all activities where vigorous extension of the leg(s) is required to give vertical force (e.g. in most lifts, throws and jumps), or the sequence of joint action and force direction in all arm strike activities. These broad principles are, in the main, based on common sense and a knowledge of anatomy and mechanics. However, many principles have grown simply from experience and observation. For example, it is debatable whether coaching points such as 'keep your eye on the ball' in racket games, cricket, volleyball and baseball, or 'keep your head down' when playing a golf shot or kicking a ball, grew from an extensive knowledge of anatomy or mechanics!

Whether principles grow from theory or from experience, one is always drawn to the same conclusion that our system of levers must be considered in its entirety when creating technical models and, thereafter, suggesting coaching advice. The sciences of kinesiology and biomechanics have grown from applied anatomy and mechanics. The coach, who wishes to create a deeper reservoir of information as a basis for establishing technical models and for studying their development, should take time to study these sciences.

Formerly when coaches wished to experiment beyond existing technical models, it came down to trial and error and the occasional casualty. Today, new models specific to an athlete can be trialled via computer-generated hologram imagery. Varying degrees of adjustment to speed, range, direction, force and synchronisation of one or several joint actions may be built into the model and performance outcomes analysed before introducing the athlete to the technique.

REFERENCES FOR PART 1

Bammes, G, *Complete Guide to Life Drawing*. Kent, UK: Search Press Ltd. (2011)

Grimm, H, *Grundriss der Konstitutionsbiologie und Anthropometrie 3. Auflage*. Berlin: Volk und Gesundheit. (1966)

Harre, D. *Trainingslehre*. Berlin: Sportverlag. (1973)

Harre, D. *Principles of Sport Training*. Berlin: Sportverlag. (1986)

Kapandji, I. Λ. *The Physiology of the Joints. Vol. 1: The Upper Limb*. London: Churchill Livingstone. (2007)

Kapandji, I. A. *The Physiology of the Joints. Vol. 3: The Spinal Column, Pelvic Girdle and Head*. London: Churchill Livingstone. (2008)

Kapandji, I. A. *The Physiology of the Joints. Vol. 2: The Lower Limb*. London: Churchill Livingstone. (2010)

Marcusson, H. *Das Wachstrum von Kindern und Jugendlichen in der Deutschen Demokratischen Republic*. Berlin: Akademie Verlag. (1961)

Rasch, P. J. and Burke, R. K. *Kinesiology and Applied Anatomy*. 3rd edn. Philadelphia, PA: Lea & Febiger. (1968)

Reader's Digest. *The Family Health Guide*. London: Reader's Digest. (1972)

Sharp, Craig. Some Features of the Anatomy and Exercise Physiology of Children, Relating to training. IAAF. NSA Vol. 14:1 (1999)

Tittel, K. *Beschreibende und Funktionelle Anatomie Des Menschen*. Jena: Urban & Fischer. (1963)

BIBLIOGRAPHY

Bar-Or, O. *The Child and Adolescent Athlete*. Oxford: Blackwell Science. (2005)

Blazevich, A. J. *Sports Biomechanics: The Basics: Optimising Human Performance*. London: Bloomsbury Sport. (2013)

Clarke, H. H. *Application of Measurement to Health and Physical Education*. 4th edn. Upper Saddle River, NJ: Prentice Hall. (1967)

Cooper, J. M. and Glassow, R. B. *Kinesiology*. St Louis, MO: C. V. Mosby. (1972)

Craig, T. 'Prevention is the only cure'. *3rd Coaches' Convention Report*. (1972)

Drake, R., Vogl, A. W. and Mitchell, A. W. M. *Gray's Anatomy*. London: Churchill Livingstone, (2010)

Dyson, G. H. G. *The Mechanics of Athletics*. 7th edn. London: University of London Press. (1977)

Fleishman, I. E. *The Structure and Measurement of Physical Fitness*. Upper Saddle River, NJ: Prentice Hall. (1964)

Hay, J. G. *The Biomechanics of Sports Techniques*. Upper Saddle River, NJ: Prentice Hall. (1973)

Hopper, B. J. *The Mechanics of Human Movement*. London: Crosby, Lockwood, Staples. (1973)

Jeffries, M. *Know Your Body*. London: BBC Publications. (1976)

Kelley, D. L. *Kinesiology: Fundamentals of Motion Description*. Prentice Hall, NJ: Upper Saddle River. (1971)

MacConaill, M. A. and Basmajian, J. V. *Muscles and Movements: A Basis for Human Kinesiology*. Baltimore, MD: Williams & Wilkins. (1969)

MacKenna, B. R. and Callender, R. *Illustrated Physiology*. Edinburgh: Churchill Livingstone. (1998)

McGinnis, P. M. *Biomechanics of Sport and Exercise*. Champaign, IL: Human Kinetics. (2013)

Margaria, R. *Biomechanics and Energetics of Muscular Exercise*. Oxford: Clarendon Press. (1976)

Muscolino, J. E. *Kinesiology: The Skeletal System and Muscle Function*. St Louis, MO: Elsevier Mosby. (2011)

Netter, F. H. *Atlas of Human Anatomy*. Philadelphia, PA: Elsevier Saunders. (2011)

Nourse, A. E. *The Body*. 3rd edn. Amsterdam: TimeLife International. (1972)

Provins, K. and Salter, N. 'Maximum torque exerted about the elbow joint'. *Journal of Applied Physiology* 7: 393–8. (1955)

Rasch, P. J. *Kinesiology and Applied Anatomy*. 7th edn. Philadelphia, PA: Lea & Febiger. (1989)

Scott, M. G. *Analysis of Human Motion*. 2nd edn. New York: AppletonCenturyCrofts. (1963)

Spence, D. W. *Essentials of Kinesiology: A Laboratory Manual*. Philadelphia, PA: Lea & Febiger. (1975)

SVUL *Abstracts of the 5th International Congress of Biomechanics*. Helsinki: SVUL. (1975)

Tricker, R. A. R. and Tricker, B. J. L. *The Science of Movement*. London: Mills & Boon. (1968)

Winston, R. *Body: An Amazing Tour of Human Anatomy*. London: Dorling Kindersley. (2005)

PART 2
THE LIVING MACHINE

The analogy is often made of athlete and machine. The 'machine' in this case must develop increased efficiency of energy expression and energy production in the athlete's pursuit of competitive advantage. Moreover, the 'machine' is actively involved in the development process.

In part 1, the skeletal and muscular systems were seen as the basic structures which give final expression of energy when programmed to do so via the central nervous system (discussed in part 3).

In part 2, the production of energy to give those structures movement is considered in detail, as is the collective involvement of several other systems. The digestive system processes the nutritional content of the athlete's diet to produce not only energy for bodily function, but also the various materials necessary for maintenance, repair and growth. The oxygen transporting system combines the respiratory and circulatory systems in its role of carrying oxygen and fuel to the working muscle where chemical energy is converted to mechanical energy. To permit all systems to function, there must be a dynamic stability of the body's internal environment. This is afforded by the fluid systems and endocrine system.

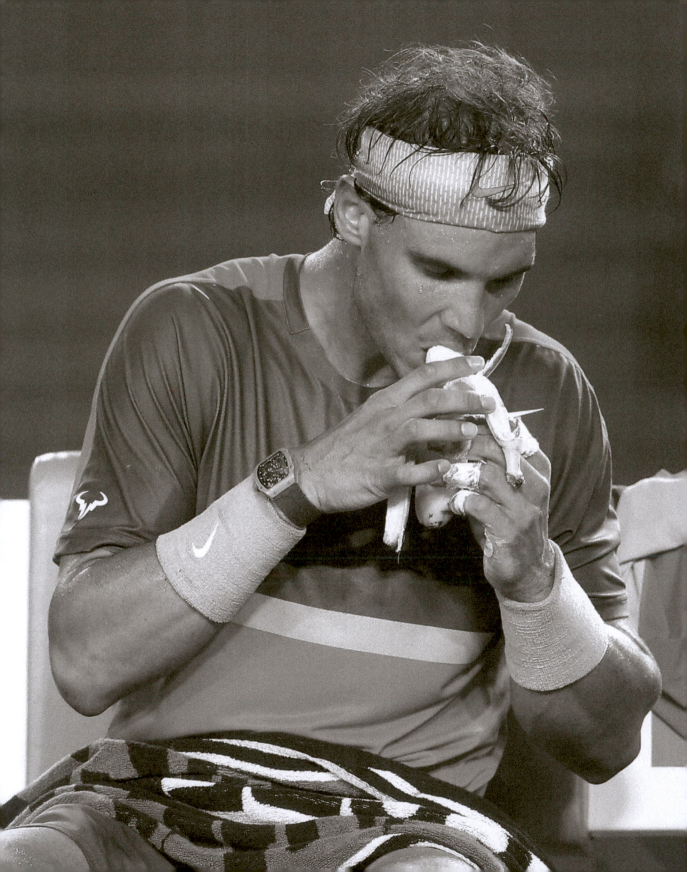

4 NUTRITION

The connection between the foods we eat and our functional capacity has been the subject of considerable interest for at least 3000 years. Biblical injunctions concerning the diet are numerous and, in other religions and cultures, food taboos and rituals may often be traced to this connection.

One of the first accounts of how meat might influence muscular work was recorded in Greece around the 5th century BC. The normal diet of the time was vegetarian but two athletes turned carnivorous and the result was an increase in body bulk and weight. Thereafter, the belief that meat would make up for loss of muscular substance during heavy work gained considerable ground. Even today, the intrusion of scientific half-truths has reinforced this belief and many athletes will not go without meat during preparation for competition. The reason for the popularity of such half-truths and beliefs may be summed up by Astrand (1967): 'The fact that muscles are built of protein makes it tempting to conclude that ingestion of excess protein stimulates muscle growth and strength.' While lack of certain foodstuffs may bring about a decrease in functional capacity, or even illness, it has yet to be proved that excessive consumption of foodstuffs will increase functional capacity.

The energy value of food is measured in kilocalories (kcal) (see p. 41). Foods vary in their calorie content: 1g carbohydrate yields 4kcal, 1g lipid yields 9kcal, 1g protein yields 4kcal. A detailed account of the day's activities can help establish the athlete's daily kilocalorie expenditure. For quick reference, the energy cost of various activities is often standardised (table 4.1). In sport, not only should we ensure appropriate kilocalorie intake, but also quantity of carbohydrate, protein and lipid (table 4.2).

Energy needs depend on activity, age, gender and build. Most energy is used when the muscles are working during breathing, digestion, circulation, exercise, etc. A balanced diet should provide correct nutrition and, ideally, the same amount of energy that is expended in activity. Foods are classified according to their nutritional value:

MACRONUTRIENTS

- Carbohydrates provide the body with energy.
- Lipids provide stored energy.
- Proteins supply material for growth and repair of body tissues.

MICRONUTRIENTS

- Mineral elements contribute towards growth and repair and essential body chemistry.
- Vitamins regulate the body mechanisms.
- Phytonutrients support the immune system.

WATER

- Water is essential in all body functions (74 per cent lean body mass; 65–75 per cent body volume).

Activities	120 lb	140 lb	160 lb	180 lb	200 lb	220 lb	240 lb	260 lb	280 lb
Light									
Cleaning	2.4	2.8	3.2	3.6	4.0	4.4	4.8	5.2	5.6
Playing Pool	2.4	2.8	3.2	3.6	4.0	4.4	4.8	5.2	5.6
Walking, 30 min/mile	2.4	2.8	3.2	3.6	4.0	4.4	4.8	5.2	5.6
Washing dishes	2.2	2.6	2.9	3.3	3.7	4.0	4.4	4.7	5.1
Moderate									
Aerobics, low impact	4.8	5.6	6.4	7.2	8.0	8.8	9.5	10.3	11.1
Cycling, 10 mph	3.9	4.5	5.1	5.7	6.4	7.0	7.6	8.3	8.9
Kayaking	4.8	5.6	6.4	7.2	8.0	8.8	9.5	10.3	11.1
Mopping, Vacuuming	3.4	3.9	4.5	5.0	5.6	6.1	6.7	7.2	7.8
Mowing lawn, power mower	4.3	5.0	5.7	6.5	7.2	7.9	8.6	9.3	10.0
Playing golf, no cart	3.9	4.5	5.1	5.7	6.4	7.0	7.6	8.3	8.9
Skateboarding	4.8	5.6	6.4	7.2	8.0	8.8	9.5	10.3	11.1
Snowmobiling	4.8	5.6	6.4	7.2	8.0	8.8	9.5	10.3	11.1
Walking, 15 min/mile	4.8	5.6	6.4	7.2	8.0	8.8	9.5	10.3	11.1
Walking, 20 min/mile	3.2	3.7	4.2	4.7	5.3	5.8	6.3	6.8	7.3
Water aerobics	4.3	5.0	5.7	6.5	7.2	7.9	8.6	9.3	10.0
Hard									
Aerobics, high impact	6.7	7.8	8.9	10.0	11.1	12.3	13.4	14.5	15.6
Circuit training	7.7	9.0	10.2	11.5	12.7	14.0	15.3	16.5	17.8
Cross-country ski machine	6.7	7.8	8.9	10.0	11.1	12.3	13.4	14.5	15.6
Moving furniture	5.8	6.7	7.7	8.6	9.6	10.5	11.4	12.4	13.3
Playing raquetball, casual	6.7	7.8	8.9	10.0	11.1	12.3	13.4	14.5	15.6
Rowing, moderate	6.7	7.8	8.9	10.0	11.1	12.3	13.4	14.5	15.6
Skiing, downhill, moderate	5.8	6.7	7.7	8.6	9.6	10.5	11.4	12.4	13.3
Swimming laps, moderate	6.7	7.8	8.9	10.0	11.1	12.3	13.4	14.5	15.6
Weightlifting, vigorous	5.8	6.7	7.7	8.6	9.6	10.5	11.4	12.4	13.3

TABLE 4.1 Energy expenditure of different activities expressed as kcal/minute against bodyweight (adapted from Blair et al., 2001)

The majority of foods only become usable after their complex structure has been broken down into simpler forms. This process begins in the mouth when food is cut and ground up by the teeth and mixed with saliva. Digestion of most foods begins at this stage, due to the presence of enzymes. The stomach, a muscular bag which contracts rhythmically, continues the churning and digestive process by adding its own enzymes in the juices it secretes, and there are others later in the digestive corridor in the duodenum (part of the small intestine).

Activities	120 lb	140 lb	160 lb	180 lb	200 lb	220 lb	240 lb	260 lb	280 lb
Very Hard									
Cycling, 12-14 mph	7.7	9.0	10.2	11.5	12.7	14.0	15.3	16.5	17.8
Cycling, 16-19 mph	11.6	13.4	15.3	17.2	19.1	21.0	22.9	24.8	26.7
Cross-country ski	8.7	10.1	11.5	12.9	14.3	15.8	17.2	18.6	20.0
Mountain biking	8.2	9.5	10.9	12.2	13.5	14.9	16.2	17.6	18.9
Playing basketball	7.7	9.0	10.2	11.5	12.7	14.0	15.3	16.5	17.8
Playing racquetball, competitive	9.6	11.2	12.8	14.4	15.9	17.5	19.1	20.7	22.2
Playing tennis	7.7	9.0	10.2	11.5	12.7	14.0	15.3	16.5	17.8
Playing volleyball	7.7	9.0	10.2	11.5	12.7	14.0	15.3	16.5	17.8
Rowing, vigorous	11.6	13.4	15.3	17.2	19.1	21.0	22.9	24.8	26.7
Running, 8 min/mile	12.0	14.0	16.0	17.9	19.9	21.9	23.8	25.8	27.8
Running, 10 min/mile	9.6	11.2	12.8	14.4	15.9	17.5	19.1	20.7	22.2
Stair climber machine	8.7	10.1	11.5	12.9	14.3	15.8	17.2	18.6	20.0
Step aerobics	8.2	9.5	10.9	12.2	13.5	14.9	16.2	17.6	18.9
Swimming, vigorous	10.6	12.3	14.1	15.8	17.5	19.3	21.0	22.7	24.4
Walking, 12 min/mile	7.7	9.0	10.2	11.5	12.7	14.0	15.3	16.5	17.8

Sport/discipline	k calories kg/day	Carbohydrate kg/day	Fats kg/day	Protein kg/day
% contribution of macronutrients to daily kcal intake of athletes	100%	65–75%	15–25%	10%
Speed elastic strength: e.g. sprints, jumps, gymnastics, racket games, volleyball, baseball, related field sports roles	3,500–5,000	8	15%	1.5–2.0
Strength endurance: e.g. middle distance, swimming, rowing, skating, downhill skiing, related field sports roles	4,000–6,000	8–10	20%	1.5–2.0
Strength: e.g. weightlifting, throws, wrestling, related field sports roles	6,000–8,000	6–8	25%	2.0–2.5
Endurance: e.g. long distance, langlauf, 90 mins+ efforts	4,000–7,000	10	25%	1.5

TABLE 4.2 General picture of athletes' diets

MACRONUTRIENTS
Carbohydrates

As their name suggests, these are compounds of carbon, hydrogen and oxygen. Carbohydrate is the principal constituent of the normal diet and, generally speaking, it meets most of the body's energy requirement. Carbohydrates occur in several forms – the simple sugars or monosaccharides, and the complex sugars, i.e. disaccharides, trisaccharides, etc. Simple sugars are often regarded as 'empty calories' and the recommended balance in the diet should be 60–65 per cent complex sugars to 40–35 per cent simple sugars.

Simple sugars
Major monosaccharides

The most common in normal diet are the hexoses (six carbon atoms).

Glucose: as the end product of carbohydrate digestion, glucose is the main form of carbohydrate used by the body and is the major fuel required to provide energy. It occurs naturally in sweet fruits.

Fructose: similar to glucose in terms of its carbon, hydrogen and oxygen composition, fructose is apparently absorbed more readily than glucose and, being independent of insulin, is not associated with the 'rebound hypoglycaemia' sometimes caused by too rich sugar foods, such as sweets and chocolate. Its value as a fuel, then, might be countered by its implications for coronary heart disease and the possibility of acidosis caused by increased blood lactate when consumed in large quantities. It is found in honey, sweet fruits and maize.

Galactose: though similar to glucose, galactose is found in different sources, mainly yeast, liver and human milk.

Complex sugars
Disaccharides

Sucrose: this sugar is found most commonly in the diet. It's found in maple syrup, treacle, white, brown and demerara sugar. Digestion breaks it down to glucose and fructose. Sucrose is a valuable energy source but, unfortunately, it encourages the activity of oral bacteria responsible for tooth decay. Figure 4.1 illustrates the chemical structure of sucrose and other disaccharides.

Lactose: during digestion lactose, which is the starch found in milk, is broken down to glucose and galactose. Milk has a very high nutritional value, although recent research has indicated an apparent 'lactose intolerance' in some individuals.

Maltose: this sugar is found in malt extract. Malt is the product of heating and drying germinated barley (a necessary link in the brewing and distilling processes). Digestion breaks maltose down to glucose only. Malt extract is a most valuable source of energy for the athlete.

Trisaccharides and tetrasaccharides

These sugars occur less frequently in foods than monosaccharides and disaccharides. The trisaccharides are found in peas, beans, and in both root and green vegetables. The tetrasaccharides are found in such foods as

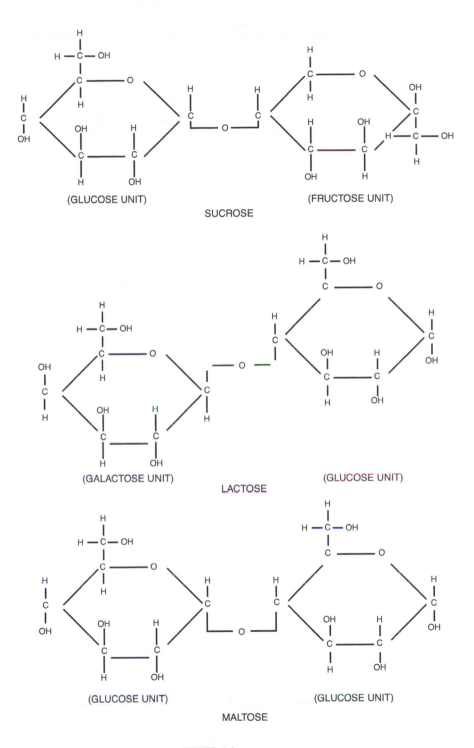

FIGURE 4.1 Disaccharides

the meat substitutes used by vegetarians. Little importance is attached to the trisaccharides and tetrasaccharides as energy suppliers and, since they are difficult to break down and may cause indigestion, their intake is not recommended for the athlete.

Polysaccharides

Starch: the principal energy source and the product of cereals. It might be thought of as the stored energy of vegetables. The digestive system breaks down the starches to maltose, which itself is broken down to glucose. Sources of starch are legion, ranging from bread to rice to pasta. Heating breaks down the starch molecules to smaller compounds called dextrins.

Glycogen: this sugar is to animals what starch is to vegetables. It is referred to as 'stored glucose' in the athlete, and is found in the liver and muscle. When released it is a readily available fuel source as glucose in muscle. It is the glycogen reservoir that the liver accesses in its vital function of maintaining levels of blood glucose, which is the *only* fuel for the brain.

Cellulose: Though of very little food value to the body, cellulose gives plants their rigid structure and provides essential fibre in the diet. Western diets tend to be low in fibre, a fact that is of some concern to nutritionists, for it is a most vital component of diet. Intestinal health is dependent on a regular flow of nutrients and expulsion of waste. Fibre in the diet ensures this. Fruit and vegetables are key resources, as are high-fibre bran breakfast cereals. Natural bran is favoured here as it expands on its journey through the digestive system, whereas most other breakfast cereals shrink.

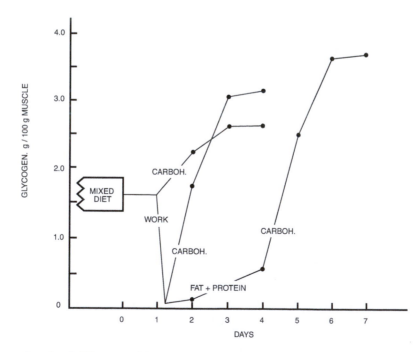

FIGURE 4.2 Glycogen 'overshoot': different possibilities of increasing the muscle glycogen content (from Saltin and Hermansen, 1967)

The body is well-equipped with regulatory mechanisms which discourage the immediate absorption of food substances once saturation level has been reached. However, this mechanism can be bypassed according to Saltin and Hermansen (1967) who advanced the 'glycogen overshoot' theory. It is believed that this has considerable significance for the long duration endurance athletes who must have high reserves of energy. Applying this theory one week before a major competition, the athlete depletes glycogen stores by hard training and then is deprived of carbohydrate for four or five days. On the final days before the major competition, the athlete takes a very rich carbohydrate diet. The result is that the amount of available glycogen in the body is much higher than would normally be the case (figure 4.2). This may not, however, be an ideal situation for the long endurance athlete (see p. 64). Such 'carbo-loading' still has an important place in distance running, but now it is programmed as a 'non-stop' boost, i.e. during the final three days of the taper, the carbohydrate intake is substantially increased (but not the total calories).

FATS (TRUE CHEMICAL NAME = LIPIDS)

Fats, like carbohydrates, are composed of carbon, hydrogen and oxygen, but the quantity of oxygen is considerably less in fats. Fats are certainly the most concentrated source of energy of all foodstuffs, yielding twice as many kilocalories, weight for weight, compared with carbohydrates. The provision of stored energy is probably their most important role in nutrition. However, they are also valuable in maintaining body temperature in, for example, the subcutaneous fat layer of sea or lake swimmers, and protecting vital organs (e.g. kidneys) with layers of fat or adipose tissue, as well as contributing in the provision of those fatty acids essential to health and in providing a transport medium for the fat-soluble vitamins.

Lipids, as fats (solid) and oils (liquid) are broken up into tiny globules by bile salts secreted by the liver. These act on fats like a detergent on an oil slick and in this form the fats may more readily react with chemicals similar to those involved in carbohydrate digestion. Even the substances of fat digestion which have not been completely broken down may pass through the gut wall to be carried, in lymph along the lymphatic system, to a point in the region of the chest where they are emptied into the blood.

The liver plays a most important role in the metabolism of fats. It may convert available glucose into fat and then into other usable substances in the body. Our fat stores, then, may be derived from excessive carbohydrate intake, or from fats and oils (figures 4.3 and 4.4). Fats belong to a much larger biochemical family known as lipids. The family is described below, but not all members have nutritional significance.

Triglycerides (acyl glycerols)

Triglycerides are also converted from dietary carbohydrates so the quality and quantity of dietary carbohydrates have a substantial consequence on the body's fats profile. The most common of these is triacylglycerol, or triglyceride or 'neutral fat'. Most edible fats and oils consist of compounds of glycerol (commonly known as glycerine) plus fatty acids. The main reason why, say, lard differs from nut oil or cream, lies in the different types or proportions of fatty acids which combine with glycerol. When three fatty acids combine with glycerol, the compound is triglyceride (figure 4.5).

Fatty acids may consist of long chains of carbon atoms which have two hydrogen atoms attached to each carbon atom (figure 4.6). When all the carbons in a fatty acid chain are linked by single bonds, the fatty acid is said to be *saturated* with hydrogen bonds. If the chain contains one (mono) or more than one (poly) it is *unsaturated* (figure 4.7).

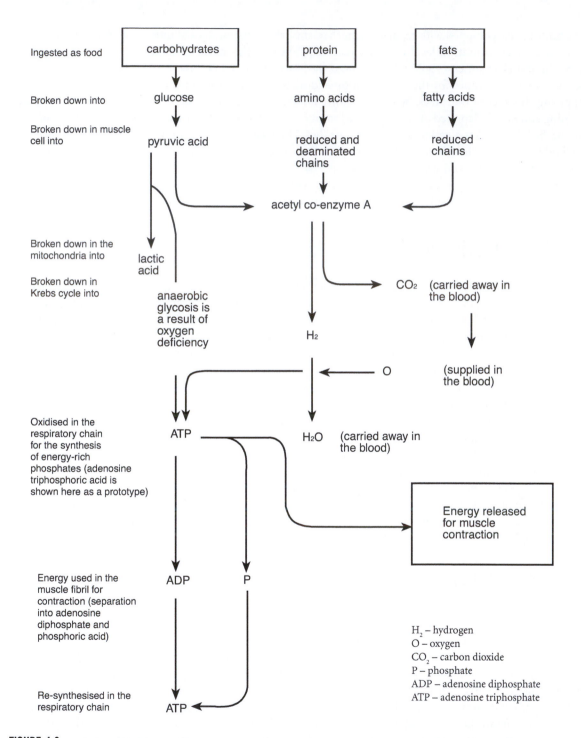

FIGURE 4.3 Metabolism of nutrients and their conversion into ATP, which when broken down to ADP provides energy for muscle contraction (the conversion of food into energy)

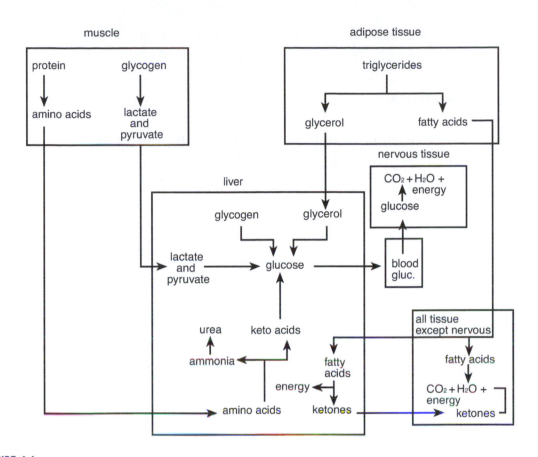

FIGURE 4.4 Summary of metabolism of stored foods as a source of energy (i.e. in fasting) (from Vander et al., 1970)

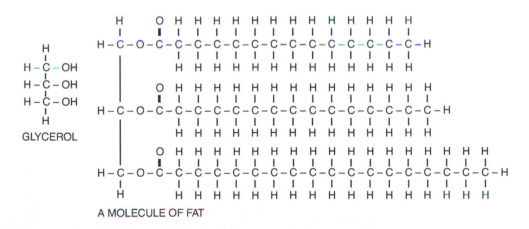

A MOLECULE OF FAT

FIGURE 4.5 Triglycerides. Such fats are called triglycerides because the compound glycerol in each molecule is attached to three fatty acid units.

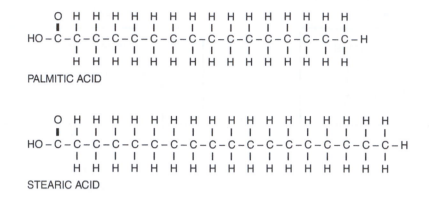

PALMITIC ACID

STEARIC ACID

FIGURE 4.6 Chemists refer to such fatty acids as saturated due to the presence of pairs of hydrogen atoms along the whole length of the chain. The two saturated fatty acids here are present in the harder fats, such as lard.

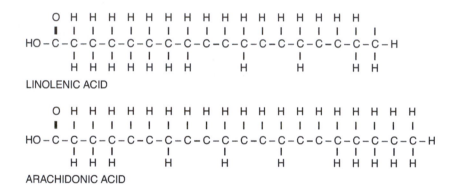

LINOLENIC ACID

ARACHIDONIC ACID

FIGURE 4.7 The existence of 'gaps' in the pairs of hydrogen atoms characterise the unsaturated fatty acids. The two unsaturated fatty acids shown here are present in fish oils.

Triglycerides occur in vegetable fats and oils, animal fats, fish oils and dairy fats. The main difference between animal fats and dairy fats, on the one hand, and vegetable fats and oils, and fish oils on the other, is that, except for palm oil and coconut oil, the latter have a much higher proportion of unsaturated fatty acids. It is well known that high blood cholesterol levels are associated with coronary heart disease and that the cholesterol level can be reduced by eating foods rich in unsaturated fatty acids. This is of considerable interest with reference to the health of the heart and circulating system/network. Table 4.3 illustrates the saturated/unsaturated fatty acid situation in several fats and oils.

Cholesterol has acquired something of a bad reputation. It is important to understand that cholesterol is an essential component of the body's chemistry. For example, steroid hormones secreted by the adrenal cortex are derived from cholesterol. Cholesterol can, however, become a problem if its content in the blood exceeds a healthy amount. Consequently, it is becoming normal practice to monitor the blood from as early as age 30 and certainly annually from the age of 40. Monitoring involves blood analysis as set out in table 4.3.

Total cholesterol	<5.0 mmol/l	(desirable)
	5.0–6.0 mmol/l	(borderline)
	>6.0 mmol/l	(high)
LDL cholesterol (low density lipoprotein)	<3.0 mmol/l	(desirable)
	3.0–4.0 mmol/l	(borderline)
	>4.0 mmol/l	(high)
HDL cholesterol (high density lipoprotein)	0.9–1,5 mmol/l	(desirable)
	<0.9 mmol/l	(low)
HDL % of total	>20	(desirable)
	<20	(low)
Triglycerides	<2.3 mmol/l	(desirable)
	2.3–4.5 mmol/l	(borderline)
	> 4.5 mmol/l	(high)

TABLE 4.3 Blood cholesterol analysis

HDL is regarded as 'good' cholesterol due to its role in protecting against disease, so higher scores are generally good. This score can be improved by increasing aerobic exercise, monounsaturated fats, fish oils and moderate alcohol, or by reducing or eliminating saturated fats, particularly hydrogenated fats and the less healthy carbohydrates.

LDL is regarded as 'bad' cholesterol because when it oxidises it lines the arteries. Oxidation of LDL results from free radicals in foods. Antioxidants (betacarotene, vitamin C, vitamin E and selenium) attract free radicals and so help prevent this oxidation process. The level of LDL can be reduced by eating the antioxidant foods listed above. Fibre and soya protein can also lower LDL. Generally, foods to cut back on or to avoid are poor quality carbohydrates and foods with a high cholesterol content.

Phospholipids: again the glycerol 'backbone' is present in this compound but only two fatty acids are attached, plus phosphate and a base containing nitrogen. The latter situation bridges the worlds of fats and proteins and, as a rule, the fatty acids are unsaturated. The phospholipids have important functions to perform in the body, ranging from fat absorption to the insulation of nervous tissue with the myelin sheath. They are not only manufactured by, and exist in, the body itself, but are also in the foods we eat. For example, lecithin is present in egg yolk and soya beans. Yakovlev (1961) has emphasised the inclusion of lecithin in the post-competition diet to aid recovery.

Sphingolipids: these compounds contain fatty acid, phosphate, choline, a complex base (sphingosine), but no glycerol. The sphingolipids are closely associated with tissues and animal membranes.

Glycolipids: there is neither glycerol nor phosphate in this compound. Instead there is a monosaccharide galactose, plus fatty acid and sphingosine. The glycolipids are found primarily in photosynthetic tissue (i.e. the leaves of plants).

Eicosanoids: arachidonic acid, a 20 carbon fatty acid (figure 4.7), is the central building block for these derivatives which include vasoactive substances such as prostaglandin and prostacyclin. Eicosanoids are critical to a number of body functions including immune response, inflammation and airway resistance.

Steroids

The basic structure of all steroids is formed from four interconnected rings of carbon atoms (figure 4.8). The steroids include cholesterol, vitamin A, bile salts, testosterone and oestrogen.

Fats in foodstuffs are primarily triglycerides, combined with small amounts of free fatty acids, phospholipids (such as lecithin) and the salts of cholesterol. Eating animal fats may cause problems associated with saturated fatty acids, but they do provide one of the most valuable sources of vitamins A and D. So, if margarine is used instead of butter, it must be composed of vegetable oils only and enriched with vitamins A and D.

The final breakdown products of fat metabolism are free fatty acids which, like glucose, are fuel for muscular activity. Recent research shows these fatty acids are the preferred fuel for the long duration endurance athletes (figure 4.9). Williams (1975) has pointed out that since this is the case, the application of the glycogen overshoot theory may not be in the athlete's interest in training. It may be better to 'train' the free fatty acid energy pathway by training in a 'fasting' state, therefore encouraging the use of free fatty acids as a fuel. However, before competition, glycogen loading is good sense even for the 5000m (Newsholme, 1994).

The right balance of dietary fats and oils is essential to good health. These fats and oils are sources of the fat soluble vitamins (A, D, E, K) and they are also required to absorb them. They keep the skin healthy and regulate body functions.

THE RIGHT BALANCE IS AS FOLLOWS:

2/3 monounsaturated fatty acids, for example:
- extra virgin olive oil;
- avocado;
- rapeseed oil;
- almonds;
- pecans;
- peanut oil.

1/3 polyunsaturated (omega 3 and omega 6) and saturated.

Each of these three (omega 3; omega 6; saturated) represent 1/9 of the daily fats and oils intake. So:

1/9 omega 3, for example:
- fish oils;
- soya bean;
- flax oil;
- walnut.

1/9 omega 6, for example:
- sunflower oil;

- corn oil;
- sesame seed oil;
- blackcurrant seeds.

1/9 saturated, for example:
- fatty red meat;
- egg yolk;
- shellfish;
- dairy products;
- poultry skins;
- hydrogenated fats (present in many margarines and cooking fats).

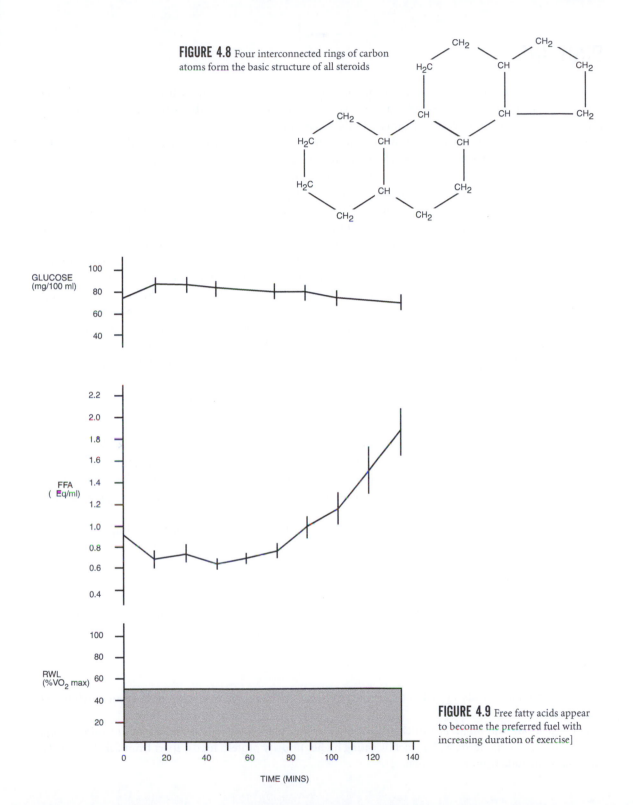

FIGURE 4.8 Four interconnected rings of carbon atoms form the basic structure of all steroids

FIGURE 4.9 Free fatty acids appear to become the preferred fuel with increasing duration of exercise]

PROTEINS

It has been pointed out that carbohydrates and fats consist mainly of carbon, hydrogen and oxygen. Protein differs in that nitrogen is an essential part of its structure and neither carbohydrate nor fats can replace protein in the diet without eventual damage to the organism.

Protein molecules are formed by linking smaller units called amino acids, which are the end product of protein digestion (figure 4.3). Differences between proteins depend on the identity, number and arrangement of amino acids. Chains of amino acids are polypeptides. If there are less than 50 amino acids, this is a peptide; if more, it is a protein. There are 25 amino acids, 20 of bio-chemical import and, of these, 10 are known as essential amino acids. They are 'essential' because the body cannot normally manufacture these amino acids at the rate required for proper functioning. The 10 essential amino acids are arginine, histidine, isoleucine, leucine, lysine, methionine, phenylalanine, threonine, tryptophan and valine.

The amino acids go via the blood from gut to liver to general circulation. The liver, again, has an important regulatory function in that it acts as a 'buffer' for amino acids, just as it does for glucose and fats. That is, if the concentration is high in the blood, the liver absorbs a large quantity into its cells. Conversely, in times of shortage, the liver releases its store. It would appear that there is a peak of circulating amino acids approximately two hours after a protein meal. Apparently, then, it is helpful, both for maintenance and repair of muscle tissue, to train at this time. It certainly does not seem advisable to train within the two hour period, or so late afterwards that the body has begun to starve, except of course in the case of the long duration endurance athletes as previously suggested. The liver is also responsible for preparing amino acids for use as an alternative energy source. However, this is a 'last gasp' mechanism and other sources of energy must be favoured.

The protein value of different foods varies quite remarkably. The disadvantages of the fat associated with meat, as pointed out by heart specialists, must be most carefully weighed against the high quality of animal protein and supply of certain vitamins and minerals. When assessing the protein value of the athlete's diet, quality as well as quantity must be taken into account. Some athletes may eat most of their daily protein in the form of potato chips rather than eggs or milk. Nevertheless, in terms of quality, the egg is the most complete protein food (table 4.4).

Because protein foods clearly vary in their quality, and some have negative health implications, it is sensible to prioritise intake.

Higher priority

Whey (the thin liquid part of milk remaining after casein, or curds, and fat are removed). Fish, tofu, soya bean, low fat cheeses and yoghurt, brown rice, oats and mixed vegetables.

Lower priority

Lean beef and other meats, eggs, full fat cheeses, nuts, pulses (beans, peas, lentils), bean sprouts, white rice, maize, potatoes.

For vegetarians, although the protein quality of individual plant foods is lower than foods of animal origin (except soya), protein needs will be met by eating higher priority protein foods, apart from fish. Some vegetarians also include whey in their diet.

	isoleucine	leucine	lysine	phenylalanine	methionine	threonine	trytophan	valine	Protein score as measure of excellence
Amino acid combination estimated as ideal for a man	270	306	270	180	144	180	90	270	100
Egg protein	428	565	396	368	196	310	106	460	100
Beef	332	515	540	256	154	275	75*	345	83
Milk protein	402	628	497	334	190	272	85*	448	80
Fish	317	474	549	231	178	283	62*	327	70
Oat protein	302	436	212*	309	84*	192	74*	348	79
Rice protein	322	535	236*	307	142*	241	65*	415	72
Flour protein	262*	442	126*	322	78*	174	69*	262	47
Maize protein	293	827	179*	284	117*	249	38*	327	42
Soya protein	333	484	395	309	86*	247	86*	328	73
Pea protein	336	504	438	290	77*	230	74*	317	58
Potato protein	260*	304	326	285	87*	237	72*	339	56
Cassava	118*	184*	310	133*	2*	136*	131	144	22

* Less than the estimated ideal proportion

TABLE 4.4 Protein value in selected foods (mg per g of nitrogen) (from Pyke, M. 1975)

Not all nutritionists agree with the daily protein intake recommended in table 4.2. For example, it is suggested the athlete in heavy endurance training would find about 2g/kg/day satisfactory, with 3g/kg/day for power/strength competitors (Wootton, 1988). Durnin (1975) has suggested that an intake of around 1g/kg bodyweight/day would be quite adequate. Although there remains confusing diversity among nutrition experts, it is reasonable for athletes to keep within the 1.5–2.5g/kg/day range (Lemon, 1991).

MACRONUTRIENTS AND ENERGY

The macronutrients yield energy originally harnessed by plants and, through them, animals. Carbohydrates and fats are the main energy providers. Proteins have a lesser role, as their main functions are to build and repair. Nutritionists have developed a rating scale that compares the capacity of different foods to increase blood glucose concentrations. This is called the *glycaemic index.*

This index indicates the increase in blood sugar over a two-hour period after consuming 50g of a food compared with 50g of white bread or glucose – the latter represents 100 per cent. A food with a glycaemic index of 45 indicates that it increases blood glucose to 45 per cent of the level of white bread.

High GI foods include:

Glucose, sucrose, cane/maple/corn syrup, honey, bagel, white bread, shredded wheat cereals, potato, corn-flakes, raisins, banana, puffed wheat cereals, carrot, white rice, white pasta, pitta bread, refined base noodles, butternut squash, watermelon, pineapple and parsnips.

Moderate GI foods include:

Wholegrain bread, pasta and noodles, muesli (no sugar), couscous, long grain brown rice, semolina, sweetcorn, rye bread, oats, new potatoes with skin, bran muffins, orange, wild rice, beetroot, spinach, lychees, mangoes, melon, dates, lentils and most beans.

Low GI foods include:

Fructose, yoghurt, peanuts, peas, soy beans, apples, peaches, pears, plums, figs, apricots, grapefruit, cherries, milk and milk products.

Consuming low glycaemic foods 30 minutes prior to exercise permits a relatively low rate of glucose absorption into the body. This eliminates 'insulin surge', yet affords a steady slow release of glucose during the exercise. This is an advantage for endurance activities.

High glycaemic index foods consumed 30 minutes prior to exercise cause increased insulin activity (insulin surge) peaking around 30–45 minutes after ingestion. Blood glucose volume likewise surges then drops off rapidly leaving an inadequate supply to meet exercise demands. This is a disadvantage in endurance activities.

In general nutrition, the emphasis must be on the moderate GI foods supplemented by a mixture which is more generous in low GI foods than high. Pre-exercise meals should be mainly low GI with moderate GI. Post-exercise should be high GI plus moderate GI. During exercise of 60 minutes duration or more, carbohydrates should be high GI. This can be achieved through specially formulated sports drinks that provide glucose and electrolytes as well as rehydration. Some people, on the other hand, are quite happy with a banana or a jam sandwich as their energy top-up and still water for their rehydration.

Knowing the glycaemic index of foods is essential to people either with diabetes mellitus type 1 (the pancreas loses its ability to synthesise insulin) or type 2 (the cells resist the effects of insulin). International travel should always be preceded by a briefing on the glycaemic index of local foods to ensure that the delicate balance of glucose intake for those with diabetes mellitus is maintained.

MICRONUTRIENTS
Vitamins

Vitamins are required for the breakdown of macronutrients. Most are the main components of co-enzymes. While they must be present in our food at a certain minimal level, the argument that mega doses will increase sports performance is yet to be proved. In fact, continued excessive intake of A, D or K may be sufficiently toxic to be life-threatening.

Water soluble

These are the B-complex vitamins and vitamin C.

Thiamine (vitamin B1): this forms part of the enzyme responsible for the breakdown of pyruvic acid in the process of releasing energy from carbohydrates. Its presence in the diet is therefore essential. Increased intake is required where there is a high energy requirement, when carbohydrate is excessive in the diet, when the diet is high in white sugar or white flour (when there is no thiamine already added), when foods relied upon to supply thiamine are heated in alkaline or neutral solutions, and when raw fish constitutes part of the regular diet. Thiamine is water soluble so some of it will be lost to the water in which the food is cooked. This applies, of course, to all water soluble vitamins. Thiamine content is high in foods such as brewer's yeast and wheat germ.

Riboflavin (vitamin B2): like thiamine, riboflavin is a component of an enzyme in the metabolism of carbohydrates, but there would appear to be no correlation between energy requirements and riboflavin. Research into the relative merits of riboflavin as a dietary supplement is inconclusive. Brewer's yeast, liver and meat extract have a high riboflavin content.

Niacin: this again is involved in enzyme activity in the metabolism of carbohydrates. However, unlike thiamine and riboflavin, niacin may be synthesised within the body through micro-organism activity in the large intestine. High quality protein, such as eggs, which are high in content of the amino acid tryptophan, provide the basis for such synthesis. Supplementing the diet with very high quantities of niacin (2–5g) reduces the concentration of free fatty acids in the blood. Niacin content is high in meat extract, yeast extract and bran.

Pyridoxine (vitamin B6): this is involved in enzyme activity in protein metabolism, but little has been revealed in research regarding the effects of excess or deficiency. Pyridoxine content is high in liver, green vegetables and in wheat germ.

Pantothenic acid: as a principal component of co-enzyme A, pantothenic acid is involved in energy production from organic acids. Liver, egg yolk and fresh vegetables contain high levels of pantothenic acid.

Biotin: this, like thiamine and folic acid, is a co-enzyme of cellular metabolism. Specifically, it forms oxaloacetic acid from pyruvic acid and the synthesis of fatty acids. Skin condition, physical and mental alertness appear related to biotin status. It is produced by bacteria in the gastrointestinal (GI) system. Biotin content is high in brewer's yeast, liver, kidneys, legumes, vegetables and egg yolk.

Folic acid (pteroylglutamic acid): this is a key substance in the formation of red blood cells and consequently is associated with vitamin B12. However, this relationship is not yet fully understood. It is also, like pyridoxine, involved in protein metabolism. Folic acid content is high in foods such as liver, oysters and spinach.

Cyanocobalamin (vitamin B12): this is essential to the maturation of red blood cells and is also involved in white cell and platelet formation. Some athletes involved in high energy demanding sports boost B12 levels by injecting large quantities of the vitamin. The athletes concerned claim certain benefits, but there is no research evidence to support these claims at present. Cyanocobalamin content is high in uncooked liver, kidneys, meat, yeast extracts, dairy products and eggs. B12 is not found in any plants, so vegans have to take it in tablet or liquid form.

Ascorbic acid (vitamin C): this cannot be synthesised or stored by the body and therefore must be supplied by the diet. It performs several roles: it aids repair of damaged tissue and the absorption of iron, it maintains healthy gums and decreases susceptibility to minor infections, and it is concentrated in some quantity in the adrenal cortex, although its exact function there is at present unknown. It has been shown that the body's ascorbic acid content falls during periods of intensive training. Moreover, when an athlete is sweating heavily, or is losing body fluids (e.g. during a common cold), ascorbic acid status in the body drops severely. Clearly, steps must be made to maintain this level, but it is not always easy. The normal diet may well supply sufficient ascorbic acid for the athlete's needs, but this is not always the case because vitamin C is easily destroyed or lost. As it is water soluble, it is often washed out of food or dissolved in cooking. Heat, processing and lengthy storage often destroy the vitamin, as does exposure to air and light (e.g. cutting an apple). All of this would appear to suggest some supplement of vitamin C to the diet. During intensive training, athletes have been known to take between 1 and 10g per day. The lower end of this range seems reasonable but is nevertheless high compared with the UK recommendations of 0.03g per day and USA recommendations of 0.06g per day. Ascorbic acid content is high in blackcurrants, green vegetables and citrus fruits.

It should be noted that due to their nature, water-soluble vitamins will simply be passed out in the urine if taken in excess and, since the athlete's needs are almost certainly greater than the recommended minimum for the general public, little harm can come of taking supplementary vitamin B complex and vitamin C, though this is not the case with the fat-soluble vitamins which can accumulate in the body.

Vitamin C, like betacarotene (provitamin A), vitamin E and selenium, is an anti-oxidant scavenging free radicals, the tissue-damaging by-products of metabolism.

Fat soluble

These are the vitamins A, D, E and K.

Retinol (vitamin A): this is only found in animal products. However, some vegetables, including carrots and the leafy green vegetables, contain substances called carotenoids which are converted to retinol during absorption through the small intestine. Being fat soluble and stable in heat, it is not exposed to the same danger of destruction by cooking as are B-complex and C vitamins. However, exposure to oxygen and ultraviolet light can reduce retinol status in foods. Retinol is involved in vision efficiency; carotenoids being found in both rods and cones. It also would appear that bone growth, the health of alimentary and respiratory tracts, and local resistance to infection are all vitamin A dependent. High dosage of vitamin A taken regularly is toxic. Fish liver oils, ox liver and sheep liver all have a high retinol content.

Betacarotene (provitamin A): may be converted into vitamin A at the rate demanded by the body's requirements for the vitamin. It is an antioxidant (see vitamin C). It is found in high quantities in green and yellow vegetables (particularly carrots, kale and spinach).

Cholecalciferol (vitamin D): essential to calcium and phosphorus absorption, cholecalciferol has a key role in development of bone and those physiological areas influenced by calcium, phosphorus and parathyroid gland activity. There are two main types of vitamin D:

- Calciferol (vitamin D2), which is formed by the ultraviolet radiation of ergosterol (a steroid found in plants such as yeast and fungi).
- Cholecalciferol (vitamin D3), which occurs naturally in substances such as egg yolk, butter and the oils of fish liver. It is also formed by the action of ultraviolet radiation on the oils present on the surface of our skins (i.e. when the skin is exposed to sunlight).

Like retinol, vitamin D in excess is toxic. Vitamin D content is high in foods such as egg yolks and vitamin-enriched produce such as margarine.

Tocopherols (vitamin E): vitamin E inhibits breakdown of those fatty acids that assist in cell membrane formation. It is also involved in forming erythrocytes, DNA and RNA, wound healing and normal neural system function and structure. It is an antioxidant (see vitamin C). It is found in high quantities in wholegrain seed, oils and eggs.

Vitamin K (phylloquinone, menaquinone): while the role of vitamin K is clearly involved in blood clotting, no obvious role is played by the vitamin in enzyme systems. It is very difficult to assess whether or not we require vitamin K in our food or whether sufficient is manufactured within our own bodies. Vitamin K is readily inactivated on exposure to light. Of the vitamin K derivatives, vitamin K1 is found in green vegetables, and vitamin K2 in bacteria.

Phytonutrients/phytochemicals

These are a group of compounds that occur naturally in fruit and vegetables. They have become the subject of debate as they are of benefit to the immune system and are as important to health as vitamins. The bitter taste in some vegetables is due to the presence of these compounds.

The phytonutrients include:

- **Carotenoids:** watercress, broccoli, spinach, yellow squashes, red peppers, carrot, pumpkin, tomato skin
- **Indoles:** Brussels sprouts and cabbage varieties
- **Isothiocyanates:** broccoli, Brussels sprouts, cabbage varieties.

Minerals

The body requires certain minerals in relatively large amounts. These are listed here as major minerals. Other minerals are needed in relatively small (or trace) amounts. These are listed here as minor minerals.

Major minerals (need more than 100mg/day)

Calcium: this performs several very important functions in the body, namely:

- the formation of bones and teeth;
- the initiation of muscle contraction;
- blood clotting;
- as part of the composition of blood;
- certain enzyme activity.

Vitamin D and protein aid calcium absorption, while phytic acid (see iron), oxalic acid (as in rhubarb and spinach) and fats inhibit calcium absorption. While the well-balanced average diet should supply sufficient calcium, and the body will readily adapt to reduced supplies, the athlete is often advised to drink an extra daily pint of (skimmed) milk or to take calcium tablets in order to ensure that calcium levels do not become too depleted due to strenuous training, especially in the case of women endurance competitors who may suffer from osteoporosis.

Calcium content is high in foods such as dried skimmed milk, whitebait and hard cheese.

Phosphorus: this is found in foodstuffs and in the body as phosphate. It has many functions in the body, chiefly:

- formation of bones and teeth;
- energy production (ATP and ADP);
- as an essential component of blood;
- as an essential inclusion of certain enzymes and hormones.

The average well-balanced diet will provide ample phosphate for the body's needs. Phosphorus content is high in cheese, brains, meat and fish.

Potassium: like table salt, potassium is a key mineral in the maintenance of the body's internal environment, but its role is mainly within the cell, whereas salt works outside the cell. While most diets offer an ample supply of potassium to meet the body's needs, it would appear that when training is so severe and prolonged that cellular proteins are beginning to break down, then the potassium levels in the body are reduced. However, like so many of the areas under discussion here, the body is well-equipped to increase potassium absorption from foodstuffs in order to restore status quo. Soya flour, dried milk, dried fruit and nuts are high in potassium.

Sulphur: like potassium, sulphur is involved in maintaining acid base balance in the body. It also has a key role in liver function. Sulphur is found in high quantities in dried vegetables, fruits, meats, poultry and fish.

Sodium: performs a balancing act with potassium in the process of action potential across cell membranes; acid base balance, osmolality and body water mineral balance. Sodium rich foods are fruits, vegetables and sodium chloride (table salt).

Sodium chloride (table salt): this is the most important soluble mineral of the diet, and is the main component of the extracellular fluid. Consequently it is very important that the sodium concentration of the extracellular fluid is closely monitored. Athletes losing more salt than usual, due to increased perspiration when in a hot environment, must increase salt intake above that provided by the normal diet. Thus preparations such as 'slow sodium' and various electrolyte drinks are included in special diets for athletes exposed to this situation. Ham, corned beef and cheese all have a high salt content.

Chlorine: is involved in the body's water mineral balance, principally in its combination with sodium as sodium chloride. It also influences membrane potential. Foods rich in chlorine are fruits, vegetables and table salt.

Magnesium: like calcium and phosphorus, is involved in the development of bones and teeth. It also has a critical role in certain types of nerve impulse transmission. Calcium 'switches on' while magnesium 'switches off '. Foods rich in magnesium are wheat germ and green leafy vegetables.

Minor minerals (need less than 100mg/day)

Iron: the element of iron is essential for production of haemoglobin carried in red blood cells (erythrocytes). If there is insufficient haemoglobin, the oxygen carrying capacity of the blood is reduced and it is reasonable to assume that the athlete's functioning capacity is also depleted. This condition is known as anaemia and by far the most common (but not the only) cause is a lack of dietary iron. In these circumstances, ferrous compounds may be taken as dietary additives. However, the body will only absorb what it needs and reject the surplus. Many endurance athletes have suffered from so-called sports pseudo-anaemia, which is a condition where the total quantity of haemoglobin in the blood is high but the concentration is lower than normal, due to a relatively greater increase in blood plasma. The reduced concentration will, however, keep blood viscosity low and consequently aid the rate of flow to and from muscle (Williams, 1975). Although, generally speaking, athletes, women and growing children have greater iron requirements than other members of the population, it is inadvisable to supplement normal dietary iron without medical advice. Regular blood counts for athletes are recommended. Vitamin C aids iron absorption and it is thought that protein may also assist. However, where diets are very high in bran cereals content, the phytic acid found in the outer husks of the cereals may prevent iron absorption by forming an insoluble compound. Iron content is high in green vegetables such as spinach, watercress and cabbage, in liver, black pudding, red meat, kidney, and in yeast.

Fluorine: serving a most vital role in the healthy growth of bones and teeth, fluorine, like its fellow halogen iodine, is involved in the functioning of the thyroid gland. Furthermore it is now well established that fluorine protects teeth from decay. Fluoridised drinking water, tea and saltwater fish contain quantities of fluorine.

Copper: is essential to the healthy development of the nervous system, especially in the composition of the protective myelin sheath. It is also a component of certain metabolic enzymes. It is present in meat.

Selenium: functions with vitamin E as an antioxidant. Together with betacarotene and vitamin C they complete the 'antioxidant cocktail'. It is present in seafood, meats and grains.

Iodine: is vital to the efficient production of the hormone thyroxine by which the thyroid gland controls the body's metabolic rate. Consequently, any lack of iodine in the diet must have serious and far-reaching effects. Where soils are rich in iodine, the plants nourished by that soil are rich in it too. In regions where soils have poor levels of iodine, potassium iodide is added to cooking salts to make up for this deficiency. Iodine content is normally highest in foods such as saltwater fish, vegetables and milk.

Chromium: has a key role in glycolysis. It is present in legumes, cereals and organic meats.

Manganese: is involved in bone growth, forms part of certain enzymes and is found in the blood and liver.

Molybdenum: is a co-factor for several enzymes critical to bodily function. It is present in animal fats, vegetable oils, meats and wholegrain.

Cobalt: is vital to the formation of vitamin B12. The pancreas contains a high concentration, which is used on demand by the body to synthesise insulin and certain other enzymes essential to the digestion of carbohydrates and fats. It is found in leafy green vegetables, liver and other foodstuffs, which are vitamin B12 sources.

Water

The body is 60 per cent water and it is essential to keep it that way! Different parts of the body account for different percentages. So, for example, 80 per cent of blood is water; 75 per cent of the brain; 22 per cent of bone; and 10 per cent of fat stores. We lose a considerable amount of water each day through perspiration, exhaled air and urine. The problem for most people is that their environment, diet and activity cause them to lose more water than they realise. Air conditioning at home, in offices, cars, airplanes, etc.; heating systems; warm climates; vigorous exercise; nervous tension; all contribute to dehydration or loss of water. We can add to the problem by consuming alcohol and caffeine.

Feeling thirsty is a reminder to top up but, unfortunately, this occurs only when we are down by around 2 per cent. We need to deal with things much earlier than this. Urine should be clear, like water, not yellow. People who are persistently in a dehydrated state are seriously compromising their performance capacity.

For most people, being hydrated means taking in around 1.5 litres of water per day. Athletes need around 2.5 litres but when competition periods are extended, and/or when hot and/or humid, they may need around 3.5 litres.

THESE GUIDELINES MAY HELP ENSURE A HEALTHY LEVEL OF HYDRATION

- Don't wait until you are thirsty to drink water, drink throughout the day.
- Drink small amounts regularly rather than a large amount occasionally.
- Have access to bottled water throughout the day, for example in the car, on your desk, in the plane, etc.
- Drink still water rather than carbonated, it is absorbed more easily.
- Drink water before, during and after exercise.
- Don't gulp water; sip it.
- Avoid tap water as it often contains extra chlorine or fluoride.
- If perspiring a lot during prolonged exercise you may be losing a lot of minerals in your sweat. Try one of the drinks that not only rehydrate, but replace minerals and contain glucose to top up the energy reservoir.

NUTRITIONAL SUPPLEMENTS

Nutritional supplements include a wide and varied range of products. The purpose of these is to improve health; and/or reduce the catabolic consequence of exposure to the challenge of adapting to the general and specific stressors of personal lifestyle; and/or prevent particular pathological conditions. They are useful and sometimes even essential therapeutic aids. Without doubt, they are widely used by athletes, often in the belief that they will enhance performance as ergogenic aids. This is only acceptable if they are:

- safe (of no threat to health);
- legal (within the laws of anti-doping policies);
- effective (on the basis of valid studies).

This said, if such products actually enhance performance, affording competitive advantage, their use would be ethically improper and should be prohibited, even if they are not contravening anti-doping laws. Most athletes will use nutritional supplements to achieve regeneration or recovery so that quality and quantity of training units can be increased per unit of time in order to persistently pursue improved competition performance levels. They would argue that this puts them beyond the edge of the ethical issue since it is training, not nutrition, which is affording them competitive advantage.

As our understanding of nutrition continues to expand and change, new advice is being suggested to enhance our health. So, for example, prebiotics, which are similar to fibre, promote the growth of healthy bacteria in the colon. These are naturally present in asparagus, onions, leeks, garlic, chicory, banana, dandelion leaves, Jerusalem artichokes, barley, rye and wheat. They are also available in commercially produced supplements. Another example is probiotics, such as acidophilus culture in yoghurt-like drinks, which help colon bacteria replace unhealthy bacteria that commonly cause disease. Again, such supplements do not raise

Supplement	Proposed advantage	Proven advantage
Amino acids: arginine, lysine, ornithine	Stimulate release of HGH; promotes muscle growth	?
Branched chain amino acids, glutamine	Stimulate release of HGH; increased pain tolerance; accelerating regeneration process	✔
Antioxidants: beta carotine, vit. C, vit. E, selenium	Reduce muscle damage from uunwanted oxidative processes following high intensity muscle activity	✔
Aspartates	Potassium and magnesium in salts of aspartate (a non-essential amino acid) improve performance and reduce muscular and central fatigue	✘
Bee pollen	Increases energy levels, enhances physical fitness	✘
BetaHydroxyBeta-Methylbutyrate (HMB)	Prevents or retards muscle damage and reduce proteolysis (muscle protein breakdown) associated with high intensity strength training	?
Boron	Increases serum testosterone levels	✘
Brewer's yeast	Increases energy levels	?
Carbohydrate gels	Prevents hypoglycaemia, increases carbohydrate metabolism	✔
Carnitine	Increases lipid catabolism, spares muscle glycogen	✘
Choline	Increases acetylcholine to increase strength or lecithin to decrease body fat	✘
Chromium	Potentiates insulin action, promotes muscle growth via enhanced amino acids uptake	✘
Colostrum	Helps tissue growth and repair, stimulates immune system	✔
Creatine (synthesised from amino acids)	Increases creatine phosphate in muscles; increases energy source and stimulates muscle growth	✔
Cyanacobalamine (Vit B12)	Enhances DNA synthesis; increases muscle growth	?
Gamma oryzamol	Increases serum testosterone and HGH level; increases muscle growth	✘
Gelatin	Improves muscle contraction	✘
Ginseng	Improves muscle contraction (NB: some variants contain high levels of Ma Hoang [Chinese Ephedrine] which would show as pseudoephedrine [illegal] in a urine sample)	✘

TABLE 4.5 Some common nutritional supplements

Supplement	Proposed advantage	Proven advantage
Glycerol	Increases intestinal and vascular hyperhydration water; improves thermoregulation and cardiovascular function	?
Inosine	Increases ATP synthesis, increases strength, facilitates regeneration	?
Kelp	High level micronutrient source	✘
Lecithin	Prevents fat gain, aids neuromuscular regeneration	?
Liquid (increases hydration via isotonic mineral replacement drinks)	Improves thermoregulation and cardiovascular function	✔
Magnesium	Increases protein synthesis or muscle contractility, increases muscle growth and strength	✘
Medium chain tryglycerides	Increase metabolic rate, promote fat loss	?
Octacosanol	Supplies energy, improves performance	✘
Omega 3 fatty acids	Maintains cardiovascular efficiency	✔
Oxygen (pure) inhalation	Improves intense exercise and speeds recovery from intense exercise	✔
Pangamic acid (B15)	Increased delivery of oxygen	✘
Phosphate	Delays muscle fatigue. Increases VO_2 max and ventilatory threshold	?
Phosphatidy-lserine (PS)	Diminishes ACTH and cortisol release without effecting HGH release, thus modifying the body's neuroendocrine response to stress (bovine derived possibly more effective than soya derived)	✔
Royal Jelly	Increases strength	✘
Saline infusion	Improves thermoregulation and cardiovascular function	✔
Smilax	Increases serum testosterone levels; increases muscle growth and strength	?
Sodium bicarbonate or sodium citrate	Increases blood buffering capacity	✔
Spirulina	Rich protein source	✘
Ubiquinone (CoQ.10)	Increases oxygen uptake	
Yohimbine	Increases serum testosterone levels; increases muscle growth and strength; decreases body fat; alpha2 adenoreceptor blocker	✘

✔ probable or certain   ? possible   ✘ probably not

ethical issues, but because they are designed to adjust how the body functions, all athletes should check these or, indeed, any supplement with the relevant people or agencies.

There have been increasing numbers of athletes testing positive for banned substances, despite the fact that they have apparently not wittingly taken them. The problem is that some supplements have additives which, on their own, and/or in combination with additives within an athlete's total diet of supplements and/ or due to the nature of training workloads, may be converted by the body's chemistry to something quite different. In other words, what has come out is not what the athlete believed had gone in. In light of this, in the interest of avoiding accidents which could have serious implications for the athlete's health and career, the 'package' of supplements in use at any time must be approved by relevant authorities. Manufacturers also have a responsibility to code their products in the context of anti-doping laws to help avoid 'accidents', where athletes and/or coaches have simply not understood the biochemical terms used in product descriptions.

Nutritional supplements include those listed in table 4.5, these are all legal substances. It is not intended to be a comprehensive list, but covers the more 'popular' areas.

Maughan, Greenhaff and Hespel (2011) have examined emerging trends in supplementation, two are worth mentioning here:

Creatine: The breakdown of creatine phosphate within the muscles gives athletes an initial burst of energy at the start of exercise. In recent years, many athletes involved in sprint, or multiple sprint sports, have used creatine supplementation as a means of boosting the body's stores of creatine, and consequently improving performance during repeated, high intensity activities. Scientists generally recommend a 'load' phase, when 5g of creatine are taken four times a day for 4–5 days, followed by a 'maintenance' phase, when much lower dosages are consumed for a period of up to six months. While creatine supplementation does work for some individuals, this may not be the case for everyone, and abdominal discomfort and weight gain are potential side effects which may outweigh any performance benefits. Furthermore, long-term excessive consumption of creatine may be harmful to the liver and kidneys.

Carbogels: In endurance sports such as marathon running, carbohydrate gels are an increasingly popular supplement. Containing a concentrated mix of carbohydrate, most provide around 100 calories of energy – sufficient for approximately 1 mile of running – and are used to supplement the body's stores of muscle glycogen during endurance activities. In an event such as a marathon, a general guideline is that no more than four or five carbo gels are required during a race, and should be consumed with water to prevent dehydration and gastro-intestinal distress.

There are other areas of supplementation that are most definitely not on the menu. They are banned substances and their use is considered as 'doping'.

DOPING

Doping is the use by, or distribution to, an athlete of certain substances which could have the effect of improving artificially the athlete's physical and/or mental condition and so augmenting his athletic ability (IAAF definition).

The World Anti-Doping Agency (WADA) was established in 1999, and today has responsibility for policing the World Anti-Doping Code across the globe. WADA is jointly funded by the Olympic movement and governments, and within the Code there are a number of substances and procedures that are banned within elite sport. The Code is updated on a regular basis, and at a national level, it is administered by national anti-doping organisations (NADOs). So, for example the NADO in the UK is UK Anti-Doping (UKAD) and in the USA is USADA. In both cases government level decisions were made that anti-doping should not rest with the national organisation funding elite sport due to potential conflict of interest.

Drug testing programmes operate across the range of sports. They vary in detail from country to country and from one international sporting body to another. In principle, however, they are there to ensure a level playing field for all athletes. Testing is based on the presence of the drug in a urine sample. That presence constitutes an offence, irrespective of the route of administration. Some sports are moving to blood samples rather than urine samples.

WADA's work is making progress in establishing the consistency of programmes across sports and nations and has broken important ground in creating an 'Athlete Biological Passport' (ABP). The underlying principle of the ABP is to monitor selected performance related biological variables over time that indirectly represent the effects of doping rather than trying to detect the doping substance or method itself.

DOPING CLASSES

There are six classes identified by WADA.

A   Stimulants (to increase alertness, reduce fatigue), for example amphetamines (in some tonics), ephedrine (in some cold cures), and caffeine (in tea, coffee, cola).

B   Narcotic analgesics (to manage pain) for example aspirin (in Veganin – short-term painkiller), codeine (in Benylin and other cold remedies).

C   Anabolic steroids (to speed recovery, improve competitiveness, increase muscle bulk) for example nandrolone (present in small amounts in some bodybuilding supplements), stanozolol.

D   Beta-blockers (to manage tension) for example stenolol, propranolol, oxprendol (normally in medicines for hypertension, cardiac dysrhythmias, etc.).

E   Diuretics (to manage [lose] bodyweight) for example amiloride, benzthiazide, bumetanide (present in proprietary brand diuretics).

F   Peptide hormones and analogues.
- Human chorionic gonadotrophin (similar to anabolic steroids) for example Pregnyl (medications related to hypogonadism).
- Corticotrophin (ACTH) (to increase blood levels of corticosteroids) for example tetracosactrin, synacthen (medications related to adrenocortical insufficiency).
- Human growth hormone (HGH: Somatotrophin) (to increase muscle hypertrophy, reduce effects of ageing process) for example Humatrope, Norditropin (medications to encourage growth).
- Erythropoetin (EPO) (to increase erythrocyte volume/aerobic capacity).

Doping methods

Blood doping (endurance athletes)

Blood transfusion of erythrocytes or related products which contain erythrocytes. The blood can be drawn from the same person (autologous) then reinfused later, or drawn from another person then transfused to the athlete (nonautologous). In some areas of this practice, the blood is drawn following altitude training then reinfused before a key championship event.

Pharmacological, chemical and physical manipulation

This covers the use of substances and methods which alter the integrity and validity of urine samples used in doping controls, for example catheterisation, urine substitution, etc.

Classes of drugs subject to certain restrictions

Different sports may ban different drugs, or there may be laws outside sport within which athletes must operate.

Alcohol is not prohibited by the IOC, but a governing body may test for breath/blood alcohol levels. Marijuana is not prohibited but may contravene civil laws. Local anaesthetics, if medically justified, may be used, but only local or intra-articular injections may be administered, although *not cocaine* as this is a banned drug. Corticosteroids may only be used for topical use (aural, opthalmological and dermatological; local or intra-articular injections; or inhalational therapy [allergic conditions, asthma etc.]), otherwise, they are banned.

Coaches should be committed to ensuring that athletes understand the critical role that nutrition plays in the performance development process. They must also be aware of the detail of their athlete's nutrition. This is part of the athlete's preparation. Without that knowledge it is not possible to relate performance to training and development. Without that knowledge athlete and coach can unwittingly expose themselves to the terrible consequence of an athlete's positive drugs test result. If the coach feels that his understanding of nutrition is limited, then he must have access to a nutritionist/sports scientist in his support team to interpret the situation for coach and athlete so that there is a joint responsibility which may be exercised in ensuring the athlete's nutrition is safe, legal and effective.

Food allergies

It is strongly recommended that all athletes be tested for sensitivity to the range of substances which may bring about an allergic reaction. Skin test or hair follicle tests may be used to uncover sensitivity to pollen, animal dander and foods – including certain drugs taken for medication. Such sensitivities should not be trivialised; an allergic reaction may be hay fever or asthma at one end of the spectrum, or anaphylactic shock or even death at the other. With athletes experimenting more and more with nutrition and supplementation, and with foreign travel and, therefore, different foods and water becoming a regular feature in our lives, there is greater risk of exposure to a nutritional content to which there could be sensitivity and/or an allergic reaction. Once tests are interpreted, the athlete will know what foods or combination of foods to avoid and carry with him relevant permitted medication should problems arise. Such information must be available to the doctor responsible for the athlete's medical welfare or supervision in his sport.

Nutritional guidelines for athletes (pre, during and post-exercise)

Against this general nutritional background the following may help in dealing with the more specific aspects of training and competition:

1. Nutrition, like most of what we require to be effective in our lives, is a matter of balance. It is traditionally best illustrated in this diagram – the food pyramid (figure 4.10). It is founded on a base of making sure that we have a daily fluid intake of at least 1.5 litres. After that it is about the ratio of one food type to another. This said, Noakes (2002) has urged caution in what constitutes 'balance'. For example, for those who are insulin resistant, type 2 diabetes is a significant risk for high carbohydrate intake over 20–30 years. He also rightly points out that changes in agricultural practice over four decades may have changed such things as gluten content of cereals and grains bringing with that the risk of gluten related illness. Certainly for people with allergies, it would be sensible to avoid cereals and grains where it is clear that there have been additives or genetic modification or there has been refinement of the original. Volek and Phinney have added to Noake's questioning of high carbohydrate diets by suggesting that there is a case for a high fat/oils diet for athletes plus substantially reduced carbohydrate intake. It would appear, then, that sport nutrition in this respect is being re-examined, that concepts are changing and that the food pyramid's dimensions may change with them!

2. General points for daily intake. In proposing the following, should athletes find it difficult to remain lean on this interpretation of the food pyramid yet are in strenuous exercise programmes, they may be insulin resistant and would be advised to raise protein and fat/oils intake and reduce carbohydrates to below 200 grams per day. Whatever, they should seek medical advice to check if they are insulin resistant.

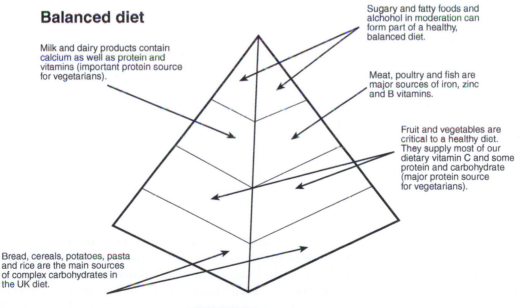

Balanced diet

Milk and dairy products contain calcium as well as protein and vitamins (important protein source for vegetarians).

Sugary and fatty foods and alchohol in moderation can form part of a healthy, balanced diet.

Meat, poultry and fish are major sources of iron, zinc and B vitamins.

Fruit and vegetables are critical to a healthy diet. They supply most of our dietary vitamin C and some protein and carbohydrate (major protein source for vegetarians).

Bread, cereals, potatoes, pasta and rice are the main sources of complex carbohydrates in the UK diet.

FIGURE 4.10 Food pyramid

Breakfast	High fluid (especially water)
	Cereals (natural bran is best)
	Fruit
	Easily digested light protein (not fried – especially if there is training in the morning)
	Low and moderate GI carbohydrates if training in the morning
	Moderate GI if training or competing in afternoon/evening
Snacks	Fruit, vegetable, cereal bars, water/fruit juice/mineral replacement drinks
Lunch	High fluid (especially water)
	High GI carbohydrates if training in morning
	Low and moderate GI if training or competing in afternoon/ evening
	Rich protein – especially egg/cheese, etc. if training in morning
	Easily digested light protein if training or competing in the afternoon/evening
	Fruit and vegetables
	Build in fats/oils
Snacks	Boost carbohydrates – low and moderate GI before evening competition
	High fluid intake (especially water)
Dinner	Rich protein if after training or competition
	High GI and moderate GI carbohydrates if after training or competing
	High fluid intake – especially if there has been a lot of sweat loss in training or competition
	Build in fats/oils
	Fruits and vegetables
	(Try to have dinner normally no later than 19.30)
Supper	Normally this meal is post evening competition
	High GI and moderate GI carbohydrates
	High fluid intake
	Easily digested, light protein
	Fruit and vegetables
	(Eating late is poor preparation for a good night's sleep – so this is essentially a light meal. However, breakfast the next morning may be boosted with a richer protein intake.)

We each have our own preferences for our daily nutrition routine, so we will have our own variations from breakfast to supper. However, these general principles should be built into our daily routine.

3. Maintaining recommended daily allowance (RDA) of micronutrients is important for athletes due to the wear and tear of persistent training and competition. Although small, this varies according to age, gender and the impact of combined physical, intellectual and emotional stressors. Status can be checked via cell analysis.

4. Micronutrient supplementation in the form of antioxidants, multivitamins and mineral tonics is pursued by around 75 per cent of all athletes, although studies do not confirm performance benefit. It is possible that high performance athletes; all athletes involved near the limits of quality and quantity training and competition; athletes operating for long periods in extreme environments; athletes recovering from health problems; and athletes whose total profile of lifestyle stressors is testing the limits of their capacity to adapt and, therefore, causing health problems, will require some level of supplementation. They should

seek the advice of a nutritionist in designing a strategy for what and how much to take, and also the frequency of days on/off supplementation.

5. In recent years the use of 'energy drinks' and 'sports drinks' has become widespread within elite and recreational sport. Each has a different role and, if used in the wrong context, can have a detrimental rather than positive effect on performance.

 Energy drinks tend to have a high concentration of carbohydrate (normally glucose) and in many cases often also contain caffeine. Energy drinks frequently contain in excess of 15 grams of carbohydrate per 100ml of fluid, and while the added caffeine does not provide energy, it acts as a stimulant and has been shown to enhance alertness and focus. Energy drinks are not recommended for use during exercise, since their high carbohydrate concentration reduces the rate at which fluid is absorbed, but may be used as a means of supplementing solid food consumption before or after an event. Many energy drinks have not been manufactured for use during sport, and are developed as a means of providing an energy boost during the day, or late into the evening. As such, they should be used with caution during sport and not as a substitute for a healthy, high carbohydrate diet.

 Sports drinks tend to fall into two basic categories: isotonic and hypotonic. Isotonic drinks have a carbohydrate content of between 4 and 8 grams per 100ml of fluid (often referred to as a concentration of between 4% and 8%). They also contain electrolytes, and in particular sodium and potassium, which are included to replace electrolytes that are lost through sweating. Scientists have shown that an isotonic concentration optimises the rate at which both fluid and energy are absorbed by the body during exercise, and as a result they are commonly used during many endurance activities and team sports. Hypotonic drinks have a concentration of carbohydrates below 4 per cent, but still contain electrolytes. They have been designed for shorter duration activities, where energy replacement may not be crucial, but when combatting dehydration remains important. Their lower calorific content also makes them popular with individuals wishing to exercise and lose weight.

6. Carbohydrate should be taken 3–6 hours before competition, or the maximum quality/quantity exercise which takes athletes to their limit. If it is to be taken within an hour of the competition or exercise, it should be less than 100g, within 30 minutes of starting, and be followed by warm-up or light activity.

7. In trained long-endurance athletes, reducing training and increasing the dietary carbohydrate to more than 10g/kg/day for three days prior to competition increases the muscle glycogen stores to their maximum value. This regime is not suitable for those preparing for intense exercise (e.g. for sprints, soccer, tennis).

8. Where training or competition lasts 90 minutes or more, taking carbohydrate delays fatigue, so enhancing performance. The carbohydrate can be taken during the activity or approximately 30 minutes before the anticipated time of fatigue. Around 30–60g/hour carbohydrate is required, whether in liquid or solid form; if solid, it must have a high glycaemic index value, for example banana, honey.

9. In some sports, athletes are required to perform prolonged exertions on consecutive days (e.g. tour cycling), or to perform in high-frequency back-to-back pressure competitions (e.g. World Cup soccer/rugby), or to train several times per day for 6–8 days at a time. Such demands require rapid regeneration by optimising the recovery process, particularly in reference to glycogen synthesis, hydration and muscle tissue repair.

Glycogen synthesis

- The optimal rate of replenishing carbohydrate is 0.7g/kg/hour, preferably in liquid form of glucose, glucose polymer or sucrose. If solid, it must have a high GI value. Adding protein to liquid carbohydrate may increase rate of glycogen synthesis.
- Animal fats intake should be reduced by replacing with vegetable oils.
- During competition or training periods of more than 90 minutes, glycogen and fluid replenishment is necessary – especially where there is high fluid loss due to heat, air conditioning, etc. Fluids should be ingested at a rate of 1 litre/hour and the carbohydrate concentration kept around 6g/litre to optimise carbohydrate and fluid delivery.
- Post-exercise carbohydrate ingestion should commence within 15 minutes of concluding the activity. To delay can reduce the rate of glycogen synthesis (e.g. delaying for two hours can reduce the rate from 7mmol/kg/hour to less than 3mmol/kg/hour). Even under optimal conditions it takes at least 20 hours (5% per hour) to re-establish glycogen stores.
- When training or competing on consecutive days, muscle glycogen must be replenished between the bouts of activity. This can be done in 24 hours, but if there is muscle damage, for example via eccentric exercise (e.g. high volume or intensity running, jumping, weight training/lifting); or body contact/impact (e.g. rugby, soccer, American/Australian rules football, ice hockey), the glycogen synthesis rate can decrease. This is due to white blood cells (WBC) competing for blood glucose in their endeavours to repair the damaged tissue. This process, however, takes around 12 hours, so early and regular carbohydrate intake through these 12 hours should make sufficient glucose available to the muscle, despite increasing competition from WBC for its use.
- Active recovery/warm down should be kept at low intensity (less than 35% VO_2 max) to avoid reducing glycogen stored in fast-twitch muscle.

Hydration

- Although, as mentioned under 'water', still drinks are more beneficial than carbonated for rehydration, the difference is not conclusive for electrolyte replacement. As suggested above, however, there is a case for keeping to still drinks when it comes to glycogen synthesis.

Muscle tissue repair

- Highly trained athletes exposed to prolonged periods of persistent training and competition loads have increased protein catabolism. It is very unlikely that protein ingested in their diet falls below the levels indicated in table 4.2.

However, the process of repair/regeneration may require support via taking appropriate protein foods such as eggs, milk, brewer's yeast, fish, meat/poultry, liver, and avoiding poorer protein foods such as rice, soya, gelatin and related foods. Cooking method is also important, so boiled, stewed, grilled and poached foods should replace fried and roasted.

10. Caffeine in coffee, tea and colas taken in a normal social context will not expose athletes to the risk of a positive drugs test result. A positive test (according to the IOC) would require 12mg per ml of caffeine in the urine (15mg per ml – National Collegiate Athlete Association, USA). It is estimated that two cups of brewed coffee (100–150mg caffeine) or five cups of regular tea (30–75mg caffeine) or six 12oz colas (32–65mg caffeine) will yield urine levels of 3–6mg per ml.

11. Alcohol impairs coordination, disturbs fluid balance and interferes with temperature regulation. It cannot be considered a sensible inclusion in an athlete's diet. Post-activity beers may be argued as contributing to fluid replacement (but alcohol dehydrates), or to aid relaxation, yet it can have quite the opposite effect! There are healthier ways to rehydrate and relax. The athlete's body is his vehicle for expressing the performance his training hours deserve. Why abuse it?

12. Finally, following extensive review of the diets of athletes, it is perfectly clear that the vast majority over-estimate their nutritional requirements. In part, this is borne of the attitude of leaving nothing to chance – 'if something is good for you, more of it is better'. That is simply not true. Over-eating causes more rapid ageing and health risks than a well-balanced diet. In fact, periodic 'fasting' prolongs the life of certain animals, giving them a younger biological age. This practice is also used to 'detox', flushing out the toxic by-products of the food we eat.

The best advice is to keep within the nutritionist's rules for a healthy diet – especially in terms of calories; review nutritional status periodically via nutrition diaries and cell analysis, and stay in the middle weight range for your height and sports discipline.

SUMMARY

With the exception of the days preceding, during or following periods of training at the athlete's limit of load quality and quantity or competition, a regular well-balanced diet should supply his nutritional requirements. Calorific requirement demanded of the athlete's lifestyle should match calorific input from macronutrients; protein content will fall within the range associated with the nature of the sport and growth and repair needs; micronutrients will meet the athlete's needs which are above normal due to the wear and tear of his lifestyle; water intake will ensure that hydration remains at an appropriate level. Special diets may be designed in preparation for the high demands of glycogen stores to fuel the activity; during the activity to replace spent glycogen and reduce the rate of dehydration; and afterwards to restock glycogen stores and rehydrate; to replace reduced levels of micronutrients and speed regeneration and repair. Relevant nutritional supplementation must be considered and responsibly applied following consultation involving athlete, coach, nutritionist and, occasionally, medical adviser. No supplementation should be taken without that consultation and without it being approved as safe, legal and effective. Care should be taken to avoid foods which may have an adverse effect on the absorption of other nutrients (e.g. raw fish, raw egg albumen).

Athletes and coaches must know which substances, products and methods are listed as banned. They must understand *why*, both at the health and ethical levels. They must live within the laws of the WADA anti-doping programme because this is the most comprehensive of all the anti-doping programmes. They must do so not just because they have to, but because they want to.

REFLECTIVE QUESTIONS

1. When athletes leave school and enter university or college they may have difficulty maintaining a well-balanced healthy diet. Often they may look to nutritional supplements. What advice in these areas should you give in a presentation to first year students joining university/college sports clubs?

2. Discuss schools of thought on carbohydrate intake in high performance sport including advantages and disadvantages of a diet rich in foods containing unrefined complex carbohydrates such as cereals and grains.

3. If vitamins and micronutrients play an important role in energy release, why not 'mega-dose' with supplements to enhance exercise performance?

4. You are leading a team preparing to compete at an international tournament in India. Describe your nutritional advice, including hydration, from departure and what provisions you suggest should be taken with the team.

5. Describe a rationale for the nutritional strategy you would propose rather than excess protein, for a person who wishes to increase muscle mass through a heavy strength training programme.

5 THE OXYGEN TRANSPORTING SYSTEM

DEFINITION, FUNCTIONS AND EFFECTS

The various nutrients available to the body by the metabolism of foodstuffs must be transported to the sites where they are used or stored. This transport is provided by a remarkable fluid which also carries oxygen, hormones and chemicals; it is a buffer solution; it removes waste products from the tissues; aids temperature control; and helps maintain fluid balance. This fluid is the blood.

Blood

The volume of blood in the body varies from person to person and will increase with training, but it is approximately as follows: men 75ml/kg bodyweight; women 65ml/kg bodyweight; children 60ml/kg bodyweight. The composition of blood is quite complex, but is summarised by figure 5.1.

Cells
Erythrocytes (red blood cells)
Erythrocytes (red blood cells) are formed in the bone marrow at an equal rate to their destruction (haemolysis); this means approximately 2–3 million cells per second. Red cell formation is stimulated by *hypoxia* (oxygen deficiency – see p. 280) and *erythropoietin*, a glycoprotein also known as haemopoietin or erythrocyte stimulating factor (ESF) which is produced in the kidneys. Intravenous injections of renal extracts or glucocorticoids stimulate red cell formation and it has been suggested that testosterone derivatives increase erythropoietin formation.

The average erythrocyte count in men is 5.7 million/mm^3 and in women and children it is 4.8 million/mm^3. The red colouring is due to its haemoglobin content, which is a combination of a protein (globin) and a red pigment (haematin). Muscle haemoglobin is called myoglobin. The red pigment contains iron, which readily combines with oxygen. This combination is a very loose affair and the oxygen can be just as easily 'disconnected' or cast free. Herein lies the oxygen transporting property of blood and the obvious importance of dietary iron. However, excessive iron will not increase the oxygen-carrying capacity of the blood. Iron absorption is tightly controlled by the body's requirements. When these are met, absorption through the intestine wall ceases and the excess iron is expelled in the faeces.

In men, the average haemoglobin (Hb) content is 15.8g/100ml blood, while in women it is 13.9g/100ml blood. To be more precise, normal values may be found within the range 14–18g/100ml blood for men and 11.5–16g/100ml for women. As 1g of fully saturated haemoglobin combines with 1.34ml oxygen, so haemoglobin may be used as an index of the oxygen-carrying capacity of the blood. Occasionally haemoglobin content is expressed as a percentage, but this can be a little confusing since 100 per cent may be normal for

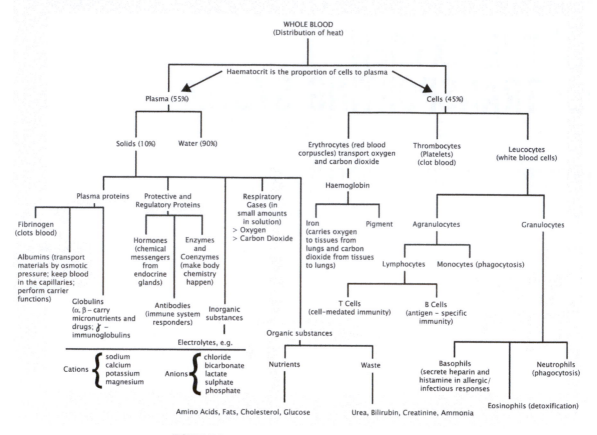

FIGURE 5.1 Summary of blood composition and function

one investigator but not for another. Moreover, there appears to be different 'normal' values according to age, gender, nationality, geographic location, and so on. Consequently, one must check the meaning of 100 per cent before evaluating the haemoglobin count of an athlete.

The idea of a normal range seems much less problematic. Information on haemoglobin status is presented in the Edinburgh Royal Infirmary Bioprofile, as in table 5.1. Reading the haemoglobin line, the athlete appears to be relatively low in the range and consequently we can assume that the oxygen carrying capacity of the blood is also low. The second line tells us why it is low. The mean corpuscular haemoglobin concentration (MCHC) is an index of the iron status of haemoglobin and here it is clear that the athlete requires some kind of iron therapy suggested by a doctor.

Normal range	You
Haemoglobin: men (14–18), women (11.5–16)	12.9
MCHC (mean corpuscular haemoglobin concentration): 32–36	32.2

TABLE 5.1 Information sent to an Edinburgh girl who ran 800m and 1500m

Training increases the total amount of haemoglobin in the body and this can be assessed by evaluating the red cell volume and haemoglobin count. Periodically the erythrocyte count may rise by 5–10 per cent with sustained work, but this is normally temporary and due to an imbalance of body fluids. However, training has a more variable effect on MCHC and it has been shown that many top endurance athletes have a tendency to iron deficiency (anaemia). This may be due to dietary deficiency, iron loss in sweat, damaged erythrocytes, etc., but may also be part of the adaptive process to ensure a higher speed of oxygen provision to the muscle. Endurance training will increase the blood *volume* by 15–30 per cent, but this hypervolaemia is usually accompanied by a 5–10 per cent fall in erythrocyte and haemoglobin concentration.

Finally, haemoglobin plays an essential part in the removal of carbon dioxide from the tissues to the lungs.

Leucocytes (white blood cells)

The leucocytes (white blood cells) are comprised of the following:

Granulocytes: *neutrophils* – involved in resistance to infection they multiply when there is an infection in the body or when there is local inflammatory reaction brought about by dead or dying tissue. The glucocorticoids increase the number of circulating neutrophils but their ability to migrate into the tissues is reduced, with consequent loss of resistance to infection. The destruction of bacteria by neutrophils is possible because the neutrophils are capable of phagocytosis ('cell eating'); *eosinophils* – collect at sites of allergic reaction and it has been suggested that they limit the effects of substances such as histamine. The level of circulating eosinophils is reduced by the glucocorticoids; *basophils* – have a much smaller share of the leucocyte population (table 5.2), and relatively little is known of their physiological function. They contain heparin and histamine and may be connected with preventing clotting. Glucocorticoids lower the number of circulating basophils.

Agranulocytes: *monocytes* – like the neutrophils they help remove bacteria and debris by active phagocytosis in the battle against infection. They act against bacteria after the neutrophils, thus forming a second line of defence. The corticosteroids have a similar effect on monocytes and neutrophils; *lymphocytes* – involved in the processes of immunity. They are formed principally from lymphoid tissue. The glucocorticoids decrease the number of circulating lymphocytes and the size of the lymph nodes.

Type of cells	Average number of cells per micro litre of blood	
Neutrophils	5400	
Eosinophils	160	
Basophils	40	
Lymphocytes	2750	
Monocytes	540	
Erythrocytes	(male) 4.8×10^6	(female) 5.4×10^6
Platelets	300,000	

TABLE 5.2 Composition of the blood's cell volume

It is worth bearing in mind that these defence manoeuvres require an expenditure of energy in addition to the weakness caused when the 'enemy' infection has gained ground. Training is never recommended during this battle unless the infection is very slight. The problem does not end here, however, because even when the battle has been won, the reserves have been depleted and must be allowed to recoup. Consequently the coach must scale down all training until the athlete feels that things are back to normal.

Thrombocytes (platelets)

The thrombocytes (platelets) are very small bodies which are fragments of giant cells called megakaryocytes. When the walls of blood vessels are damaged, platelets adhere to the injury site and secrete materials contained in their granules. This adhesion and secretion is the action of clotting. The number of circulating platelets is increased by glucocorticoids.

The role of the glucocorticoids has been previously mentioned to draw attention to some of the microphysical effects of stressors. Stress increases adrenocorticotrophic hormone (ACTH) activity (see chapter 8), which in turn raises the amount of circulating glucocorticoids. Why this occurs is still unexplained, but these microphysical effects may ultimately cause the major physical problems of high blood pressure, coronary disease, etc. (figure 5.2). This is the reason for the concern for the health of 30–45-year-olds constantly exposed to stressors of business, professional life, and so on.

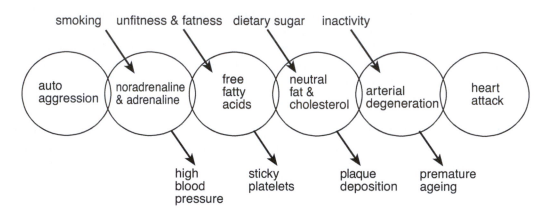

FIGURE 5.2 Factors which contribute to the possibility of a heart attack. Carruthers referred to this situation as 'knitting a heart attack' (from Carruthers, 1971).

Plasma

Approximately 55 per cent of the blood volume is a straw-coloured fluid called plasma. It is made up of over 90 per cent water, and under 10 per cent solids. The solids are made up as follows:

Plasma proteins

These are comprised of: albumins – they carry materials to sites of need or elimination (e.g. minerals, ions, fatty acids, amino acids, bilirubin, enzymes, drugs); globulins – the α1, α2, and β1, β2 globulins carry micronutrients and are carriers for drugs. The l globulins are immunoglobins or antibodies which generally protect the body against bacteria, viruses and toxins; fibrinogen – aids blood clotting. (The fluid 'squeezed' from a clot is serum.)

Protective and regulatory proteins

- **Hormones:** (see chapter 8).
- **Antibodies:** produced by the immune system to fight antigens (foreign agents) invading the body.
- **Enzymes and coenzymes:** most chemical reactions occurring in the body are regulated by the catalytic action of enzymes and/or coenzymes. The chemicals which undergo change in an enzymically catalysed reaction are called substrates for that enzyme.

Inorganic substances

These are principally the electrolytes:

- **Cations** (positively charged) – sodium, potassium, calcium and magnesium
- **Anions** (negatively charged) – chloride, bicarbonate, lactate, sulphate and phosphate.

They also include copper, iodine, iron and lead. Lactate is the end product of the lactic anaerobic energy pathway. Normal levels are 1–1.8mmol/litre, but in prolonged intensive exercise, this can rise to 20mmol/litre. Due to its ease of diffusion, blood lactate gives a reasonable picture of lactate concentration in muscle. Peak lactic acid concentration in the blood is not achieved until several minutes after activity.

Respiratory gases

Plasma contains small amounts of inspired oxygen and carbon dioxide in sodium and as bicarbonate being transported out of the body via the lungs.

Organic substances

Nutrients: – amino acids (see chapter 4)
 – fats and cholesterol (see chapter 4)
 – glucose (see chapter 4)

Waste: – urea, from the breakdown of protein. This varies in line with protein in the diet.
 – creatinine, from the breakdown of body tissues
 – ammonia, formed in the kidneys from glutamine brought to it in the blood. This varies with the quantity of acids which are neutralised in the kidney.
 – bilirubin; during destruction of erythrocytes by the reticuloendothelial system at the end of their 120 day life, haemoglobin is released and both iron and globin are split off and bilirubin is formed.

Other substances are present in minute amounts in plasma, but are not listed here in detail.

Among the properties of blood already listed is its function as a 'buffer solution'. A buffer solution contains a weak acid or alkali and a highly ionised salt of the same acid or alkali. The presence of the highly ionised salt maintains the pH balance of the solution when it is exposed to an influx of acid or alkali substance (see chapter 7, page 119).

Biochemical analysis of blood can probably give the clearest picture of the status of an athlete's body chemistry, short of biopsy techniques. Advancements in technology allow analysis of blood to test over 100 parameters of a given sample of blood in 60 seconds.

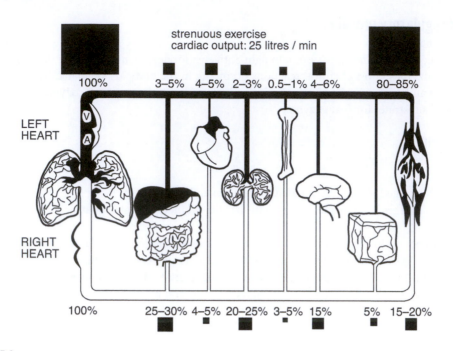

FIGURE 5.3 Astrand and Rodahl illustrate the circulation 'picture' with great clarity in this extract from *A Textbook of Work Physiology* (1986). The figures indicate the relative distribution of the blood to the various organs at rest (lower scale) and during exercise (upper scale). During exercise the circulating blood is primarily diverted to the muscles. The area of the black squares is proportional to the minute volume of blood flow.

To fulfil its tasks, the blood must be:

- pumped around the body (heart);
- contained in tubes/vessels through which it is pumped (blood vessels);
- taken to a source of oxygen (lungs);
- taken to a source of fuel (gut, liver);
- taken to areas where oxygen and fuel are used (tissues);
- loaded with waste (tissues);
- unloaded of waste (lungs, kidneys).

Astrand and Rodahl's (1986) diagram of circulation helps to give the overall picture (figure 5.3).

The heart

The heart is a muscle which, by its contraction, pumps blood round the body to all areas to meet the needs of the moment. For example, at rest, the gut has a lot of blood to cope with digestion and the acceptance of nutrients for transporting to storage or circulation. During exercise the blood is directed to where it is needed, i.e. the muscle for mechanical and physiological work, and the skin for temperature control.

The continuous pumping of the heart also returns 'used' blood, carrying increased carbon dioxide back to

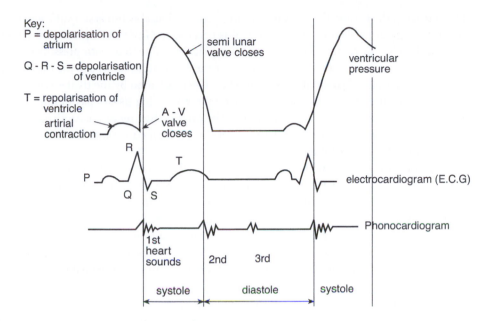

FIGURE 5.4 The relationship between the contraction patterns and mechanisms of the heart, the ECG and the heart sounds (from Guyton, 1990)

the lungs, where the excess carbon dioxide is unloaded and oxygen supplies are replenished. Blood is carried from the systemic circulation through the vena cavae into the right atrium. There is no valve on entry, as thickening and contraction of muscle prevents backflow. It then passes through the tricuspid (A–V) valve into the right ventricle, then through the pulmonary (semilunar) valve into pulmonary circulation – offloading carbon dioxide and taking on oxygen. From the lungs via the pulmonary veins it enters the left atrium. Again, there is no valve. It then passes through the mitral (A–V) valve into the left ventricle, then back into the systemic circulation through the aortic (semilunar) valve then via the aorta. Electrocardiograms (ECGs) are frequently used to assess the status of the heart's contractile mechanisms, but may also be used in laboratory testing work to provide an accurate heart rate assessment. Figure 5.4 shows the relationship between the ECG, blood pressure, heart sound, and ventricular pressure. The ECG is recorded on a printout form or on an oscilloscope. Changes in the T-wave have been noted when the athlete is experiencing high level stressors in training or competition (Carlile and Carlile, 1960).

Blood pressure

Blood pressure is also used as a guide to the efficiency of the heart and blood vessels. Normal values are 120mmHg/80mmHg. This means at systole (i.e. when the heart thrusts its contents from the left ventricle into the aorta which takes the oxygen-rich blood to the tissues) the pressure is 120mmHg, and at diastole (i.e. when the left ventricle is being refilled) the pressure is 80mmHg. These pressures, especially the systole, rise in the first few minutes of exercise, but gradually fall over the following 30 to 45 minutes. Other blood pressures of interest are those of systole and diastole at the right ventricle which send oxygen-depleted blood along the pulmonary artery to the lungs. These pressures are 25mmHg and 7mmHg, to avoid damaging the lungs.

When the blood reaches the tissues, the pressure has dropped considerably but is still sufficient to squeeze the fluids through the capillary walls into the tissue. This is because the *hydrostatic* pressure is lower in the tissue than in the capillaries. The return of the fluid to the capillaries is due to *osmotic* pressure generated by albumen in the blood. This may be thought of as a 'thirst' for fluid. The fluid returns to the capillaries and is pressed back towards the heart by hydrostatic pressure. The oxygen required by the tissues is removed from the blood at capillary level and the carbon dioxide formed by the working tissues passes into the capillary to be carried back to the right heart, then on to the lungs. The cycle is then repeated. Any 'spillover' of fluid between capillary and tissue goes into the lymphatic system to be drained off into circulation at another point, or into the body's extracellular fluids.

The volume of blood pumped out with each contraction of the heart muscle is known as the stroke volume. The number of heart beats per minute is called the heart rate. Compared with untrained people, training of the oxygen transporting system at a given workload lowers the athlete's heart rate on recovery from that workload, as well as at rest. The highly trained endurance athlete may have a range from approximately 40 beats per minute to 200 per minute. At the latter rate, the heart is apparently 'failing' because there is insufficient time to fill the volume of the ventricles. As a consequence, the stroke volume is reduced to much less than maximum. (In top male endurance athletes maximum is approximately 220ml; resting = 80ml.) As we grow older, maximum heart rate reduces. Astrand and Christensen (1964) suggest 210/minute at the age of 10, 180/minute at 35 years of age and 165/minute at 65 years of age.

Cardiac output is the total volume of blood pumped out by the heart per minute. This is the product of heart rate × stroke volume. Astrand et al. (2003) state that 'cardiac output during standard exercise repeated during a course of training … is maintained at the same level'. This implies that stroke volume increases with training (since heart rate decreases).

The blood vessels

The blood vessels are best presented in diagram form, as illustrated in figure 5.5 showing the complete 'circuit'.

A healthy blood vessel network is essential to life. It is fundamental, then, that its health is regularly monitored. Of course there will be debate on when to commence monitoring but as early as 30 years may be sensible. As a minimum four measures should be taken – total cholesterol, HDL, LDL and serum triglycerides. (See chapter 4 and table 4.3 for more information.)

These four measures represent a valuable 'early warning system' for coronary heart disease. They are even more effective if a coronary calcium score is measured as this gives assessment of coronary event risk.

It is also sensible to consider a lifestyle of good practice in how to keep the network healthy! Key factors are: no smoking; moderate alcohol, with frequent alcohol-free days; white meat and fish more than red meat and processed meat; vegetable oils rather than animal fat; supplementation of omega 3, 6, 9 oils; low cholesterol foods in general; exercise three–four days per week, 30–60 minutes at a time; de-stressing activities such as meditation.

The lungs

The lungs provide the large surface area necessary for the exchange of oxygen (passing into the blood) and carbon dioxide (passing out of the blood). Before it reaches the tiny alveoli, air is warmed, moistened and cleansed as it passes via the nose and mouth through the trachea, bronchi and bronchioles. Finally, exchange

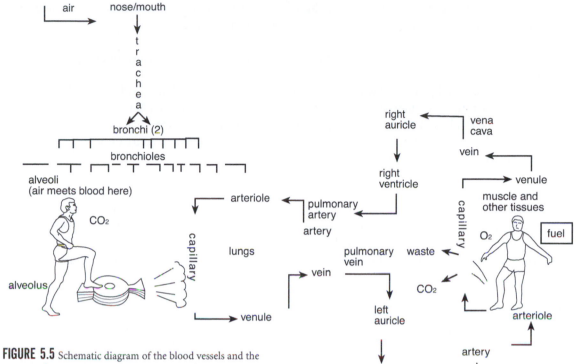

FIGURE 5.5 Schematic diagram of the blood vessels and the passage of oxygen from outside the body, to the working muscle

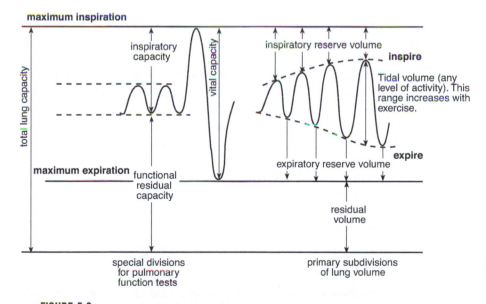

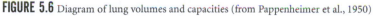

FIGURE 5.6 Diagram of lung volumes and capacities (from Pappenheimer et al., 1950)

of gases takes place between the alveoli and the pulmonary capillaries. Certain measures of lung capacity are frequently used to assess the efficiency of the breathing mechanisms (figure 5.6).

- Vital capacity is the maximal volume of gas that can be expelled from the lungs following a maximal inspiration.
- Inspiratory capacity is the maximal volume of gas inspired from the functional residual capacity.
- Functional residual capacity is the volume of gas remaining in the lungs when the respiratory muscles are relaxed.
- Expiratory reserve volume is the volume of gas expired from the functional residual capacity.
- Residual volume is the volume of gas which remains in the lungs even after forced expiration.
- Total lung capacity is the sum of the vital capacity and residual volume.

In women, the lung volumes are approximately 10 per cent smaller than for men of the same age and size. Training for aerobic endurance may increase vital capacity. Vital capacity decreases with age and although this is clear in the over 40s, the exact commencement of this decline is normally in the early 30s, but is variable according to the individual concerned.

Vital capacity is greatest among endurance athletes – in Stockholm an Olympic medallist in cross-country skiing recorded 8.1 litres.

Gut and liver

It has been pointed out that many of the end products of digestion are absorbed from the intestine into the blood, which carries these products to storage or further processing and then carries required nutrients into general circulation. Concentration of blood flow in this area of the circulatory system is much greater at rest than it is during exercise (figure 5.3). Prior to competition, emotional excitement causes an increased flow of adrenaline, an arresting of the digestive process, and a very obvious problem if a meal has been eaten too recently.

The liver performs a number of functions:

- It maintains a supply of glucose to the blood.
- It is the most vital organ of metabolism.
- It is a storage organ, holding glycogen, fat, proteins, some vitamins, and other substances involved in blood formation, and blood itself. These substances are released and reserves replenished as the need arises.
- It synthesises plasma proteins and heparin.
- It secretes bile which is necessary for the absorption of fats and the fat soluble vitamins A, D, E and K.
- It is involved in the formation and destruction of erythrocytes, and in the protection of the body against toxic invaders (e.g. through oxidation of alcohol and nicotine).

The liver has responsibility for making potential energy available to the tissues in the form of glucose. Its efficiency in this role *must* be maximum in exercise. Consequently it is wrong to make demands of the liver to oxidise, say, alcohol, while energy provision is required.

The tissues

The main tissues of interest to those involved in training theory are the muscles, which are dealt with in detail in chapter 6.

Elimination of the waste products of exercise

The principal waste products of exercise are urea, carbon dioxide, water, metabolites other than lactate, and lactic acid itself. The main fate of urea and water is to be filtered through the kidneys and expelled from the body. Carbon dioxide is carried in the blood to the lungs, where it passes into the alveoli and is then expelled from the body. Metabolites other than lactate are disposed of first by oxidation. The oxygen required for this purpose is referred to as that which repays the alactic oxygen debt (i.e. as in creatine phosphate anaerobic energy pathway.)

LACTIC ACID IS ELIMINATED AS FOLLOWS

1. The muscle lactate is disposed of first by oxidation to pyruvate, and then by dissimilation to carbon dioxide and water.

2. Some of the blood lactate is then taken up by the liver which reconstructs it to glycogen, via the 'cori cycle' (see chapter 6, page 107).

3. The remaining blood lactate diffuses back into the muscle, or other organs, to be oxidised then dissimilated. Such oxidation of lactate causes formation of carbon dioxide, the fate of which is mostly the reconstitution of blood bicarbonate, before being excreted by the lungs.

It should be noted that lactate cannot be oxidised in the blood stream itself. Moreover, it appears that the reconstruction of glycogen from lactic acid is not possible in human muscle.

MAXIMAL OXYGEN UPTAKE

Maximal oxygen uptake (VO_2 maximum) is the body's maximal aerobic power and is defined as 'the highest oxygen uptake the individual can attain during physical work breathing air at sea level' (Astrand and Rodahl, 1986). Oxygen uptake is the difference in oxygen content between the air inspired and the air expired, expressed in ml/kg bodyweight/minute. In other words it is the amount of oxygen required by the body to fulfil its functions at a given time. Obviously more oxygen will be required in severe exercise and so oxygen uptake will increase. However, a point is eventually reached where the body can take up no more oxygen. At this point the value is referred to as the maximal oxygen uptake.

Evaluation of the athlete's VO_2 maximum is the best criterion of his status of aerobic efficiency. In table 5.3, Swedish statistics give the ranges for certain groups of athletes.

The highest recorded improvements of VO_2 maximum are between 15 per cent and 20 per cent. Improvement is made possible by increasing the efficiency of the oxygen transporting system. The principal areas for possible improvement are as follows:

1. The heart. Stroke volume can be increased by specific endurance training, as can the capacity to raise the maximum heart rate.

2. The blood. The oxygen-carrying capacity of the blood can again be increased by specific training. Both total mass of erythrocytes and total haemoglobin may be increased. Ekblom's (1972) 'blood doping' demonstrated the artificial increase of the blood's oxygen-carrying capacity.

3. The muscle. The difference between the oxygen content of artery and vein (e.g. before and after the muscle accepts fuel and oxygen from the capillaries) is known as the arterio-venous oxygen difference (a-vO$_2$). Increasing the size and number of mitochondria (the oxygen users) of muscle, and the density of capillaries in muscle by specific endurance exercise, will increase the value of a-vO$_2$, as will the increase in myoglobin, the muscles' own internal oxygen transport system.

A relationship between heart rate, per cent VO$_2$ maximum, and blood lactate concentration is suggested by table 5.4. However, because heart rate does not increase linearly over the full range of exercise intensity but is close to this over a given range, this relationship can only represent an approximation.

	Male	Female
400m	63–69	52–58
800–1500m	74–77	52–58
3000m	77–82	
Cross country	72–83	55–61
Normal	38–46	30–46

TABLE 5.3 VO$_2$ max ranges for Swedish athletes according to competition distance (ml/kg body wt/min)

Lactic acid mg/100ml blood	% VO$_2$ max.	Heart Rate	Scale of intensity
25	50	130	low
30	60	150	light
70	75	165	high
90	90	180/190	submaximum
100	100	190+	maximum

TABLE 5.4 Relationship of blood lactate concentration, % VO$_2$ max and heart rate (adapted from Suslov, 1972)

ACCLIMATISATION AT ALTITUDE

In the mid 1960s the problems of competing at altitude raised questions about the possible advantages of training at altitude (see p. 280). At altitudes such as that of Mexico City (2.3km, 7500 feet), there is a reduced partial pressure of oxygen (pO$_2$) due to reduced barometric pressure, thus there is a lower pressure forcing oxygen into the blood in the lungs. The partial pressure at any point is obtained from the formula:

pO$_2$ = % oxygen concentration of dry air × (barometric pressure - 47)
(47 = partial pressure of water vapour)

THE OXYGEN TRANSPORTING SYSTEM 99

Thus, with a constant oxygen concentration of 20.94 per cent dry air, table 5.5 shows the pO_2 at different altitudes.

Altitude		Pressure, mmHg	kPa	pO₂ tracheal air, mmHg	kPa
m	ft				
0	0	760	101.3	149	19.9
500	1640	716	95.5	140	18.7
1000	3280	674	89.9	131	17.5
1500	4920	634	84.5	123	16.4
2000	6560	596	79.5	115	15.3
2500	8200	560	74.7	107	14.3
3000	9840	526	770.1	100	13.3
3500	11,840	493	65.7	93	12.4
4000	13,120	462	61.6	87	11.6
4500	14,650	433	57.7	81	10.8
5000	16,400	405	54.0	75	10.0
6000	19,690	354	47.2	64	8.5
7000	22,970	308	41.1	55	7.3
8000	26,250	267	35.6	46	6.1
9000	29,530	230	30.7	38	5.1
10,000	32,800	198	26.4	32	4.3
19,215	63,000	47	6.3	0	.0

TABLE 5.5 Calculations of pO_2 based on dry conditions for average temperature at altitude when the temperature at sea level is 15°C (59°F) and the barometric pressure is 760mmHg (101.3kPa). The tracheal air represents inspired air saturated with water vapour at 37°C (98.6°F). There would only be water molecules in the trachea at this point (abbreviated from Astrand, Rodahl, Dahl and Stromme, 2003).

Hypoxia is more an effect than a fact at altitude because the chemical composition of the atmosphere is almost uniform up to an altitude of over 20,000 feet. Also, at altitude, with the reduced barometric pressure, there is a reduced air resistance, implying an advantage to speed activities. The force of gravity is also reduced, suggesting an advantage where relative strength or maximum strength is critical. Air temperature and humidity are on the whole lower and this increases the loss of water via respiration, causing problems in endurance sports, intermittent but long duration team games, and so on. Finally, ultraviolet radiation is more intense so competition or training during hours when the sun is high should be avoided.

THE IMMEDIATE EFFECTS OF EXPOSURE TO ALTITUDE ARE:

- increased breathing rate, even at rest
- increased heart rate (tachycardia)
- giddiness
- nausea
- headache
- sleeplessness
- greater arteriovenous oxygen difference
- decreased VO_2 maximum
- rapid increase of haemoglobin concentration in first few days.

The total effect of these adjustments is a reduction of work capacity, but the degree of reduction can vary between individuals.

The long-term effects of continued exposure to altitude are:

- Increased erythrocyte volume (increased erythropoietin secretion due to hypoxic effect).
- Increased haemoglobin volume and concentration.
- Increased blood viscosity.
- Continued lower VO_2 maximum.
- Decreased tolerance of lactic acid.
- Reduced stroke volume of the heart.
- Increased capillarisation in the muscle.

It is clear that training at altitude is sound preparation for competing at altitude and that altitude performances will improve as adaptation continues.

Although debate continues as to the value of altitude training for enhancing performance at sea level, the balance of practical experience supports the view that there are advantages to a carefully managed programme (see also p. 280).

SUMMARY

Although blood is referred to as the oxygen transporting vehicle, it is also the principal means of transporting to the tissues the fuel and materials essential for maintenance, repair and growth, and of transporting waste from the tissues to disposal sites. The effectiveness of this vehicle is enhanced by increased functional capacity of heart, lungs, blood vessels and blood, combined with more efficient use of oxygen, fuel and various materials at the sites where they are required. Blood also transports heat from muscle to skin.

Increased efficiency of the overall oxygen transporting system implies increased working capacity, which itself implies more value from training units for the athlete and more life in the years of the non-athlete.

Specific training will increase efficiency of the system and it is therefore self-evident that both athletes and non-athletes should adopt such training.

Periodic blood analyses are acknowledged to be valuable aids to evaluate body chemistry and are recommended for athlete and non-athlete alike. In addition, it is suggested that VO_2 maximum, blood pressure and blood lactate (for a given workload) be similarly tested to establish a broad picture of oxygen transporting system efficiency, relative to the physiological demands of a sport.

The 'anaerobic threshold', or onset of blood lactate accumulation (OBLA point), is also a critical measure. The OBLA point gives an indication of the workload (on cycle, canoe or rowing ergometers, or on a treadmill) at which the body just starts to seriously use anaerobic energy with the probability of a rapid build-up of lactic acid in the blood.

Knowing the heart rate at which this happens can help a competitor to optimise aerobic training by working appropriately just under the OBLA point, i.e. just below the anaerobic threshold. The anaerobic threshold may sometimes be determined without blood sampling – by noting alterations in breathing patterns during a maximum aerobic test.

REFLECTIVE QUESTIONS

1. What are the normal value ranges for blood volume, plasma volume, haemoglobin concentration and haematocrit? How do these values change with endurance training? Discuss the advantages and disadvantages of such change.

2. How do heart rate, stroke volume and cardiac output change during incremental increase to VO_2 max? Are responses different after endurance training? If so, what are they and how might they affect performance?

3. An athlete attempts to perform a maximum lift in the standing press. After straining to achieve it, he comments: 'I feel a bit dizzy and see spots before my eyes.' Suggest a plausible physiological explanation. What action would you propose to prevent this?

4. Weightlessness over a tour of duty in the International Space Station has implications for the cardiovascular system. Discuss the differences for the system between weightlessness and normal gravity. Would there be a difference between male and female astronauts? If so, what? What exercise programme would you consider appropriate for astronauts when in space?

5. List all the improvements in cardiovascular function after endurance training and arrange these to demonstrate potential cause and effect relationships to VO_2 max.

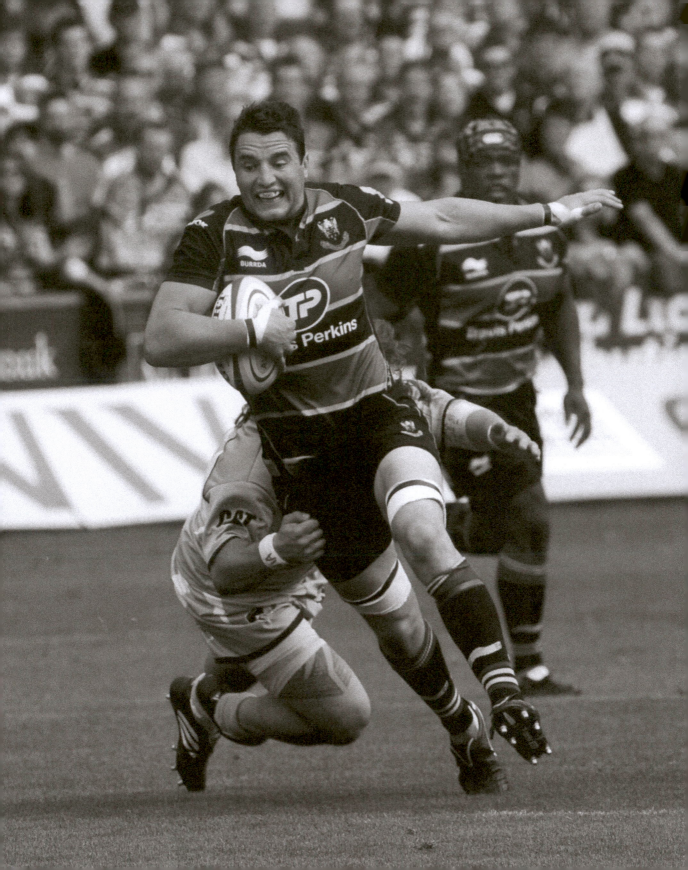

6 THE WORKING MUSCLE

On arrival at the muscle, the fuel is combusted with or without oxygen as the muscle converts chemical energy to mechanical energy. Before examining the working parts of the muscle, the various 'energy pathways' should be explained.

THE ENERGY PATHWAYS

The energy pathways are each designed to reform (or reconstitute) the compound adenosine triphosphate (ATP). It is the breaking down of this compound which provides energy for cell function. This breakdown may be expressed as an equation (figure 6.1), in full, or diagrammatically as the symbolic removal of P from ATP to produce ADP + P.

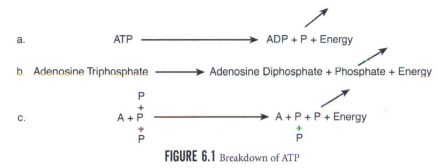

FIGURE 6.1 Breakdown of ATP

The production of this vital compound, which has been referred to as 'the energy currency of life', may be effected by one of three pathways – creatine phosphate anaerobic energy pathway (CrPEP), lactic anaerobic energy pathway (LAEP) and the aerobic energy pathway (AEP).

Creatine phosphate anaerobic energy pathway (also known as alactic anaerobic energy pathway)

In the muscle there is a store of a compound, creatine phosphate (CrP), which consists of creatine plus a large number of phosphates. If, after ATP is broken down to ADP, a phosphate was added to ADP, thereby reconstituting ATP, then the process of energy production could be continued. A store of phosphates would be required for this, and that is where CrP comes in. As ATP breaks down to ADP, a phosphate may be drawn from the CrP store to make ATP. This process may be continued until the CrP store is exhausted. The hydrolysis of CrP to resynthesise ATP is regulated by the enzyme creatine kynase.

$$ATP \rightarrow ADP + P + Energy$$
$$ADP + P^* \rightarrow ATP + Creatine$$

There is approximately three to four times the amount of CrP as ATP in the muscle. It permits athletes to work at high intensity for 10–15 seconds with little lactic acid production. Some 25–30 seconds recovery is required for resynthesis of approximately half of the CrP–ATP energy stores. These energy compounds in the muscle are sometimes known as phosphagen stores and this refers to CrP plus ATP. Short, intermittent bursts of activity, for example, in football, basketball, hockey, rugby, lacrosse, hurling, fencing, or sprints up to 200m on the track, will call upon this pathway. Training can develop CrPEP capacity to some extent. This would involve short intervals of maximum effort (5–10 seconds) with long rests (one minute).

Lactic anaerobic energy pathway

This energy pathway involves the breakdown of glycogen (glycolysis) in the absence of oxygen, with the resultant formation of ATP plus lactate (lactic acid and associated products). This pathway is therefore referred to as the lactic anaerobic energy pathway.

THE CHEMICAL REACTION MAY BE SUMMARISED AS FOLLOWS:

$$Glycogen + P + ADP \rightarrow ATP + Lactate$$
(1 Unit)   (3 Units)

The accumulation of lactate will terminate use of this energy pathway after 40–50 seconds maximum effort. Consequently it is the pathway called upon principally by athletes whose sports demand high energy expenditure for up to approximately 60 seconds, and those in 'multiple sprint sports' such as squash, ice hockey, rugby, lacrosse, hurling, sprint cycling, 400m track and 100m swim. Thereafter, there must be a progressive recruitment of an alternative energy pathway. It is known that exposure to lactic anaerobic stressors in training will increase the athlete's ability to utilise this pathway. It should be said that such training must be based on the sound foundation of training to develop the aerobic energy pathway.

Aerobic training produces cellular adaptations which increase the rate of lactate removal, so lactate accumulation impacts at a higher level of exercise intensity. For untrained, healthy people the threshold for commencement of lactic accumulation is around 55 per cent VO_2 max. A trained athlete can be as high as 75 per cent VO_2 max. Blood lactate threshold is also known as 'onset of blood lactate acid' (OBLA). The trained athlete can also tolerate 20–30 per cent higher blood lactate levels than the untrained athlete, partially due to a 20 per cent increase in activity of the glycolitic enzyme, phosphofructokinaise.

Aerobic energy pathway

This pathway involves the oxygen transporting system and the use of oxygen in the mitochondria of the working muscle for the oxidation of glycogen or fatty acids. Due to this pathway's dependence upon oxygen, it is referred to as the aerobic energy pathway. This is involved in prolonged work of relatively low intensity and is of increasing importance the longer the sport's duration. Taken to its logical conclusion, only lack of fuel (together with overheating and dehydration) will end an exercise of several hours' duration involving this pathway. The chemical reaction may be summarised as:

1 unit glycogen + P + ADP + O_2 = 37 units ATP + CO_2 + H_2O
1 unit free fatty acids + P + ADP + O_2 = 140* units ATP + CO_2 + H_2O
* *Approx.*

This pathway may be developed by specific training.

It will be seen from the 'rates of exchange' of free fatty acids and glycogen to ATP, that the free fatty acids appear the most favourable currency. However, about 8 per cent more oxygen per calorie is needed if the energy comes from fat sources. The very poor exchange rate of glycogen in lactic anaerobic exercise is only one factor contributing towards the phenomenon known as 'oxygen debt'.

THE BEST WAY OF EXPLAINING THIS IS TO ILLUSTRATE THE SITUATION WITH AN EXAMPLE:

- 22.4 litres of oxygen are required to remove 180g lactic acid
- 180g lactic acid from glycolysis yields 55kcal
- aerobic glycolysis yielding 55kcal requires 11.0 litres oxygen

Thus, if the lactic anaerobic pathway is used, 100 per cent interest must be paid on the debt. This is referred to, naturally, as the lactic oxygen debt. There also exists a CrP debt. The 'bill' here, looks like this:

refill of oxygen stores (blood, myoglobin)	= 1.0 litres oxygen
elevation of temperature and adrenaline concentration	= 1.0 litres oxygen
increased cardiac and respiratory involvement	= 0.5 litres oxygen
breakdown of ATP and CrP	= 1.5 litres oxygen
TOTAL	= 4.0 litres oxygen

So, in addition to the oxygen debt created by the lactic energy pathway, there is a CrP debt which must be repaid irrespective of the energy pathway used. Repayment of these debts will, of course, rely on an efficient system to aid recovery, which implies a well-developed oxygen transporting system. Consequently it is fundamental to athletes in all sports that the aerobic pathway is trained.

It would appear that the fuelling system for combustion in aerobic exercise varies according to its duration and intensity. In prolonged aerobic exercise the preferred fuel is free fatty acids because the glucose stores (glycogen) are limited compared to the very large fat stores. Unlike glycogen, fatty acids can only be used in the aerobic pathway, whereas in higher intensity exercise involving aerobic and anaerobic pathways, or exclusively anaerobic, the preferred fuel is glycogen.

The contribution of aerobic and anaerobic systems to energy output varies with the duration of the activity concerned. Astrand and Rodahl (1986) has represented this diagrammatically (figure 6.2). It must be emphasised, however, that it is not sound to deduce from these statistics that the ratio of training time should vary proportionately. The aerobic system is the fundamental basis of all endurance sports and there are few

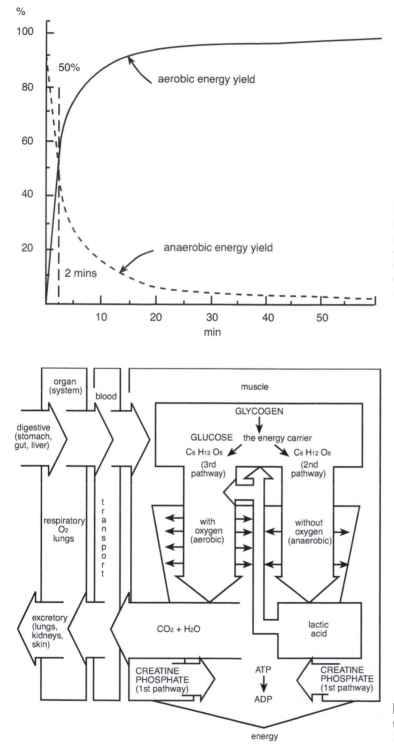

FIGURE 6.2 Astrand's classic representation of % of total energy yield from aerobic and anaerobic pathways, during maximal efforts of up to 60 min duration, for an athlete of high maximal power for both types of energy production (from Astrand and Rodahl, 1986).

FIGURE 6.3 Schematic summary of the three pathways (from Jäger and Oelschlägel, 1974)

sports which do not make demands of endurance capacity, even if only to ensure quicker recovery within and between training units. A sound aerobic basis will enable the athlete to be exposed to more frequent specific stressors as stimuli for specific adaptation.

The three energy pathways are summarised diagrammatically in figure 6.3, but before leaving this area, it might be useful to include a brief glossary of expressions often used concerning energy production.

Glycogenolysis: the conversion of glycogen to glucose, mainly in the liver, for use as a fuel.

Glycolysis: the oxidation of glucose or glycogen to pyruvate or lactate, the latter two substances being intermediate steps in energy production.

Glycogenesis: the synthesis of glycogen from glucose.

Gluconeogenesis: the formation of glucose or glycogen from noncarbohydrate sources (e.g. glycerol, glucogenic amino acids and lactate).

Tricarboxylic acid cycle: also referred to as citric acid cycle, or Krebs cycle, this is the final common pathway of carbohydrate, fats and protein oxidation to carbon dioxide and water.

Hexosemonophosphate shunt: an alternative system to the tricarboxylic acid cycle and is a side branch of glycolysis. Also known as the pentosephosphate cycle, it produces NADPH which provides reducing power and free energy during anabolic reactions.

Cori cycle: the release of lactate from muscle into the circulation for uptake by the liver and conversion to glucose. Consequently, it is central to the lactic–anaerobic energy pathway.

Alanine cycle: the release of alanine (and amino acid) from muscle into the circulation for uptake by the liver and conversion into glucose. It becomes important towards the limits of the aerobic-energy pathway in long-term, high intensity exercise – providing 15–20 per cent of the energy requirement.

Figure 6.4 gives a general picture of fuel production.

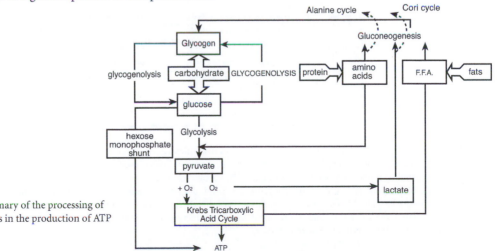

FIGURE 6.4 Summary of the processing of energy fuel sources in the production of ATP

THE MUSCLE

The breakdown of ATP to ADP supplies the energy that is required to cause the muscle to contract, or shorten. By shortening, the muscle pulls on the tendons which are attached to the bony levers. It now remains to explain the mechanisms involved in muscle contraction and in initiating ATP/ADP breakdown.

The muscle consists of many muscle fibres which, if examined under a light microscope, have a striped or striated appearance (figure 6.6c). To each muscle fibre is attached the endplate of a motoneuron.

The motoneuron is the nerve cell which finally controls skeletal muscle and the 'endplate' is its attachment to the muscle fibre. A motoneuron and the muscle fibres it supplies is called a motor unit. Occasionally a fibre may be supplied by more than one motoneuron, but as a rule only one motoneuron is involved.

Where very fine movement is required, there may be as few as five fibres to one neuron (e.g. the muscles of the eye). On the other hand, when gross movement is required, as in the thigh, the ratio may be one neuron to several thousand fibres. The motoneuron is housed in the anterior (ventral) part of the spinal cord and signals pass from here along a tendril-like arm, the axon, at the end of which are branches to which are attached the endplates (figure 6.6). These in turn are attached to a specific number of muscle fibres. The axon is for the most part surrounded by a myelin sheath, which is 'pinched' at intervals like a string of linked

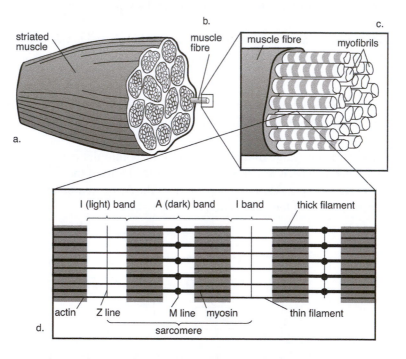

FIGURE 6.5 The striated muscle (a), is composed of muscle fibres (b), which appear striated (striped) under the light microscope. Each muscle fibre is made up of myofibrils (c), beside which lie cell nuclei and mitochondria. The striated appearance of the myofibril arises from the repeated light and dark bands. A single unit of this 'repetition' is a sarcomere (d). This consists of a Z line, an I band, an A band which is interrupted by a lighter zone (the H-band, which is devoid of action filaments), another I band – then the next Z line. In the centre of the H-band, M-lines cross the myofibril. These bands, in turn, arise from the overlapping of actin and myosin filaments (from Huxley, 1958). The sarcomere is the actual unit of contraction in the muscle fibre, which contains tens of thousands of both sarcomeres and mitochondria (for aerobic energy).

sausages (figure 6.6). The pinched areas are known as the *nodes of Ranvier* and due to their presence the nerve impulses can pass more quickly along myelinated axons than non-myelinated axons. It is believed that this is due to a saltatory conduction (jumping) of the impulse from node to node.

Each muscle fibre consists of bundles of myofibrils beside which lie the nuclei of the muscle cells and mitochondria. The striations noted in the fibre are, in fact, striations of the massed myofibrils. If a closer examination is made of the light and dark bands of the myofibril, the actual contractile mechanism is revealed (figure 6.5). The contractile unit, bound by the Z lines, is the sarcomere. As the actin filaments attached to opposing Z lines slide past the myosin filaments towards each other, the Z lines are drawn closer together. The sarcomeres of a single myofibril are joined end to end and all sarcomeres in that myofibril will contract at one time giving a total shortening of that myofibril. Moreover, the 'signal' to contract, which arrives via the axon and endplate at the muscle fibre, causes the whole fibre to contract. Thus, when the signal is sent, contraction of the fibre is brought about by the contraction of all its myofibrils, and the myofibrils contract as a result of the shortening of their sarcomeres.

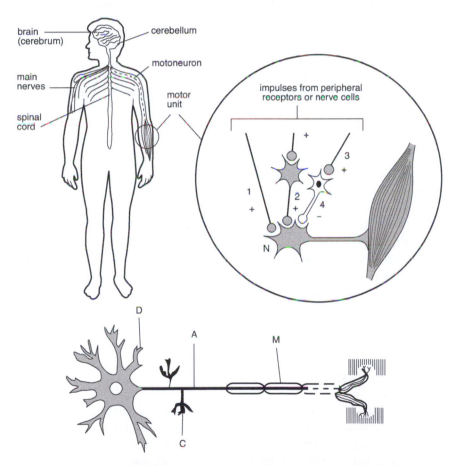

FIGURE 6.6 The motoneuron N, in the spinal cord can be excited (+) directly (1) or via an interneuron (2). Thus, an impulse is propagated in the nerve fibre, and the muscle is stimulated – causing muscular activity. Other nerve terminals can prevent the motoneuron from being stimulated. Schematically, nerve end (3) stimulates interneuron nerve cell (4), which is inhibitory. The lower diagram shows a motoneuron: A, axon; C, collateral; D, dendrite; M, myelin (from Schreiner and Schreiner, 1964).

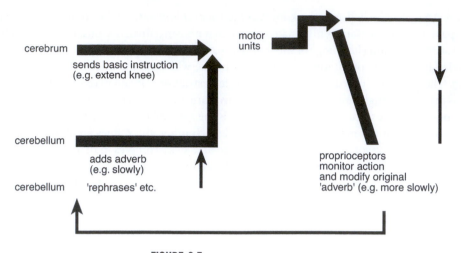

FIGURE 6.7 Control of muscular action

It should be pointed out that the 'all or none law' applies to muscle fibre contraction. When the signal to contract arrives at the endplate, the whole muscle fibre contracts to the limit of its capacity. On the other hand, when there is no signal the muscle fibre assumes its resting length. Thus, there are no gradations of contractile force at the muscle fibre level. Contractile force is graded by the selective involvement of an appropriate number of motor units. The selective involvement is controlled by the central nervous system. This system brings a directive from the cerebrum and this directive is modified or qualified by the proprioceptor mechanisms. Thus, recruitment of the appropriate number of selected motor units for a given task is learned and the muscle concerned is programmed to contract (figure 6.7).

When the impulse to contract arrives at the sarcolemma of the muscle fibre, it passes rapidly to every sarcomere. Within each sarcomere, running longitudinally, there exists a system of tubules known as the sarcoplasmic reticulum. The sarcoplasmic reticulum contains calcium ions and when the impulse arrives the calcium ions are released. This initiates an enzyme reaction with myosin, which causes the breakdown of ATP to ADP, thus releasing the energy to slide the actin and myosin past each other and bring about contraction of the myofibril. The calcium ions are returned to the sarcoplasmic reticulum by active pumping of its membranes. In the meantime, ADP is reconstituted to ATP via the CrP stores. Here then, among the small pockets of glycogen and scattered mitochondria, is the final product of that process which was started by eating and digesting a meal.

Types of muscular activity

Having gone into such detail in order to explain the mechanism of contraction, it should be said that the researcher rather than the coach is concerned with the microstructure of the muscle. It has become fashionable for the coach to consider the complex detail, described above, under the umbrella term 'the contractile component' of muscle. In popular terminology then, the contractile component is joined both in parallel and in series with 'the elastic component' (figure 6.8). That part of the elastic component in parallel comprises such elements as connective sheaths and structural proteins, while that part of the elastic component in series comprises the tendons. The elastic component can be stretched and consequently develop tension due

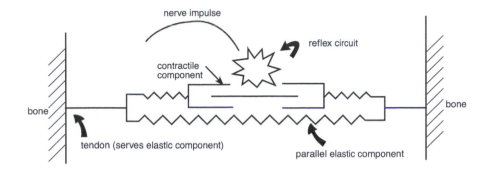

FIGURE 6.8 Schematic representation of the contractile and elastic components plus reflex mechanisms in muscle

to its elastic resistance to that stretch. This, in effect, is the second mechanism in the muscle's contribution to contractile force. It is effective in those activities which involve voluntary muscle contraction and elastic recoil (e.g. running jumps, hopping, rapid agilities).

There is one other mechanism which may add to the efficiency of the overall force expression of contractile and elastic components. This is the myotonic reflex.

Both muscle and tendon are equipped with reflex systems. Approximately 90 per cent of the tendon receptors are accommodated in the musculotendinous junction, while the remainder are in the tendon itself. The stimulus of stretch in this system effects the reflex response of inhibiting the contractile mechanism, thus allowing the muscle to lengthen and therefore relieving the degree of stretch in the tendon and musculotendinous junction. The muscle fibres are equipped with muscle spindle receptors. Their stimulus is the lengthening of the muscle fibre, the response being a stimulus to the muscle to contract, as elicited by the 'knee jerk' reflex.

It is reasonable to assume that in physical activity the reflex response to contract has an overall lower threshold than that to lengthen. The net result of this reflex activity is a more vigorous contraction of a given muscle when it is forcefully stretched (e.g. in the take-off leg in long jump). This 'net reflex' is the myotonic reflex and its existence now provides the athlete with a third contribution to a summated contractile force, although its activation can be harmful, e.g. in too vigorous, bouncy, dynamic stretching exercises (as opposed to safer slow stretch). Only when the technical model of an activity is appropriately structured can all three systems (contractile component, elastic component and myotonic reflex) be summated.

The speed of contraction of a muscle will vary inversely with the force opposing it. Thus maximal speed is achieved when the muscle has no force resisting its action and zero speed is achieved when the immovable object is encountered (figure 6.9). Maximum strength training is aimed at increasing the quantity of force required before zero speed is reached, while speed training is aimed at acquiring even higher speeds from existing maxima by assisting the movement via motivation, facilitation, learning, etc. If we consider the muscle actions of the athlete in figure 6.10 it is clear that some muscle actions will be dynamic (cause movement at joints) while others will be static (cause no movement at joints). In any given activity, there is a specific pattern of static and dynamic contraction carefully synchronised to meet the demands of that activity. The specific role of a given muscle within the total scheme of the specific pattern is referred to as *auxotonic*.

It should be noted that dynamic and static muscle activity may be subdivided into special classifications. *Dynamic* may be concentric, i.e. overcoming a resistance or load (e.g. quads shortening in raising a squat

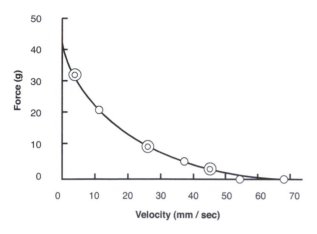

FIGURE 6.9 Force–velocity curve of tetanised muscle at 0°C. Abscissae: force (g wt). Ordinates: velocity (mm per sec). Small circles: experimental points. Large circles: points 'used up' in fitting the theoretical curve. Agreement between theory and experiment is significant only at other points on the curve (Wilkie, D.)

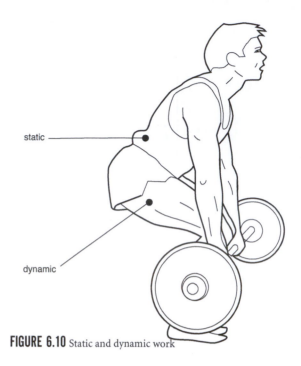

FIGURE 6.10 Static and dynamic work

bar); or eccentric, i.e. yielding to a resistance or load (e.g. quads lengthening in lowering a squat bar). *Static* may be maximum, i.e. meeting an immovable object; or sub-maximum, i.e. the role of the postural muscles in holding the spine in position when standing.

In any activity where muscular contraction arrests eccentric contraction prior to concentric contraction (e.g. when muscle contraction stops you yielding to a load before it will allow you to overcome it), the point at which the eccentric movement stops is known as the point of *amortisation* of muscle. In many technical textbooks the phase during which a limb is being forced to yield prior to this point is referred to as the amortisation phase. Examples of this are in the take-off leg in long jump, in the arms in various agilities in gymnastics, etc. The duration of time in the amortisation phase, and at the point of amortisation, is critical to the efficient contribution of combined force from both contractile and elastic components. It must be emphasised that the eccentric action is *dynamic* in the amortisation phase. If it is passive, then kinetic energy, which has been derived from an approach run or preparatory movement, will be absorbed and the only force available for the ensuing movement will be from the contractile component alone. This is seen when a trampolinist 'kills' the recoil of a trampoline, when a skier 'damps' the undulations of the ski slope and when the testee in the jump-reach test is not permitted a preliminary movement. This whole area should be clearly understood if the coach is to develop specific training exercises for sports demanding this type of muscle activity.

Types of muscle fibre

The study of the muscle's contractile properties usually examines the muscle not only longitudinally, but also through a transverse section. By using muscle biopsy techniques and applying histochemical staining, three categories of human muscle can be identified, based on stain shading – from dark to light with an intermediate shade, depending on the fibre's concentrations of different types or isoforms of myosin ATPase:

- **Slow-twitch (type I)** fibres stain dark.
- **Fast-twitch (type IIb, also now called type IIx):** fibres remain light in colour.
- **Fast-twitch (type IIa)** fibres fall between the light and dark shade.

The size theory of motor unit recruitment states that type I are recruited first before the smaller IIb or IIa.

Yet another classification is differentiating between fusiform and pinnate fibres. Fusiform are arranged in parallel along the longitudinal axis of the muscle. Pinnate fibres are arranged at angles and are shorter and offer great force producing capabilities over shorter ranges.

Putting all this together suggests that the muscle 'architecture' involved in a given movement will change the force development pattern during shortening or lengthening as movement occurs. This will be visited again in chapter 14.

The implication of fibre differentiation is shown in the many studies of muscle fibre population in various groups of athletes (e.g. see Dahl and Rinvik, 1999). Golnick's (1973) classic study illustrates this, showing that specific enzyme activity is involved in speed training (PFK: Phosphofructokinase) and endurance training (SDH: Succincdehydrogenase) and that the percentage of slow-twitch fibres is related to endurance demand (table 6.1).

	Type I	Type IIa	Type IIb/IIx
Biochemistry	SO	FOG	FG
Oxidative capacity	High	Medium/high	Low
Calcium capacity	Low	Medium / High	Low
Glycolytic capacity	Low	High	High
Myosin ATPase	Low	High	High
Colour	Red	Pink	White
Contractility	Slow twitch	Fast twitch	Fast twitch
Relaxation	Slow	Fast	Fast
Fibre structure			
Capillaries/mm²	High	Medium	Low
Fibre diameter	Small	Medium	Large
Mitochondrial volume	High	Medium	Low
Function	S	FR	FF
Fatigue resistance	Low	Medium/High	High
Force potential	Low	Medium	High

Key: SO = slow, oxidative; FOG = fast, oxidative, glycolytic; FG = fast, glycolytic; S = slow contracting; FR = fast contracting, fatigue resistent; FF = fast contracting, fast fatiguing

TABLE 6.1 Summary of properties of muscle fibre types

Athlete	(Aerobic) (slow) units of succinate dehydrogenase	% slow-twitch fibres	(Anaerobic) (fast) units of phospho fructokinase
Long-distance runner	8.03	75	15.07
Middle-distance runner	5.14	65	26.53
Sprinter	3.95	26	28.34

TABLE 6.2 Relationship of event to percentage slow-twitch fibres and enzyme concentration (adapted from Golnick, 1973)

It is very clear, even from our limited understanding of neuromuscular function, that specific training will make many areas of this complex system more efficient. Greater force of muscle contraction can be developed, sophisticated recruitment of motor units may be learned, and energy systems may be trained to meet the specific demands of sports activities.

EPIGENETICS

Yet we remain in the dark as to the reason why the effect of a training stimulus while working for one athlete may not work for another. Our DNA (deoxyribonucleic acid) is a molecule that provides the genetic instructions needed for the development of an organism. DNA molecules exist alongside each other as long strands which form a 'double helix' within the cells. Portions of the DNA molecules provide 'codes' that determine the function of cells, and these are often referred to as a gene. These genes are inherited, but can be activated by the cell's internal environment, or changed by the sequence in which the DNA molecules lie (known as the genotype). In recent years, the study of epigenetics has investigated the way in which the genotype can be changed by external factors, (and not – as in genetics – by inherited factors). For example, exposure to a particular type of training, or a changed nutritional regimen, may 'switch on' a particular gene, causing an adaptation or change within the cell and muscle. Conversely, there may be no change, and as a result certain individuals may be 'non-responders' to a particular type of training or diet. Scientists studying epigenetics are examining whether genetic markers' can be used to identify individuals who may – or may not – respond to specific types of training, which would give a greater insight into the potential for the long term development of an athlete in a particular sport.

SUMMARY

The three energy pathways are: creatine phosphate anaerobic energy pathway; lactic aerobic energy pathway; and aerobic energy pathway.

Extent, intensity and duration of exercise variously dictate which pathway or pathways are involved. Consequently this shapes decision making in training programmes to prepare athletes for the energy demands of their sport. Muscle activity may involve reflex mechanisms and elastic component in addition to the contractile component according to the specifics of technical models.

Muscle is composed of three types of fibre: type I (slow, oxidative); type IIa (fast, oxidative, glycolytic); type IIb/IIx (fast, glycolytic). These characteristics are relevant to endurance and speed in competitive sport and within the muscle architecture of a given movement. Muscles may have a dynamic (concentric or eccentric) role or a static (postural operating maximally or submaximally) role and should be developed for their role within that architecture.

A training stimulus may produce intended training effect in one athlete but not in another. The study of epigenetics may afford clearer guidance in fitting training stimuli more accurately to the specifics of a given athlete's training response.

REFLECTIVE QUESTIONS

1. Why can the fibre type of a muscle influence muscle energy metabolism?

2. Athletes with spinal cord injury can receive artificial electric stimulation to their paralysed muscles and, when used in training, experience muscle hypertrophy. Apart from the aesthetic implications, what other benefits may derive from increasing the muscle mass of their lower limbs and what are some possible problems that may arise?

3. What are the changes in muscle fibre type proportions that can be expected for either endurance or muscular power? Discuss advantages and disadvantages of designing training programmes with this in mind.

4. Explain why muscle pH affects the recovery of creatine phosphate (CrP). Why might an increase in aerobic endurance training improve the rate of recovery?

5. Some sports physiologists believe that measuring VO_2 max is not as suitable for equating exercise intensities and metabolic responses to exercise between individual athletes as is OBLA. Discuss the basis of that opinion; and your view on which is better (and why).

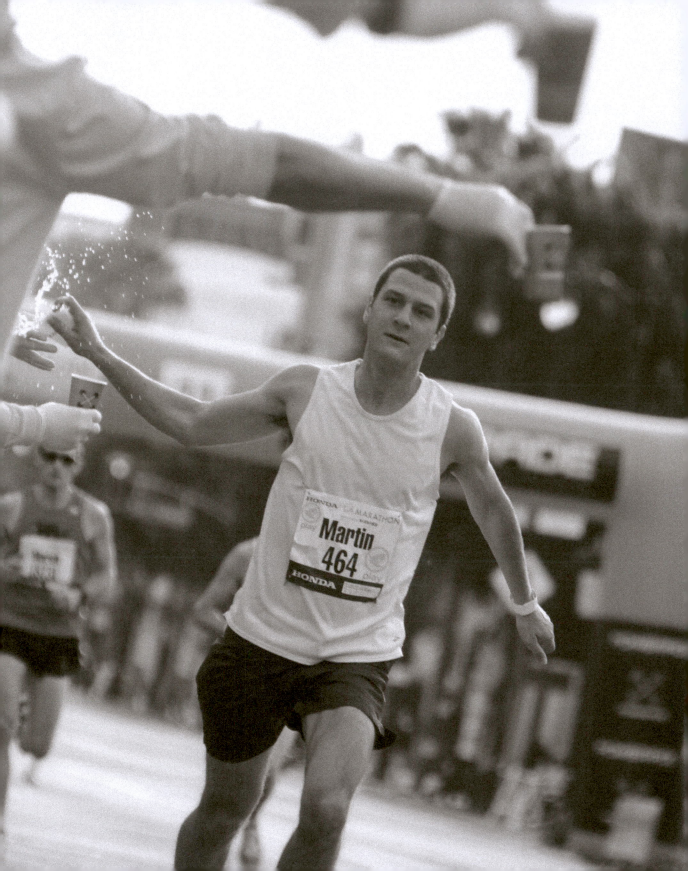

7 THE FLUID SYSTEMS

HOMEOSTASIS

The body is composed of tissues and the tissues are composed of cells. Each cell has fluid in it (intracellular) and outside it (extracellular, mainly interstitial – in between cells). Provided the various concentrations of substances in the extracellular fluid are controlled, the cells will continue to function efficiently. However, stressors bombard the body and threaten the integrity of the cell–organ–fluid cycle within it. 'Stress' is embarrassment of this cycle, evidenced by greater urgency of activity within the cycle. It is therefore essential that the body maintains a certain constancy of its internal environment to ensure that the composition of extracellular fluid is not threatened. This process is called *homeostasis*. The functions of all organs in the body, with the exception of the reproductive organs, are directed towards the goal of homeostasis. Should the various tissues which comprise each organ fail in their highly specialised contribution towards homeostasis, the cells bathing in the extracellular fluid will be damaged and reduce the organic functioning capacity. The situation may be summarised as follows:

- Total body function relies on the efficient functioning of the organs.
- The organs' function relies on the efficient functioning of their tissue cells.
- The cells' function relies on the constancy of the composition of the extracellular fluid.
- The extracellular fluid is given constancy (homeostasis) by the efficient functioning of the organs.

Figure 7.1 illustrates the total fluid in the body, as well as indicating its relationship to blood composition and volume.

Water, through specific bodily fluids, serves several functions:

- It provides the body's transport and reactive medium.
- It is the vehicle for transporting nutrients, gases and for eliminating waste in urine and faeces.
- Because of its heat stabilising qualities, it absorbs substantial levels of heat with minimal temperature change.
- Gaseous diffusion only takes place across moistened surfaces.
- It affords structure and form to the body.

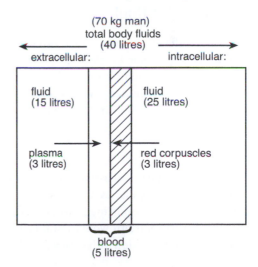

FIGURE 7.1 Distribution of body fluids

SPECIFIC FLUIDS: COMPOSITION AND FUNCTION
Blood

This has already been discussed in some detail (see chapter 5). Approximately 90 per cent of the blood is fluid – most intracellular (e.g. within the blood cells), some extracellular (e.g. the plasma). The latter has a higher amino acid concentration than other extracellular fluid, especially albumin, which is an important factor in keeping plasma inside the capillary blood vessels.

Interstitial fluid

This is that portion of the extracellular fluid outside the blood vessels (e.g. total extracellular fluid, excluding plasma). This fluid includes that in which the cerebrum and spinal cord bathes (cerebrospinal fluid), the fluid in the abdominal cavity, the joint capsules (synovial fluid), the pleural envelope about the lungs, and in the eyes.

Intracellular fluid

This is the fluid inside each cell containing many chemicals and electrolytes responsible for functional efficiency of the cell. Various mechanisms are 'built into' the cell membrane. The mechanisms allow movement of sodium *out* of the cell and potassium and phosphates *into* the cell. Also found in this fluid are glucose, oxygen, carbon dioxide, amino acids and lipids. From previous discussion (see chapter 5), it will be recalled that fuel is combusted with or without oxygen to provide energy for cellular function, leaving substances such as carbon dioxide and lactate which pass through the cell membrane with the assistance of one of the membrane mechanisms already mentioned. These products are then carried in the intra or extracellular fluids of the blood, to be 'blown-off ' or oxidised as the case may be. Oxygen travels the reverse route.

Extracellular fluid

This fluid differs from intracellular principally in its electrolyte concentration. These differences of concentration are responsible for electrical potentials across the membrane of the cell. If these electrical potentials did not exist, it would be impossible for nerve fibres to conduct impulses or for muscle to contract. In addition, the extracellular fluid provides a system for the transport of nutrients and other substances. It may help to recall that plasma and lymph are both extracellular fluids.

Lymph

This has already been discussed with reference to the white cells' role in the body's immune system. The walls of the lymphatic capillaries are freely permeable to protein and approximately 95 per cent of protein, lost from the oxygen transporting system each day, is returned via the lymphatic vessels. If these plasma proteins were not returned, death would result in 12–24 hours. Consequently it has been suggested that the single most important function of lymph is its role in returning plasma protein to circulation.

Acid-base balance and pH

Maintaining the acid-base balance of the body's fluids is critical to homeostasis and ensures the optimal metabolic functioning and general regulation of the body's physiology.

Acids ionise in solution, releasing hydrogen ions (H^+). Examples in the body include carboxylic acid, citric acid, and phosphoric acid.

Bases (alkalis) accept H^+ to form hydroxide ions (OH^-) in aqueous solutions. Examples in the body include sodium and calcium hydroxide.

The pH refers to the concentration of H^+. Solutions with relatively more OH^- than H^+ have a pH above 7.0 and are referred to as basic or alkaline. Solutions with more H^+ than OH^- have a pH below 7.0 and are referred to as acidic. Distilled water has a pH of 7.0, so $H^+ = OH^-$. Figure 7.2 is a picture of the pH scale from 0–14, with examples.

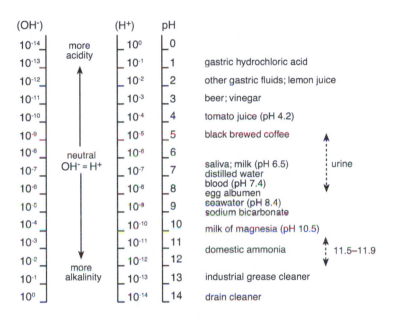

FIGURE 7.2 Examples of pH values

Very narrow pH ranges are highly specific to given body fluids. Extreme changes in pH produce irreversible damage to enzymes.

Buffers are chemical and physiologic mechanisms which prevent changes of H^+. There are three buffering mechanisms:

- Chemical buffers – for example, carbolic acid and sodium bicarbonate.
- Ventilatory buffer – the respiratory centre increases breathing rate in response to an increase in H^+ in body fluids.
- Renal buffer – the kidneys continually excrete H+ to maintain acid-base status of body fluids.

In prolonged high intensity exercise, large amounts of lactate enters the blood from active muscle. At exhaustion, blood pH can approach 6.8. Only after conclusion of exercise does blood pH stabilise and return to 7.4.

Fluid accumulation

Occasionally fluid collects at certain sites in the body. A fluid collection is known as an *oedema*. If this occurs in a potential space (e.g. joint space) it is known as an *effusion*. Several things may cause this. For example, infection can cause a blockage of the lymphatics (drainage system) in a potential space, through the accumulation of dead white cells. Trauma caused by a knock or strain may also cause an effusion, which may be reduced by applying ice packs or cold water to the affected region. Again, hormonal factors can elicit fluid retention. For example, the female hormone oestradiol triggers retention of fluid. Fluctuation in bodyweight in the course of the female menstrual cycle is mainly attributable to ebb and flow of the body's fluid volume.

Oedema, effusion, or fluid retention, may lead to discomfort, for example swollen joints, and possible influence on relative strength, as well as reduction of functioning capacity. The phenomenon may even constitute a serious health threat if it exerts pressure on blood vessels. Consequently, medical advice should be sought to discover the cause.

Fluid loss

The kidneys, in addition to filtering approximately 1700 litres of blood in 24 hours and rejecting the blood's waste products in soluble form in the urine, are the key agents in controlling expulsion or retention of body fluid. In other words, they are the principal regulators of the body's fluid volume and concentration. If the body's salt-water balance is disrupted, water must be retained in the body or a greater concentration of salts must be expelled (or both) to restore equilibrium. This imbalance can be caused by internal or external conditions, for example, the high sweat rate required to cool the body by evaporation in a hot environment or through persistent exposure to air conditions or the considerable loss of fluid via sweat, urine, 'running nose', etc., which accompany upper respiratory tract infections such as the common cold. Since a greater proportion of water than salts and electrolytes is lost in the first instance, intracellular and extracellular fluid concentration, and ultimately blood concentration, increases. The consequent increased osmotic pressure causes (**1**) release of anti-diuretic hormone (ADH) from the posterior pituitary which *increases reabsorption of water* by the tubules of the kidney, and (**2**) withdrawal from circulation of the hormone aldosterone which is secreted by the cortex of the suprarenal gland and this *decreases absorption of salt* by the tubules of the kidney (figure 7.3).

When there is excessive water intake, ADH levels are lowered, another hormone angiotensin is formed locally, and aldosterone levels are raised thus diluting and increasing the volume of urine expelled. When body fluids are being reduced, it is self-evident that athletes must increase fluid intake to replace what has been lost and to relieve the body of the increased burden on its regulatory mechanisms (see also 'Water', page 74). Moreover, where periods of sweating are prolonged, not only must fluids be replaced but also electrolytes and salts. Fortunately there are several electrolyte solutions commercially available to the athlete (see chapter 4).

The athlete should be aware of those substances which will increase fluid loss and therefore reduce his ability to combat the stressor of heat. These substances include xanthines such as coffee (caffeine) and tea (theophylline), excess sucrose, alcohol, and drugs involving mercurial compounds, chlorothiazide, Diamox, etc. Certain antibiotics are actively excreted by the tubules of the kidney, and athletes are normally advised to

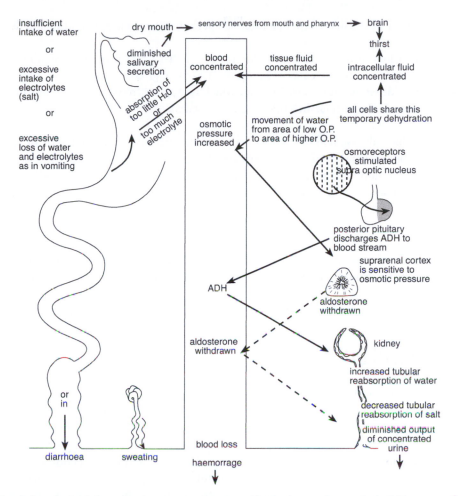

FIGURE 7.3 Regulation of water balance showing measures that restore blood volume and restore body fluids to normal osmotic pressure (from MacKenna and Callender, 1998)

increase fluid intake when taking them. Air-conditioned residential, working and exercising environments, and in air travel can have a profound dehydrating effect.

Intentional dehydration has been attempted by athletes to reduce bodyweight and therefore increase relative strength. This practice is fraught with dangers, not least of which is the impairment of function due to electrolyte imbalance. If weight must be reduced for some reason, then medical advice must be taken. Of course 'dieting' has been pursued, often very successfully, with the view to reducing weight while maintaining or even increasing normal body function. The following observations on the subject should be noted.

1. Dehydration techniques, using diuretic drugs, are most certainly not recommended for athletes.

2. Dehydration techniques, via reduction in fluid intake, may only be considered valid if under medical supervision and then only for short periods.

3. 'Slimming diets' must be considered over an extended period, rather than for rapid weight decrease.

4. Initial rapid weight loss in dieting is largely due to loss of that water previously required to store the glycogen now liberated to provide energy (3g water for each 1g glycogen). When the stored glycogen is called upon to provide energy, it releases its water which is expelled from the body. Unfortunately, when the 'slimmer' returns to the normal diet, this weight is replaced.

5. Any diet *must* include all essential nutrients to support the high metabolic demands of the athlete or the relevant metabolic demands of the non-athlete. While an increase in protein intake will increase metabolic rate (to the slimmer's advantage), and a reduction in carbohydrate intake will certainly affect weight loss, it would be fundamentally wrong to avoid carbohydrate completely since muscle and nerve cells rely on carbohydrate for their metabolism. A return to a balanced diet, but scaled down, is the moral of the story.

6. Some athletes, such as crew members in sailing, of course, wish to increase weight. The ingestion of certain approved drugs can do this, but it is mainly through fluid retention. This cannot be considered a healthy practice, nor should it be recommended for athletes. In the medium term, weight gain may be better pursued by digesting more calories. In the longer term, muscle may be increased.

TEMPERATURE REGULATION

Average body temperature is 37°c (rectal) and 38.6°c (oral) it fluctuates over a 24-hour cycle and changes if hungry, sleepy, in a cold/hot environment or when physically active or stressed. The athlete's problem is maintaining body temperature within the limits which permit him to function efficiently, which is at a body temperature of 37.5–38.5°C. In certain conditions the problem is to avoid overheating (hyperthermia). This can be avoided by the loss of body heat to the external environment and the reduction of heat gain from that environment. This will occur when training or competition takes place in a very hot/dry or hot/humid climate. On the other hand, the problem may lie at the other extreme where the athlete must avoid losing body temperature to the external environment and insulate against the low temperature of that environment. This will occur when, for example, sailors are exposed to dampness and extremely low temperatures for long periods of time. This may lead to the condition of exposure or hypothermia.

The balance between heat production and heat loss will be maintained when the sum of the factors to the left of figure 7.4 equals the sum of factors to the right.

Heat production	Heat loss
1. Basal metabolism	5. Radiation
2. Muscular activity (including shivering	6. Convection and conduction
3. Effect of body temperature on cells	7. Evaporation (convection)
4. Hormonal effect on cells (thyroxine and adrenaline)	8. Respiration, micturition and defecation

FIGURE 7.4 Factors contributing to the balance between heat production and loss at rest

1. Basal metabolism

The metabolic rate is the measure of the rate at which energy is released from foods. It is therefore the rate of heat production by the body, which is measured in kilocalories. Basal metabolic rate is this measurement when the athlete is at his most rested state, i.e. without temperature stressors, etc. It is determined by the inherent rates of chemical reactions in the cell and the amount of thyroid hormone activity in the cells. The basal metabolic rate is generally expressed in terms of kilocalories per square metre body surface per hour. Several factors influence metabolic rate, which is most closely related to the surface area of the skin:

- The basal metabolism of children is greater than that of adults because they are growing as well as coping with day to day lifestyle.
- Fasting or starvation would appear to decelerate metabolic rate. It has even been suggested that by reducing metabolic rate in this way the ageing process will be slowed down.
- Protein causes a greater increase in metabolic rate than fats or carbohydrate. On comparing diets of equal calorific value, protein can raise the metabolic rate by 20 per cent over a period of 4–6 hours, while carbohydrate and fats will affect only 5–10 per cent increase.

2. Muscular activity

Heat production of muscles accounts for 40 per cent of all the body's heat production, even at rest. During severe exercise this can rise to as much as 20 times that provided by all the other tissues put together. This is due to the oxidation of foodstuffs to meet the fuel demands necessary for ATP/ADP breakdown. The metabolic rate, in work of only a few seconds duration, may be over 40 times greater than at rest. Because babies and young children have less tolerance to increases and decreases of temperature, it is essential that they are not exposed to such.

3. Effect of body temperature on cells

The immediate effect of exposure to high temperature is to increase heat loss via sweating, etc. Metabolism is not greatly affected. If continued exposure elevates body temperature, basal metabolism increases by 7 per cent for every 0.5°C. This would have the net result of further increasing temperature. The immediate effect of exposure to low temperature is an increase in metabolic rate, and shivering further increases heat production. It has been suggested that the metabolic rate can be doubled with the involvement of shivering and that metabolic changes occurring in cold exposure may be hormonally influenced. It is possible to acclimatise both to cold and heat. Should exposure to extremes of temperature continue at a rate incompatible with adaptation to the specific stressor, and without the benefits of acclimatisation, there is a very real risk of hyperthermia or hypothermia.

4. Hormones

Thyroxine increases the rate of functioning of cell enzymes, thus increasing metabolic rate and heat production. This increase in metabolic rate may also be elicited by adrenaline and noradrenaline. The anterior pituitary gland also influences the metabolic rate indirectly via the thyrotrophic hormone which stimulates the thyroid gland.

5. Radiation

Radiation is the transfer of heat from one object to another with which it is *not in contact*. Normally, the athlete radiates more heat towards objects cooler than himself, and vice versa. The closer the two temperatures, the less will be the athlete's heat loss. Frequently, athletes express concern that heat is coming from artificial playing areas on which they are training or competing. In many cases this is not really true; in fact the athlete cannot lose all the heat he wishes to that particular playing area. Often, women athletes lose more heat than men by radiation.

6. Convection and conduction

Heat may also be lost to air and objects with which the body has contact. The cooler the air or object, the greater the heat loss. If air is continually moving past the body, warmed air (from the body's heat) is moved away to be replaced by 'unwarmed' air. The more rapidly the air moves the greater is the quantity of heat conducted from the body. Thus, there exists a combined conduction/convection heat loss due to passage of air over the body surface. Where there is a cool wind and body temperature is to be maintained, athletes should be sheltered or wear wet suits (waterproof over-suit). In water, heat is lost directly by conduction.

7. Evaporation (convection)

In addition to the small amount of extracellular fluid which continually diffuses through the skin and evaporates, the sweat glands produce large quantities of sweat when the body becomes very hot – up to two litres per hour. This process obviously increases the rate of heat loss through evaporation. As in conduction, air currents play a major role in the removal of heat by evaporation. As the air close to the body becomes saturated, new air arrives to accept the evaporating sweat. Should the air fail to be replaced, then conduction and evaporation avenues of heat loss will be reduced. The situation is more alarming when air is humid because the sweat will not evaporate. Williams (1975) says:

'In hot, dry environments, the limiting factor for heat dissipation is the rate of sweat production, whereas in hot, humid environments it is the capacity of the environment to receive water vapour, i.e. the relative humidity. In the shade outdoors the athlete will therefore be cooler than in the shade indoors, provided the air is moving. On the other hand, when temperature loss is to be avoided, the athlete should keep out of the wind and keep the body surface dry.'

Men tend to sweat at higher proportionate rates than women.

8. Respiration and expulsion of wastes

Approximately 3 per cent of heat lost at 21°C is via these avenues.

CLOTHING AND TEMPERATURE REGULATION

Clothing should be considered in light of the foregoing discussion. In a hot environment, wicking materials are preferred. These draw sweat away from the skin through capillary action and because the materials are non-absorbent, the moisture has more surface area and evaporates faster. Sportswear manufacturers have developed a range of synthetic materials for this purpose. It should also be mentioned that where competition is to be held in hot/dry or hot/humid environments, dry kit should not replace sweat-soaked kit. Fleeced wet suits are recommended where the competition environment is cold and, where appropriate, these should be worn between rounds of competitions and during warm-up. In field games and/or winter sports, thought should be given to maintaining a comfortable temperature for continued efficient activity. Above all, both skin and kit must be kept as dry as the occasion permits.

Maintaining body temperature should not be confused with the problems of exposure to strong sunlight. In the latter case, athletes should be as conscious of the need to shelter from the weakening effects of the sun as they are to maintain a body temperature compatible with efficient physical activity. When competing or training or generally being exposed to sunlight, a high UVA factor suncream or screen should be used.

Acclimatisation to temperature

The body can adapt to the stressors of dry and wet heat. The stressor of high temperature causes a decrease in endurance capacity. Should athletes be required to compete in such conditions they must therefore be exposed to a stimulus for adaptation if performance capacity is to be maintained. The adaptation to external environments, such as altitude, time shift, heat, etc., is known as acclimatisation. Buskirk and Bass (1974) have enumerated the practical aspects of acclimatisation to heat:

1. Acclimatisation begins with the first exposure, progresses rapidly, and is well developed in 4–7 days.

2. Acclimatisation can be introduced by short, intermittent exercise periods in the heat, e.g. 2–4 hours daily. Inactivity in the heat results in only slight acclimatisation.

3. Subjects in good physical condition acclimatise more rapidly and are capable of more work in the heat. However, good physical fitness alone does not automatically confer acclimatisation.

4. The ability to perform 'maximal' work in the heat is attained more quickly by progressively increasing the daily workload. Strenuous exertion on first exposure may result in disability which will impair performance for several days. Care should be taken to stay within the capacity of the athlete until acclimatisation is well advanced.

5. Acclimatisation to severe conditions will facilitate performance at lesser conditions.

6. The general pattern of acclimatisation is the same for short, severe exertion as for moderate work of longer duration.

7. Acclimatisation in hot/dry climates increases performance ability in hot/wet climates and vice versa.

8. Inadequate water and salt replacement can retard the acclimatisation process.

9. Acclimatisation to heat is well retained during periods of non-exposure for about two weeks; thereafter it is lost, at a rate that varies among individuals. Most people lose a portion of their acclimatisation in two months. Those who stay in good physical condition retain their acclimatisation best of all.

10. If it is desirable to retain acclimatisation, periodic exposures at frequent intervals are recommended and heat exposures should not be separated by more than two weeks.

It is advisable to plan acclimatisation programmes in the months before an event which requires such. Often such events also require time change and it does not make sense to be adjusting the body clock and trying to acclimatise at the same time. This represents an unnecessary drain on energy reserves.

Acclimatisation to cold is rather more difficult to study than acclimatisation to heat. This is because man normally protects himself against cold by creating his own miniature subtropical climate with increased and insulated clothing, heated accommodation, etc. 'Local acclimatisation' is known to be possible. For example, when the hands are exposed to cold for short periods over a number of weeks there is an increased blood flow through the hands, enabling them to perform their normal functions without impairment due to cold-induced numbness. While heat will be lost from the body due to local acclimatisation, at least the athlete's functioning capacity will be maintained. This type of acclimatisation is invaluable to sailors, climbers and athletes involved in outdoor winter games or games played in a cold environment. Having said this, the athlete may simply learn how to avoid becoming extremely cold through experience or advice from the technical authorities concerned in the given sport.

Warm-up

Unfortunately there is an astonishing lack of consistency in research conclusions on the physiological value of warm-up. Possible advantages might include:

- increased local muscle blood flow
- increased metabolic rate (7% for 0.5°C increase)
- increased speed of oxygen and fuel transfer to tissues
- increased speed of nerve impulse conduction
- increased speed of contraction and relaxation of muscle
- decreased viscous resistance in the muscle.

Perhaps most of the advantage derived from warm-up is psychological, due to the blend of ritual rehearsal and psycho-physiological preparation unique to each athlete. Even if this is the only advantage of warm-up, it seems ample justification for its inclusion. Pending more conclusive support for the value of warm-up, athletes should be encouraged to pursue the preparation which coach and athlete know to be relevant to the forthcoming competition or training unit. So it should be specific, not general and leave the athlete ready for what is to follow – physically, mentally and emotionally. A warm-up should not elevate body temperature above 38.5°C.

Although referred to as a warm-up, in preparation for a training unit, the content may be designed to serve as a training unit itself and focus on ensuring all joint actions are systematically exercised. Any subsequent training unit might only focus on joint actions specific to a technique or sport.

At the conclusion of a competition or training unit, athletes are frequently encouraged to 'warm down'. This normally involves light but continuous activity, where the heart rate is in the range of 120–140/minute. In pursuit of recovery from exercise-induced stress, the object is principally to raise the metabolic rate and encourage the removal of waste products from muscle through maintaining an increased rate of local blood flow. It is also a valuable period for early reflection on lessons learned from the foregoing competition or training unit.

SUMMARY

The body's fluid systems comprise blood, interstitial fluid, intracellular fluid, and lymph. Together, they serve two vital purposes. The first is to offer a medium for the transportation about the body of substances essential to normal function. To meet this, a relative stability of fluid volume and concentration must be maintained and this is primarily achieved by a balance between the kidneys and the thirst mechanism. High temperatures, infection and certain dietary inclusions are examples of threats to such stability. The second purpose is temperature control, which is seen as the balance of heat production and loss. A relative stability of body temperature is critical to physical performance. The athlete uses warm-up to attain a state of readiness and an optimal temperature for physical performance, using the capacity to adapt to the stressors of dry and wet heat to prepare for competition in climates where such stressors will be evident.

REFLECTIVE QUESTIONS

1. How should an athlete dress to play 90 minutes of outdoor tennis at $-7°C$?

2. An athlete has entered an eight hour race in the desert (at sea level $46.1°C$; 20% relative humidity) while carrying only a lightweight backpack. What do you advise he wears and what items should he take (and why) in the backpack?

3. Your soccer team is scheduled for a tournament in Singapore in what is early spring at home. Discuss how you would prepare the team for this hot, humid environment:
   a. If all preparations must be done at home.
   b. If time, money and travel are not considerations.

4. List drinks you would recommend and those you would advise against where your athletes are exposed to dehydration via air conditioning and high temperature and humidity. Give a physiological explanation for each drink you recommend or advise against.

5. The hormonal changes which regulate the menstrual cycle influence fluid retention. What relevance does this have, if any, in answering the following questions?
   a. Why do normally menstruating women catabolise more lipid at a given sub maximal exercise intensity?
   b. What are the possible bodyweight implications at different phases of the cycle?
   c. Are there differences of tolerance in thermoregulation at different phases of the cycle? If so, why?

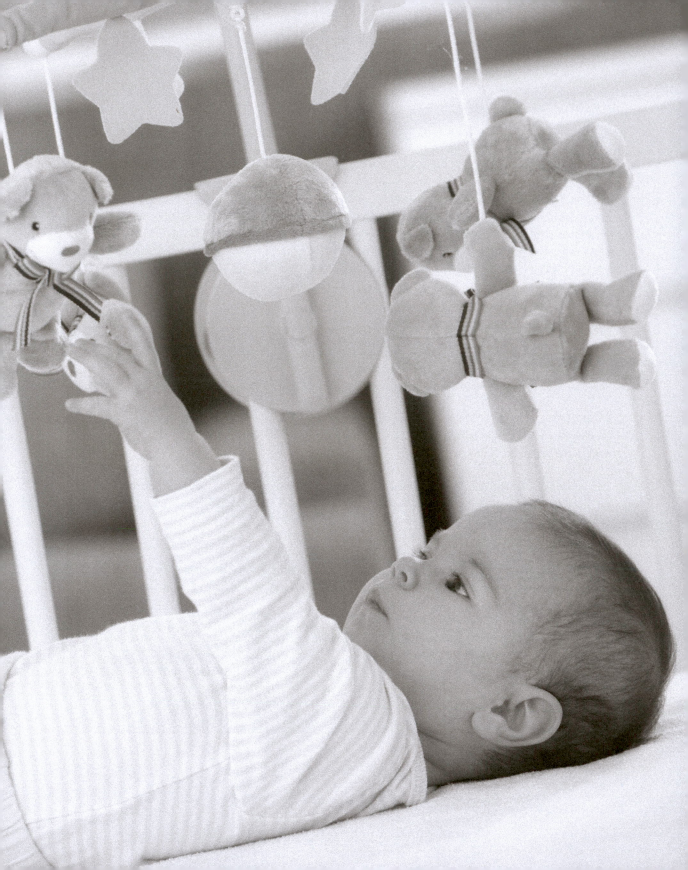

8 THE HORMONES

Hormones are highly specific chemical compounds produced in the specialised cells of the endocrine glands. Unlike, for example, the lymph system, these glands have no ducts and tubes and their secretions are transported normally in the blood. The hormones may exert both generalised and specialised effects on other tissues and organs – functions implied by the word endocrine (*endo*: within; *krinen*: to separate).

Hormones may be divided into two groups – local and general. All general hormones and the most important local hormones are reviewed here. Some general hormones affect all cells, for example growth hormone secreted by the pituitary, and thyroxine secreted by the thyroid. Other general hormones affect specific cells, for example gonadotrophic hormones secreted by the pituitary affect the sex organs. These substances perform a global function of regulation within the context of homeostasis via the fluid systems.

LOCAL HORMONES

Local hormones affect cells in the immediate vicinity of the organ which is secreting the hormone.

Acetylcholine: acts locally to promote rhythmic activity in smooth muscle (which has no nerve supply), in heart muscle, and in certain epithelial tissue (e.g. oesophagus and trachea). However, this hormone is probably best known in another capacity: acetylcholine occurs in the motor nerves which run from the spinal cord to skeletal muscles. It is the 'transmitter' substance of the skeletal system. Synthesis of acetylcholine occurs in the cytoplasm of the nerve-muscle junction, but is quickly stored in about 300,000 synaptic vesicles and secreted to effect transmission of nerve impulses across a given synapse (figure 8.1). Where chemical transmission of nerve impulses is effected by acetylcholine, these fibres are known as cholinergic. Such fibres are found in parts of the sympathetic and parasympathetic systems and in the motor fibres to skeletal muscle.

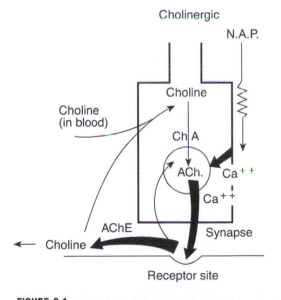

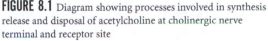

FIGURE 8.1 Diagram showing processes involved in synthesis release and disposal of acetylcholine at cholinergic nerve terminal and receptor site

Histamine: found in higher concentration in lung, intestine and skin, and those tissues which are exposed to the external environment. It would appear that histamine occurs in the tissue mast cells, the basophil cells and platelets of the blood. The exact form in which it is held in these cells is not yet known. Secretion by damaged cells anywhere in the body causes the walls of local capillaries to allow more fluid to pass through them, resulting in oedema. Histamine is released in conditions such as hay fever, and antihistamine drugs are taken to counter the unhappy effects of histamine release.

Prostaglandins: act principally on smooth muscle which contracts or relaxes according to the location, quantity and nature of the prostaglandin involved. They may cause dilation of certain blood vessels and increased heart rate through increased sympathetic nervous action. They may also stimulate or inhibit the release of free fatty acids according to whether the quantity of prostaglandins involved is low or high respectively. The prostaglandins would appear to number approximately 20 and these are divided into two categories: E-prostaglandins (PGE, or E), and F-prostaglandins (PGF, or F). Both of these groups occur in the central nervous system where their actions are stimulatory or inhibitory on individual neurons, within or without the central nervous system. The prostaglandins also appear to exert a modulatory role in nerve endings and in hormone secretion. Despite the relative infancy of research, the prostaglandins are noted here because they appear to have a role of considerable importance in the regulation of body function. They were independently identified in 1933–34 by Goldblatt and Euler, but still the world of prostaglandins is far from being completely understood.

Angiotensin: stimulates the secretion of aldosterone from the adrenal cortex, thereby promoting sodium reabsorption by the kidney. Angiotensin is also the most powerful pressor substance known, causing general constriction of the arterioles, and increasing blood pressure. This hormone also promotes secretion of the catecholamines – adrenaline (epinephrin) and noradrenaline (norepinephrin) – from the adrenal medulla. Angiotensin is formed in two parts:

- By the action of renin, secreted by the kidneys of the α2 globulin fraction of the plasma proteins, angiotensin I is formed.
- By the action of a converting enzyme on angiotensin I, angiotensin II is formed.

The majority of the 'conversion' takes place as the blood passes through the lungs. The α2 globulin is synthesised in the liver and referred to as *angiotensinogen*. Circulation of angiotensinogen is increased by the glucocorticoids and oestrogen. Angiotensin highlights the interdependence of chemicals in such complex bodily processes as homeostasis. It clearly has a key role in saltwater balance.

Kinins: cause contraction of most smooth muscle. In small quantities they reduce arterial blood pressure due primarily to dilation of blood vessels. By increasing the permeability of the blood vessels, plasma proteins are offered ease of egress. In increased quantities, the kinins facilitate the movement of leucocytes from blood to the surrounding tissues. Finally, it has been shown that the kinins stimulate the sensory nerve endings. It would appear that the plasma kinins are formed by antigen-antibody interplay.

5–HT: (serotonin, 5–hydroxytryptamine) is present in the mucosa of the digestive tract, in approximately 90 per cent of blood platelets, and in the central nervous system. 5–HT is a derivative of the essential amino acid tryptophan. The process is stimulated by an enzyme found in the digestive tract, nervous system, kidney and liver. There does not appear to be any evidence that blood platelets can synthesise 5–HT, so it is presumed that they 'collect' this hormone while passing through the digestive tract. 5–HT is a cardiac stimulant and constricts the blood vessels, especially the large veins. Associated with the latter is the raising of both systolic and diastolic blood pressure. It also increases the respiratory rate, acts as an antidiuretic, and stimulates smooth muscle and pain nerve endings in the skin. It is possible that the release of 5–HT from the blood platelets, following injury, causes pain and associated reflex actions in the circulorespiratory system. Serotonin is a neurotransmitter in the brain which may be involved in 'central fatigue' in exercise and possibly in the 'overtraining syndrome'.

Due to their proximity in the brain, it is difficult to separate the roles of those nerve terminals whose transmitter substance is noradrenaline or adrenaline (adrenergic) from those whose transmitter substance is 5–HT (serotoninergic). Consequently there is still some question over their respective physiological effects on mood and behaviour.

The adenosine group (ATP, ADP and AMP): found in all cells and the role of ATP in energy production has already been discussed (see chapter 6). The compounds decelerate heart rate and dilate blood vessels, lowering blood pressure. They also relax smooth muscle. The *cytokines* form a group of about 20 which have important effects on the immune system among other functions.

GENERAL HORMONES

The general hormones are associated with specific glands of origin (figure 8.2), and are emptied into the blood to be carried all around the body.

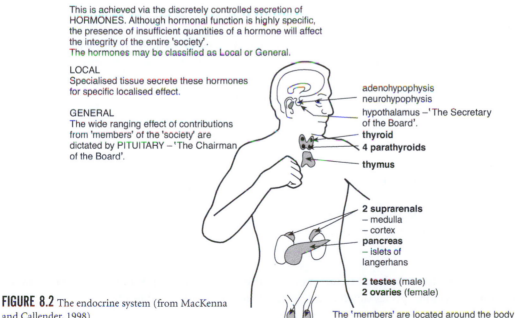

FIGURE 8.2 The endocrine system (from MacKenna and Callender, 1998)

The pituitary gland

The pituitary gland consists of two parts: the *posterior* (neural pituitary or neurohypophysis), and the *anterior* (the glandular pituitary or adenohypophysis).

Although the pituitary exerts a 'chairman's' influence over the endocrine system, its role is carefully controlled by a most diligent 'chief executive' – the hypothalamus (see p. 134), which in turn is influenced by the cerebrum.

The posterior part of the pituitary gland appears to be the 'store house' for hormones manufactured in the hypothalamus.

ADH (antidiuretic hormone or vasopressin): key role in saltwater balance has already been discussed (see chapter 7). Secretion increases with increasing exercise.

Oxytocin: produces ejection of milk from the lactating breast.
The posterior pituitary secretes these hormones from storage as required.
The anterior part of the pituitary gland has many functions which may be broadly categorised as:

- control of growth (e.g. bones, muscle)
- control of other areas of the endocrine system (e.g. thyroid, adrenal cortex)
- regulation of metabolism of carbohydrates, proteins and fats.

These functions are fulfilled by six hormones secreted by the adenohypophysis, which are as follows:

Growth hormone (somatotrophic hormone, STH, or human growth hormone, HGH): acts directly on the tissues. The following are some effects of growth hormone secretion:

- Increases the mass of skeletal muscle
- Increases lipolysis (breakdown of lipids) and increases circulating free fatty acids, offering the latter as a source of energy
- Increases bone growth
- Promotes transfer of amino acids from extracellular fluid to cells
- Increases the size of the thymus
- Stimulates RNA formation
- Inhibits carbohydrate metabolism.
  Secretion of growth hormone is increased by:
- Exercise, especially in women because oestrogen increases secretion of growth hormone
- Lowered glycogen in the blood (hypoglycaemia), or starvation
- Circulating amino acids (especially arginine)
- Extreme cold and even emotional excitement or stress
- Sleep.

Growth itself is primarily affected by heredity, nutrition, good health and the contribution of other hormones in addition to growth hormone, principally the androgens, thyroid hormones and insulin.

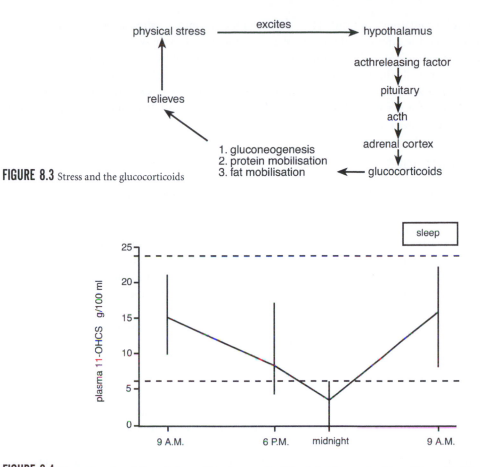

FIGURE 8.3 Stress and the glucocorticoids

FIGURE 8.4 Mean diurnal variation of plasma 11 hydroxycorticoid levels in 24 normal subjects. The vertical lines indicate the range of observations. The horizontal dashed lines show the normal range between 9 am and 10 am. (After D. Mattingly in Baron et al., 1968; Keele and Neil, 1973.)

ACTH (adrenocorticotrophic hormone or corticotrophin): causes the rapid secretion of glucocorticoids from the adrenal cortex; rapid conversion of cholesterol and its salts to pregnenolone and thence along the mineralocorticoid, or 17hydroxycorticoid, or androgen and oestrogen pathways; a fall in adrenal cortex ascorbic acid concentrations (though its role in the adrenal cortex is not clear); and stimulation of growth. The secretion of glucocorticoids under normal conditions and stress are both dependent upon ACTH secretion (figure 8.3).

ACTH is secreted according to a basic rhythm during the course of the day. The peak secretion would appear to occur during sleep before awakening, whereas the trough would appear to occur towards evening. This rhythm of ACTH secretion is reflected in plasma cortisol (figure 8.4) and is referred to as being the diurnal or circadian rhythm.

There is considerable evidence to support the theory that rhythmic control is spread over even longer periods. The rate of ACTH secretion is accelerated by disruption of homeostasis (i.e. stress).

Thyrotrophin (thyroid stimulating hormone TSH, thyrotrophic hormone): stimulates growth and acts directly on the thyroid gland to stimulate thyroxine secretion and acts directly with dietary iodine on the thyroid gland. In children increases in thyrotrophin secretion are produced by cold temperatures, but this effect is slight in adults. Normally the hypothalamus is a controller of thyrotrophin secretion and a decrease in thyroid hormone status also effects an increase in thyrotrophin secretion. Consequently this system is one of negative feedback and is effective both at pituitary and hypothalamus levels. It should also be added that it is thought that stress stimulates secretion of thyrotrophin.

Gonadotrophic hormones

Follicle stimulating hormone (FSH): stimulates ovarian follicle growth in the female and spermatogenesis in the male.

Luteinising hormone (LH or interstitial cell stimulating hormone – ICSH): stimulates ovulation in the female and testosterone secretion in the male. FSH and LH are the pituitary gonadotrophins and their inter-related role is evident in the female menstrual cycle, the central nervous system, and the hypothalamus. It is yet to be clearly shown that a similar periodicity exists in men regarding androgen secretion.

Prolactin (luteotrophic hormone LTH, luteotrophin, lactogenic hormone, mamotrophin, galactin): stimulates secretion of milk and maternal behaviour, inhibits testosterone, mobilises fatty acids.

Endorphins

The endorphins are hypothalomic neurotransmitters and are split from the large prohormone precursor molecule, pro-opiomelancortin (POMC), which is isolated from the anterior pituitary and is secreted into general circulation. Beta-endorphin and beta-lipotrophin increase with exercise and have an opiate, an analgesic effect in response to pain, and this is responsible for the so-called 'exercise high'. Endorphins have also been associated with menstrual cycle regulation and modulating the response of ACTH, prolactin, HGH, catecholamines and cortisol.

THE SECRETING GLANDS
Hypothalamus

The hypothalamus has already been suggested as assuming the role of a diligent 'chief executive' to the pituitary, and has been referred to in discussion of pituitary hormones. It receives a more generous blood supply than any other cerebral structure. It is mainly via this generous blood supply that stimuli promote the hypothalamus to secrete specific releasing agents to the pituitary, which in turn secretes an appropriate hormone from those listed above. It also manufactures the two hormones stored in the neurohypophysis and has a regulatory function in temperature control, thirst, hunger, sexual and emotional behaviour. It also exerts neuro-endocrine control of the catecholamines in response to emotional stimuli via impulses coming down from the cerebrum.

Thyroid gland

The thyroid gland secretes three hormones: thyroxine, triiodothyronine and calcitonin. The main hormone is thyroxine, although triiodothyronine is relatively more active. The function of these two hormones is similar and it has become conventional to base discussion on thyroxine.

Thyroxine performs several functions in the body:

- It is essential to normal metabolism, and the increased metabolic rate brought about by thyroxine increases oxygen consumption and heat production (calorigenesis). Thyroxine also increases dissociation of oxygen from haemoglobin.
- It is essential to the normal function of the central nervous system, but does not increase oxidative metabolism within this system.
- It is essential to normal growth and development of the body when growth hormone is secreted by the adenohypophysis. Growth hormone can only work at maximum efficiency in the presence of thyroxine. Moreover, thyroxine is vital to differentiation and maturation of certain tissues such as the epiphyses in ossification.
- The absorption of carbohydrate through the intestine reflects the level of thyroxine activity.
- High activity increases absorption and utilisation of glycogen by the tissues and increases glycogenolysis in the liver, muscle and heart, as well as increasing gluconeogenesis and insulin breakdown.
- It is involved in the regulation of lipid metabolism and is known to reduce cholesterol in the blood by encouraging its metabolism by the liver and by increasing the quantity excreted in bile.
- Excessive thyroxine causes excessive protein breakdown.
- Heart rate, blood pressure and cutaneous circulation may increase with an increase in thyroxine secretion.
- The gonads (sexual organs) function normally only when thyroxine secretion is normal. Thyroxine levels are important factors in lactation.
- The equilibrium of thyroxine secretion is also critical to normal function of the digestive tract.
- Hormone secretion increases with increasing exercise.

Calcitonin (thyrocalcitonin): inhibits the process of resorption of bone, and consequently calcitonin is secreted in response to increased concentration of calcium in the blood. Calcitonin should be considered as one of the three main guardians of calcium equilibrium in the body. The others are parathyroid hormone and vitamin D. Magnesium and phosphate are also linked with the body's calcium profile.

Parathyroid glands

The parathyroid glands secrete a hormone which promotes calcium resorption in the body.

Parathyroid hormone: secreted when there is a decrease in calcium concentration in the blood. When magnesium concentration is high, there is a decrease in parathyroid hormone secretion. Although phosphate concentration does not directly affect secretion, it is possible that it does so indirectly when, for example, high phosphate leads to lowered blood calcium levels. Parathyroid hormone acts directly on bone and kidney and it would appear that it also may have a direct effect on the intestine.

Vitamin D is essential to the direct actions on bone and probably on intestine. This vitamin also increases calcium and phosphate absorption from the intestine. Secretion increases with long-term exercise.

Adrenal glands

The adrenal glands each lie above one kidney, hence their other title – the suprarenal glands. These glands comprise an inner medulla and an outer cortex, which are, in fact, two distinct organs.

The adrenal cortex

The adrenal cortex is involved in the stress response and regulates carbohydrate, fat and protein metabolism, and also saltwater balance.

The hormones secreted by the adrenal cortex fall into three main categories, but two smaller groups of progesterone and oestradiol should also be considered (not known to have any significant feminising activity). The main groups are as follows.

The glucocorticoids *cortisol* (hydrocortisone) and *corticosterone*: promote glucose formation, hence their name. Corticosterone has little importance in man and comprises roughly a third of the glucocorticoids in blood. Consequently it is reasonable to follow convention by discussing only cortisol here. Cortisol has several functions to fulfil:

- It is essential to normal carbohydrate metabolism.
- It promotes gluconeogenesis in the liver.
- It is essential to breakdown of glycogen to glucose, by adrenaline or glucagon.
- It promotes catabolism of proteins.
- It brings about redistribution of fats via lipolysis and lipogenesis.
- In excess, it reduces the response of tissue to bacterial infection.
- It mimics (but is less effective than) aldosterone in saltwater balance and also plays an important role in maintaining blood pressure.
- It increases the blood platelet count and shortens blood clotting time.
- In excess, cortisol raises blood lipid and cholesterol levels.
- It increases acidity in the stomach and when combined with a slight increase in release of pepsin (an enzyme involved in protein digestion) it is possible that peptic ulcer formation may result.
- It promotes absorption from the intestine of fats which are insoluble in water.
- In excess it interferes with cartilage development and the reduction of epiphysial plates. This may lead to interrupted growth in children. Also in this connection, it decreases calcium absorption from the intestine and increases calcium loss in the urine.
- Increased secretion in heavy prolonged exercise only.

Finally, it is well known that cortisol is used in the treatment of certain injuries. The injury site is infiltrated with a quantity of cortisol in excess of the normal physiological level. The cortisol protects the site from damage and prevents the normal response to tissue trauma, such as histamine release, or migration and infiltration of leucocytes at the injury site. Cortisol does not actively heal the injury, but creates a favourable environment for healing. However it will be appreciated, from what has been said above, that cortisol infiltration is not without considerable risk and it is hardly surprising that sport authorities in medicine are extremely cautious in suggesting its use. For example, it has a weakening effect on collagen, as in tendons, rendering them brittle over time.

The mineralocorticoids *aldosterone* and *11-deoxycorticosterone* (cortexolone): cause retention of sodium and increased excretion of potassium in the urine. Consequently they are key agents in saltwater balance. Aldosterone is approximately 30 times as powerful as 11-deoxycorticosterone in terms of sodium retention, but it is less efficient as an agent in potassium excretion. Secretion increases with increasing exercise.

Androgen secreted by the adrenal cortex has a less masculinising effect than testosterone. It is necessary for the growth of body hair in women. The principal adrenal androgen is dehydro-epi-androsterone. As stated, the hormones of the adrenal cortex follow a circadian rhythm, but their secretion is increased by stressful stimuli. The various compounds involved are all steroids and derived from cholesterol (figure 8.5). It will be clear that several results of excess secretion of these corticosteroids are not compatible with good health and, consequently, persistent exposure to cumulative stressors which exhaust adaptive response should be avoided. In this respect, sport and physical recreation may be considered therapeutic.

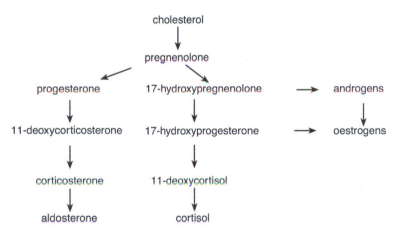

FIGURE 8.5 Possible pathways in the synthesis of steroid hormones from cholesterol (from Keele and Neil, 1973)

The adrenal medulla

The adrenal medulla secretes the catecholamines adrenaline and noradrenaline. The actions of adrenaline (epinephrine) and noradrenaline (norepinephrine) are very similar, but the latter is more efficient in raising blood pressure and less efficient in metabolic actions and in relaxing smooth muscle. Their secretion is stimulated by: physical and emotional stressors, cold exposure, decreased blood pressure, low blood glycogen, certain drugs (e.g. anaesthetics), afferent nerve stimulation, and increasing exercise.

Involvement of the catecholamines and the sympathetic nervous system in the 'fight or flight mechanism' is well known. These two independent systems provide a most efficient means of meeting emergency situations. Such means might be summarised as:

- Increase in heart rate and cardiac output, and rise in blood pressure.
- Mobilisation of muscle and liver glycogen, leading to increased blood sugar.

- Increase in metabolic rate.
- Skeletal muscle fatigues less readily.
- Relaxation of smooth muscle in the wall of the bronchioles, which leads to a better supply of air to alveoli.
- Respiration rate is raised.
- Dilation of coronary blood vessels and those of skeletal muscle, thus providing increased blood supply to those organs urgently requiring it.
- Constriction of blood vessels of abdomen; contraction of sphincters of digestive tract, ureters and sphincters of urinary bladder; inhibition of digestive tract movement and wall of urinary bladder ('butterflies' and increased micturition in pre competition).
- Dilation of pupils of eye.
- Constriction of smooth muscle of skin and cutaneous blood vessels ('goose flesh' and pallor).
- Increased ability of blood to coagulate.
- Affect on reticular formation of brain to increase memory recall, and to increase attention and concentration.

While the value of catecholamines is clearly of advantage in the fight or flight mechanism, the value is much less clear in the face of psychological and emotional stress. In fact, Carruthers (1971) sees such secretion as part of a most undesirable chain of events (figure 5.2, p. 90). They are secreted for a purpose and if not used for that purpose, they must be 'burned off ' – for example, via light aerobic exercise. Adrenaline secretion increases in heavy exercise; noradrenaline increases with increasing exercise.

The pancreas

The pancreas, in addition to its exocrine function of secreting pancreatic juice, also has an endocrine function which it fulfils via the *islets of langerhans*. There are two types of cell involved in its endocrine function:

1. Cells secrete *glucagon*, which increases blood glucose by glucogenolysis and gluconeogenesis.

2. Cells secrete *insulin* (table 8.1), which decreases blood glucose by stimulating reabsorption of glucose in the kidneys, reducing liver glycolysis and increasing glycogen formation from glucose in muscle.

Stimulation	Inhibition
Monosaccharides	Adrenaline
Amino acids	Noradrenaline
*Ketones	Insulin
Glucogen	Fasting
Growth of hormones	
* product of liver metabolism of FFA	

TABLE 8.1 Factors influencing insulin secretion via blood

The thymus

The thymus increases in size from childhood until adolescence, and thereafter progressively atrophies. This gland is responsible for the 'education' of the T-lymphocyte immune cells so that they do not attack the body's proteins. This process of clonal selection by deletion occurs through apoptosis, or induced cell suicide.

The testes

The testes have an exocrine function in the manufacture of sperm and an endocrine function in the secretion of testosterone. Testosterone, in addition to its initial role in the foetus of forming the male genitalia, is also responsible for development of the secondary male characteristics at puberty, the maintenance of some of these throughout adult life, and the male emotional profile.

Testosterone causes nitrogen retention in the body and increased synthesis and deposition of protein, especially in skeletal muscle. By this process, there can be little doubt that testosterone derivatives increase strength, given that dietary factors and training regimens are appropriate. In addition, testosterone and its derivatives promote retention of water, sodium, potassium, phosphorus, sulphate and calcium. It is mainly the retention of water which causes the considerable weight gains which are recorded in studies of the effect of testosterone ingestion.

For several years, some athletes have been known to illegally take testosterone derivatives for their anabolic effect. Anabolism is the formation of energy rich phosphate compounds, proteins, fats and complex sugars by processes which take up rather than release energy. (Catabolism = releasing energy, and metabolism = energy transformations in the body.) It would appear that the taking of such substances increases strength, promotes formation of erythropoetin, and so on. However, to do so, with or without medical advice, in pursuit of competitive advantage, is, apart from being illegal in the world of sport, also highly irresponsible. By disrupting one part of the endocrine system in this way the equilibrium of the total system is compromised. For example, the following have been advanced as possible, and in some cases are probable, additional effects of taking testosterone derivatives:

- Initial enlargement of the testes is followed by shrinkage because the high level of testosterone causes a negative feedback in the system resulting in no luteinising hormone being sent to the testes.
- The long bones mature too rapidly.
- An increase in sexual desire is followed by a decrease.
- The salt/water imbalance due to fluid and electrolyte retention may lead to kidney, circulatory and coronary disorders.
- The probability of prostate gland cancer would appear to be increased.
- There is a higher incidence of jaundice in those taking these substances.
- Liver disorders are associated with testosterone ingestion.

Several of these effects may be irreversible. Secretion increases with exercise.

The ovaries

The ovaries, in addition to discharging ova, secrete two hormones: an oestrogen known as oestradiol, and a progestin known as progesterone. These hormones are responsible for the development of female primary and secondary sexual characteristics, the growth and development of the female sex organs at puberty (e.g.

enlargement of uterus), the menstrual cycle, the physiological and anatomical changes associated with pregnancy (e.g. conversion of pelvic outlet, broadening of hips), and changes in the mammary glands.

Oestradiol: the involvement of oestradiol is very slight until puberty when the hypothalamus stimulates the adenohypophysis to secrete gonatrophins, which stimulate the ovary to discharge ova and secrete oestradiol and progesterone. Consequently, athletes may find performance fluctuation due to such changes as strength-weight ratio, alignment of femur relative to tibia, and basic metabolism undergoing gross adjustment. Figure 8.6 outlines possible weight variations in the course of the cycle. It has been suggested that the cycle should be adjusted to make 'optimum competition weight' days coincide with major competitions. Indeed, this has been achieved by administration of certain drugs. However, it is not clear what long-term effect such adjustment of this most basic rhythm will have on other rhythms. Oestradiol, in addition to its key role in the menstrual cycle and those functions listed above, also effects:

- Deposition of fatty tissue on thighs and hips.
- Growth rate of bones after puberty. It has a 'burning out' effect leading to an early growth spurt but also an early cessation. Looking at it another way, the male child grows longer, longer!
- Blood cholesterol levels are reduced by oestradiol and possibly this helps in the prevention of development of coronary heart disease.
- While testosterone increases sebaceous gland secretion and the possibility of acne, oestradiol increases water content of the skin and decreases sebaceous gland secretion.

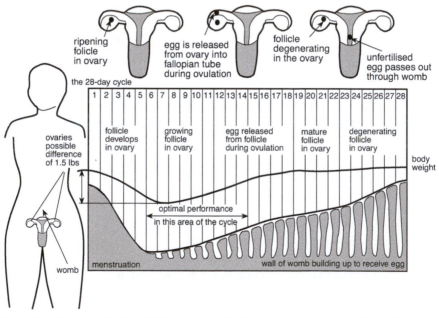

FIGURE 8.6 Menstruation. The cycle of changes which take place in the tissue lining a woman's womb culminate about every 28 days when the blood-enriched lining comes away as the menstrual flow. The changes in the womb occur in parallel to the developments in an ovary, where an egg ripens and is released at ovulation, about halfway through the cycle. The egg travels along a fallopian tube towards the womb. It is fertilised, becomes implanted in the lining of the womb, and menstruation ceases for the duration of pregnancy (adapted from Reader's Digest, 1972).

Progesterone: increases body temperature and it is thought that its secretion at ovulation is the reason for increased body temperature at that time. Combinations of these female steroids have been marketed as oral progestogens (female oral contraceptives). These oral progestogens have been used by some athletes in order to effect control of the menstrual cycle but, again, the general equilibrium of the endocrine system is exposed to the possibility of certain compromises such as weight increase, increase in emotional irritability and feelings of depression, decreased status of vitamin B6, vitamin B2, folic acid, vitamin C, vitamin B12, and of trace elements such as zinc. The depression is manageable on trying different types of 'pill', possibly with folic acid supplementation. Depending on menstrual phase, exercise increases secretion.

THE IMMUNE SYSTEM

The immune system consists of a complex, well-regulated interdependence in the grouping of hormones, cells (e.g. white blood cells; see chapter 5), and interactive adaptive mechanisms which defend the body when attacked by outside microbes – viral, bacterial and fungal; foreign macromolecules; and abnormal malignant cell growth. When infection occurs, the immune system works to reduce the severity of the condition and to accelerate repair and recovery.

Exercise, stress (emotional, physical or mental) and ill health constitute interactive factors, each impacting on the body's immune system. Each factor can independently affect immune status, immune function and, consequently, resistance to infection and disease. In the absence of adequate in-built regeneration, the collective cumulative effect of these factors expose a person to the danger of serious fitness and/or health breakdown.

Conditions from so-called 'overtraining' through to chronic fatigue syndrome are all, quite simply, cumulative stress related. The body struggles to adapt to a growing aggregate of stressors, the immune system cannot cope, and the body cannot regenerate sufficiently to regain control. It is as if the body cannot get above the base line (0) following loading and tiring (figure 21.2, p. 333).

Light moderate physical activity provides some protection against upper respiratory tract infections, compared to a sedentary lifestyle, and does not seem to increase the severity of the condition. On the other hand, intense physical activity (e.g. heavy training to exhaustion) creates a period of between three and 72 hours where resistance to bacterial and viral attack is decreased. This renders the athlete easy prey to respiratory infection, which makes its presence felt within 7–11 days.

SUMMARY

The hormones are the supreme guardians of homeostasis. They regulate organic functions through their individual and combined roles. A knowledge of hormone function is essential to a comprehensive understanding of an athlete's status, not only his level of athletic fitness but also his general health. It is possible that an athlete will receive medication in the form of ingested hormone preparations (such as oral progestogens to regulate the menstrual cycle; creams for the skin such as cortisol creams for treatment of eczema; injections such as insulin for diabetes mellitus). Consequently, it is important to understand why and how the use of these preparations will affect the integrity of the endocrine system. Medical advice must be sought to establish the implication of exposing the athlete to certain training stressors. In recent years it has been tempting to see the hormones not only as regulators of total body function, but also as possible instruments to advance athletic performance. Indeed, it is not uncommon for hormone preparations to be discussed along with the athlete's nutrition. However, the equilibrium which exists within the body is very delicate and, as yet, not completely understood. Conservation is as necessary to our internal environment as it is to the external environment and, with or without medical supervision, the pursuit of 'hormonal advantage' in sport is as unwise as it is unethical. It is clear that cumulative stress threatens the immune system. In designing the personal preparation plans of athletes, a review of the total stressor profile of the athlete's lifestyle is essential.

REFLECTIVE QUESTIONS

1. Discuss the meaning of the following statement: 'Hormones act as silent messengers to integrate the body as a unit.'

2. Create a wall chart succinctly representing the following information

Hormone producing gland	Hormone	Effects of hormone	Control of hormone secretion	Effects of hypo release and hyper release	Effects of exercise on hormone release

3. Several women members of the swimming team you are coaching have approached you for advice about the loss of their menstrual cycle. Apart from recommending that they see a gynaecologist and the team doctor, how would you explain this condition to them?

4. Very intense exercise and prolonged sub maximal exercise are associated with increased protein breakdown. What endocrinologic characteristics of exercise and recovery from exercise stimulate protein synthesis and an eventual increase in muscle mass?

5. How does exercise and training influence the body's immune system? Is such influence always positive? If negative, discuss possible reasons why. It can be the case that people in high pressure roles in business or in sport are excessively fatigued or pick up infections or viruses when they take a break from the pressure. Discuss possible endocrinologic reasons for this phenomenon.

9 PHYSIOLOGICAL DIFFERENCES IN THE GROWING CHILD

It is very easy to see training as the only stressor to which the young athlete's organism is exposed. However, this is most certainly not the case. Training is only one stressor in a complex assault on the organism which must adapt to the demands of growth and maturing function.

EFFECTS OF STRESS

As a result of multi-stressor situations, metabolic functions take place at a higher rate and the stress characteristics of circulation and respiration are quite apparent. One may rightly assume that the resistance or elasticity of the blood vessels contribute to the type of circulo-respiratory adjustments seen in youngsters in training. However, the main focus of attention should be on the heart itself and its ability to pump out blood. The measurements we are looking for, then, are *stroke volume*, *heart rate* and *blood pressure*. Consequently, considerable attention is also given to cardiac output, which is 4–5 litres at rest and over 20 litres in exercise. The increase can be affected by increasing heart rate and stroke volume. Obviously, the more blood the heart can pump out per unit of time the better it is for the athlete, so endurance training is geared in the first instance to improving cardiac output. Due to the small size of the untrained child's heart, cardiac output increase is brought about almost entirely by increased heart rate. This frequency regulation, in contrast with the volume regulation of adults and trained youths, is a particular feature of the circulation of untrained youngsters.

Research in the former German Democratic Republic (GDR) and Sweden shows a linear relationship between the heart volume and maximum oxygen uptake (VO_2 maximum) with age, from 8–18 years. However, examination of heart size on its own does not give any real indication of the performance capacity of young athletes since the normal size range is very large. The relative size of the heart compared with other morphological and functional values would, however, give some indication of performance (table 9.1).

According to Hollmann and Venrath (1962), the greatest increase in heart volume occurs at approximately 11 years of age for girls, and approximately 14 years of age for boys. The heart weight is greatest 2–3 years later. Furthermore, as young people mature, heart rate decreases while blood pressure and the range between systole and diastole increases. Training adds to these natural growth phenomena, giving greater heart volume, range of blood pressure and maximum heart rate. This provides lower functional values at rest and higher functional values under stress, i.e. an increased range of functional ability.

Muscle biochemistry in pre-puberty does not favour lactic anaerobic activity. There are significantly lower levels of the glycolytic enzyme phosphofructokinase in children compared with adults. This would suggest that 'early teens' success in sprints or endurance events may be due to aerobic and/or alactic anaerobic efficiency, or an early maturity. Attempting to 'force' anaerobesis on the pre-pubertal child is as pointless as it is unwise.

Age	Untrained		Trained		
	Boys	Girls	Boys	Girls	
11	376	349	417	392	
12	440	366	461	448	
13	483	452	508	496	
14–15	549	501	584	539	
*14–15	555.1	469.9	660.6	443.7	sprints
			620.2	498.8	middle distance
			650.9		football

TABLE 9.1 Heart volumes in ml of untrained and trained 11–15-year-olds (from Harre, 1986).

Up to 12 years of age, oxygen intake is approximately equal for boys and girls. Thereafter, girls accelerate to their maximum between 13 and 16 years of age, and boys increase their oxygen intake rather more slowly to reach their maximum at 18–19 years of age. Although it was suggested earlier that cardiac output increase is almost entirely due to heart rate increase in the child, sports physiologists now suggest that a regulation of stroke volume can be seen in trained children and youths. This manifests itself in a greater increase in systolic blood pressure, or in blood pressure range, accompanied by only a slight increase in heart rate. This is illustrated in figure 9.1 by comparison of trained and untrained boys and girls. It can be seen that heart rate for trained children is lower than for untrained. In recovery, the total time for trained children is shorter (figure 9.2).

The peak of biological adaptability in children occurs between 10 and 15 years of age, at a period when physical capacity has by no means reached its maximum. As far as developing physical ability is concerned, youth is the best time for the athlete, bearing in mind that the growing organism is required to expend considerable energy in growing and maturing. Heavy strength work and anaerobic (lactic) work are not to be emphasised in early youth, but mobility, which will almost certainly be on the decline after 8–9 years of age, must be consciously worked for where appropriate. While aerobic endurance training and general training can often be found in simple endurance sports (e.g. orienteering, paarlauf) and field games, care must, nevertheless, be taken to ensure adequate rest periods, especially where endurance training is taken to the 'controlled' environment of the track or pool. Harre has noted (1973) that 'when there has been a logical choice of training methods and due observation of the basic principles of training, functional disturbances are, as a rule, not the result of loading in training. Much more to blame here are the total stressors put upon the young athlete, and performance-diminishing features such as immoderate amount of stimuli (e.g. excessive TV watching, inadequate sleep, unsuitable diet, etc.).' On top of this, in the years 13–18, the emotional stressors of culture and the human environment with its ebb and flow of behaviour, attitudes and relationships, plus rigorous academic demands can be extremely exacting.

It is of critical importance, then, that meticulous care is exercised by all involved in a young athlete's development to monitor the balance of cumulative stressors against the athlete's capacity to cope with them. Fatigue (see chapter 23) for the growing child is not to be ignored, it is an urgent alarm call to review the stressors. Given such monitoring the ability to recover improves as the young athlete grows and as training load is responsibly and systematically increased. However, long interruptions to training result in a deterioration of this ability. A regular medical check-up, accompanied by a physiotherapy check-up, will help avoid

FIGURE 9.1 (a) Average heart rate at rest and in exercise for 12–14 yrs. Trained and untrained girls with standardised exercise loading (Harre, 1973). (b) Average heart rate at rest and in exercise for 12–14 yrs. Trained and untrained boys with a standardised exercise loading (Harre, 1986).

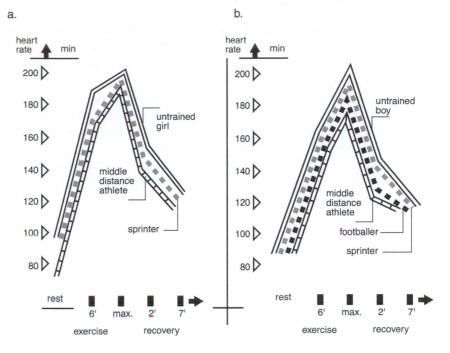

FIGURE 9.2 (a) Heart rate in the third minute of recovery for sixty-five 10–14-year-old athletes in preliminary training for speed sports (Harre, 1986). (b) Heart rate in the third minute of recovery for forty-three 10–18-year-old athletes in preliminary training for endurance sport (Harre, 1986).

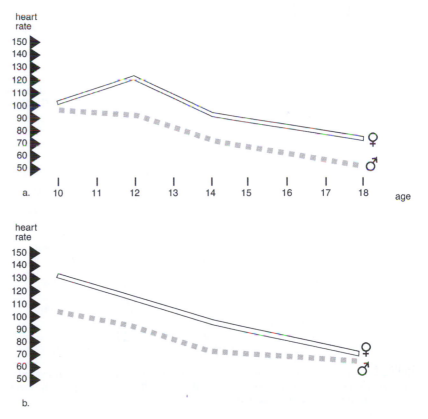

any functional problems which can arise due to excessive stressor bombardment. This done, training will always, if accompanied by careful thought, be to the athlete's benefit.

Due to the existence of natural androgenic hormone to an extent never matched elsewhere in their life, girls should be exposed to regular moderate strength training as soon as they finish their adolescent growth spurt, but before sexual maturity. Menstruation is occurring earlier now (around 13 years and 2 months – 4) than in 1890 when 15 years was the age of menarche (it may be earlier or later). The combined stressors of the relatively 'new' phenomenon of menstruation, plus growing itself, suggest avoidance of training loads which produce excessive fatigue in the early teenage athlete.

Although the importance has been stressed of regarding the child as a child and not a mini-adult (because of basic dimensional differences), many measurements and values are, in fact, proportionate to, or 'scaled down versions' of, the adult's. For example, blood volume in terms of ml/kg of bodyweight is 75 for men, 65 for women and 60 for children.

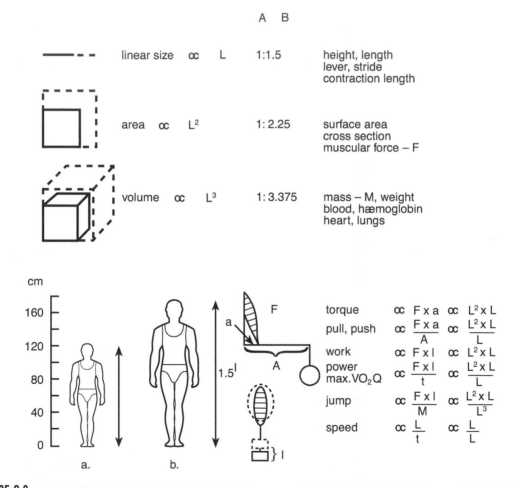

FIGURE 9.3 Schematic illustration of the influence of dimensions on some static and dynamic functions in geometrically similar individuals. A and B represent two persons with body height 120 and 180cm respectively (partly modified from Asmussen and Christensen, from Astrand and Rodahl, 1977).

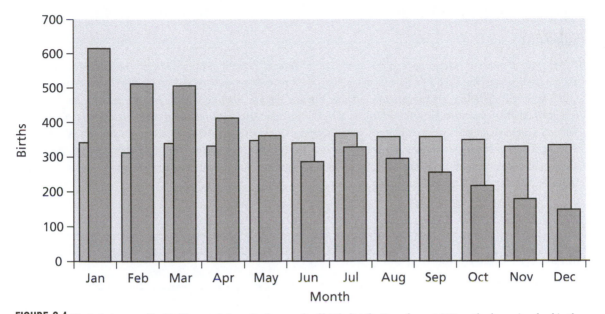

FIGURE 9.4 The 'relative age effect' is illustrated above by the month of birth distribution of over 4,000 youth players involved in the qualifying squads for U17, U19 and U21 tournaments organised by UEFA in 2010/11

Finally, in recent years research originally from 1985 by R. H. Barnsley, A. H. Thompson and P. E. Barnsley) in Canadian ice hockey has suggested a bias, evident in the high performance end of sport and academia, where participation of persons born early in the period of selection is higher than would be anticipated from a normal annual distribution of births. Conversely, there are few of those born later in the selection period. This is referred to as the relative age effect (RAE).

What appears to be happening is that, for example, young soccer players are likely to be selected for junior teams at an early age when born in January–March and consequently have a greater chance of succeeding in sport at the highest level later in life. On the other hand, those born in the latter part of the selection year, October–December, often with similar amounts of talent, are frequently overlooked by selectors at an early age and consequently have a significantly reduced chance of succeeding in elite sport (figure 9.4).

Morris and Nevill (2006) concluded, in a study of the FA 'School of Excellence' players that those born towards the end of the year are frequently unable to demonstrate their talent due to a lack of physical maturity and strength. Once overlooked, these individuals may be lost to sport altogether, while those who have been selected receive better coaching, become established within the 'system', and have a much greater chance of becoming successful in the future. The challenge for selectors and coaches is to establish programmes that identify and nurture young people on the basis of their talent, not their physical maturity, and while solutions such as quotas and narrower age bands for selection have been discussed, the danger of overlooking talented young people simply because of the time within the selection year that they are born, remains.

SUMMARY

The process of growing reaches beyond the readily observed anatomical indications. Within the athlete there are proceeding structural and functional changes which are part of the growing process. While these changes in the athlete's physiology are preparation for adult life and the possibility of a progressive intensity and extent of loading consistent with the advanced athlete's training, they also represent high-energy expenditure. Moderate exercise reflecting a varied intensity and extent of loading is essential to normal growth. Organised training for boys and girls should be introduced around 10–12 years of age. However, the coach must see the growing athlete's training as characterised by a sound programme of all-round development which does not produce exhaustion of already reduced energy reserves.

REFLECTIVE QUESTIONS

1. Design a strategy to address R.A.E in a school context, identifying possible issues and suggest possible solutions to these.

2. Discuss the arguments for and against establishing age group records (e.g. 10–14 years) for performance in marathon and maximum strength related sport.

3. Create a reference guide for coaches working with young athletes succinctly representing the following:

Function	Comparison with Adults	Implications for exercise programmes
Cardiovascular, e.g. Max cardiac output Max stroke volume Max heart rate, etc.		
Metabolic, e.g. Aerobic – VO_2 max, etc Anaerobic – HR at OBLA CrP and ATP breakdown, etc.		

4. List and discuss physiological factors which influence changes in exercise and training content for boys and girls in the final two years of primary/grade school and the first two years of secondary/high school.

5. A young female athlete you have been coaching has progressed steadily through her teens and at 16/17 years is competing with top senior women outperforming them regularly over 1500m. However, this year, at 18 years, despite normal increases in training, she struggles with training and cannot match the performances of the previous year. Discuss physiological changes that may have brought this about and why. What is your strategy for getting things back on track?

Increase	Decrease
Strength of bone	Heart rate at rest
Strength of ligaments	Heart rate at submaximal workloads
Thickness of articular cartilage	Oxygen uptake for given workload
Cross-section area of muscle	Blood lactate for given workload
Muscle strength and power	Pulmonary ventilation for given workload
Creatine phosphate and ATP in muscle	Triglycerides in blood
Myoglobin	Arterial blood pressure
Capillarisation of muscle (including heart)	Glycogen utilisation
Heart volume	Blood cholesterol
Heart weight	Risk of myocardial infarction
Myocardial contractility	Obesity–adiposity
Blood volume	Platelet stickiness
Total haemoglobin	Stress associated with physical/psychological
2,3 diphosphoglycerates	stressors e.g. humidity, altitude, emotion, etc.
Fibrolytic activity	
Maximum heart rate	
Stroke volume	
a-vO$_2$ difference at maximal workload	
Blood lactate at maximal workload	
Pulmonary ventilation at maximal workload	
Respiratory rate at maximal workload	
Diffusing capacity of lung at maximal workload	
Lean body mass	
Glycogen content of muscle	
Size and number of muscle mitochondria	
Mitochondrial activity (succinic dehydrogenase, phosphofructokinase)	
Range of joint action	
Speed of limb movement	
Tolerance to stress	

TABLE 9.2 Summary of cumulative effects of sub-maximal and maximal exercise

SUMMARY OF PART 2

Training might be thought of as the practical means of adapting the organism to certain specific demands of a sport. The systems which have been reviewed in these chapters are all involved in the adaptation process, or permit adaptation to take place. Some specific effects of training, which illustrate adaptation by the increase or decrease of certain functional capacities, are listed in table 9.2 overleaf. It should be said here, however, that no single form of training will affect all of these adaptations.

The athlete trains to compete or participate in physical activity. The demands of each sport, and the specific environment of any contest, are unique to the individual athlete concerned. Thus, when training for a given sport, the specific adaptation of that athlete's organism to meet the demands of that sport is also unique. Adaptation will also vary according to whether it is a final or a friendly competition, or at altitude or in high humidity, in pursuit or defence of a title, the location in a circadian or monthly cycle, at home or following lengthy travel, and so on.

Not every problem relating to specific adaptation will be resolved by a study of the human organism, but at least these problems can be more clearly defined and identified, even within the limits of our understanding of organic function.

REFERENCES FOR PART 2

Astrand, P. O. 'Diet and athletic performance'. *Federation Proceedings* 26: 1772–7. (1967)

Astrand, P. O. and Christensen, E. H. 'Aerobic work capacity'. In. F. Dickens, E. Neill and W. F. Wicklas (eds), *Oxygen in the Animal* Organism. New York Pergamon Press, (1964)

Astrand, P. O., Per-Olaf and Rodahl, K. *Textbook of Work Physiology*. 2nd edn. New York: McGraw-Hill. (1977)

Astrand, P. O., Rodahl, K., Dahl, H. A. and Stromme, S. B. *Textbook of Work Physiology*. 4th edn. New York: McGraw-Hill. (2003)

Baron, D. N., Compston, N. D. and Dawson, A. M. *Recent Advances in Medicine*. 15th edn. London: J. & A. Churchill, (1968)

Blair, S. N., Dunn, A. L., Marcus, B. H and Carpenter, R. A. *Active Living Every Day*. Champaign, IL: Human Kinetics. (2001)

Buskirk, E. R. and Bass, D. E. *Climate and Exercise in Science and Medicine of Exercise and Sports*. Johnson, W. R. and Buskirk, E. R. (eds). London: Harper & Row. (1974)

Carlile, F. and Carlile, U. 'T-wave changes in strenuous exercise'. *Track Technique* 2. (1960)

Carruthers, M. E. 'Biomechanical effects of psychological factors on physical performance'. Paper presented to British Association of Sports Medicine and Scottish Amateur Athletic Joint Coaching Committee Conference on Bioprofiling, Glenrothes. (1971)

Dahl, H. A. and Rinvik, E. *Menneskets Funksjonelle Anatom*. Oslo: J. W. Cappelems Forlag. (1999)

Durnin, J. V. G. A. 'Protein requirements of physical activity'. *6th Coaches' Convention Report*. (1975)

Ekblom, B., Goldbarg, A. N. and Gullbring, B. 'Convention report: Response to exercise after blood loss and reinfusion'. *Journal of Applied Physiology* 32: 2. (1972)

Golnick, P. D., Armstrong, R. B., Saltin, B., Saubert, C. W., Sembrowich, W. K. and Shephard, R. E. 'Effect of training on enzyme activities and fibre composition of human skeletal muscle'. *Journal of Applied Physiology* 34: 107–11. (1973)

Guyton, A. C. *Physiology of the Human Body*. Philadelphia, PA: Holt Saunders. (1990)

Harre, D. *Trainingslehre*. Berlin: Sportverlag. (1973)

Harre, D. *Principles of Sport Training*. Berlin: Sportverlag. (1986)

Huxley, H. E. 'The contraction of muscle'. *Scientific American* 19(3). (1958)

Jäger, K. and Oelschlägel, G. *Kleine Trainingslehre*. 2nd edn. Berlin: Sportverlag. (1974)

Keele, C. A. and Neil, E. *Samson Wright's Applied Physiology*. 12th edn. London: Oxford University Press. (1973)

Lemon, P.W. *Protein and Amino Acid Needs of the Strength Athlete*. Int J Sport Nutr. June; 1 (2): 127–45 (1991)

MacKenna, B. R. and Callender, R. *Illustrated Physiology*. 5th edn. Edinburgh: Churchill Livingstone. (1998)

Maughan R.J., Greenhaff P.L. and Hespel P. 'Dietary supplements for athletes: emerging trends and recurring themes'. *Journal of Sports Sciences* 29(suppl. 1): S57–66. (2011)

Morris, J.G. and Nevill, M. E. *A Sporting Chance: Enhancing Opportunities for High-Level Sporting Performance: Influence of Relative Age*. Official Report. Loughborough: Loughborough University. Available at www.lboro.ac.uk/microsites/ssehs/youth-sport/research. (2006)

Newsholme, E. A., Leech, T. and Duester, G. *Keep on Running: The Science of Training and Performance*. Chichester: John Wiley and Sons. (1994)

Noakes, T. *Lore of Running: Discover the Science and Spirit of Running*. Champaign, IL: Leisure Press. (2002)

Pappenheimer, J. R., Comroe, J. H., Cournand, A. et al. 'Standardisation of definitions and symbols in respiratory physiology'. *Federation Proceedings* 9: 602. (1950)

Pyke, M. *Success in Nutrition*. London: John Murray. (1975)

Reader's Digest. *The Family Health Guide*. London: Reader's Digest. (1972)

Saltin, B. and Hermansen, L. *Glycogen Stores and Prolonged Severe Exercise, Nutrition and Physical Activity*. Uppsala: Almqvist & Wiksell. (1967)

Schreiner, K. E. and Schreiner, A. *Menneskeorganismen*. 6th edn. J. Jansen (ed.). Oslo: Universitetets Anatomiske Inst. (1964)

Suslov, F. 'Views on middle and long distance training'. *Modern Athlete and Coach* 10(1). (1972)

Vander, A. J., Sherman, J. H. and Luciano, D. S. *Human Physiology, The Mechanism of Body Function*. New York: McGraw-Hill. (1970)

Volek, J. S and Phinney, S. D. *The Art and Science of Low Carbohydrate Performance*. Miami FL: Beyond Obesity Llc. (2012)

Williams, C. 'Adaptation to stressors of a changing environment'. *6th Coaches' Convention Report*. (1975)

Wootton, S. *Nutrition for Sport*. New York: Simon & Schuster. (1988)

Yakovlev, N. N. 'Nutrition of the athlete'. *Track Technique* 20–26. (1961)

BIBLIOGRAPHY

Badewitz-Dodd, L. *Drugs and Sport*. Amsterdam: Media Medica. (1991)

Bergeron, M. F. et al. 'International Olympic Committee consensus statement on thermoregulatory and altitude challenges for high level athletes'. *British Journal of Sports Medicine* 46(11): 770–79. (2012)

Bloomfield, J., Fricker, P. A. and Fitch, K. D. *Textbook of Science and Medicine in Sport*. Melbourne: Blackwell Scientific Publications. (1992)

Brewer, J. *London 2012 Training Guide – Athletics (Track Events)*. London: Carlton. (2011)

Brooks, G. A. and Fahey, T. D. *Exercise Physiology: Human Bioenergetics and its applications*. New York: John Wiley & Sons. (1984)

Browns, F. *Nutritional Needs of Athletes*. Chichester: John Wiley. (1993)

Cermak, N. M. and van Loon, L. J. 'The use of carbohydrates during exercise as an ergogenic aid'. *Sports Medicine* 43(11): 1139–55. (2013)

Cohn, E. E. and Stumpf, P. K. *Outlines of Biochemistry*. 3rd edn. New York: John Wiley & Sons. (1972)

De Vries, H. A. and Housh, T. J. *Physiology of Exercise*. 6th edn. Madison, WI: Brown & Benchmark. (1994)

Donath, R. and Schüler, K. P. *Enharung Der Sportler*. Berlin: Sportverlag. (1972)

Ehlert, T., Simon, P. and Moser, D. A. 'Epigenetics in sports'. *Sports Medicine* 43(2): 93–110. (2013)

Folk, G. E. *Textbook of Environmental Physiology*. Philadelphia, PA: Lea & Febiger. (1974)

Ganong, W. F. *Review of Medical Physiology*. 6th edn. San Francisco, CA: Lange Medical Publications. (1973)

Giampietro, M., Bellotto, P. and Cardavone, G. 'Nutritional supplements'. *NSA* 13(2): 31–3. (1998)

Grisogono, V. *Children and Sport: Fitness, Injuries, Diet*. London: John Murray. (1991)

Gunnarsson, T. P. and Bangsbo, J. 'The 10–20–30 training concept improves performance and health profile in moderately trained runners'. *Journal of Applied Physiology (1985)* 113(1): 16–24. (2012)

Harries, M. *The Oxford Textbook of Sports Medicine*. Oxford: Oxford University Press. (1994)

Harris, R. C., Sodeland, K. and Hultman, E. 'Elevation of creative in resting and exercised muscle of normal subjects by creative supplementation'. *Clinical Science* 83: 367–74. (1992)

Hausswirth, C. and Mujika, I. *Recovery for Performance in Sport*. Champaign, IL: Human Kinetics. (2013)

Houlihan, B. *Dying to Win: Doping in Sport and the development of Anti-Doping Policy*. Strasbourg: Council of Europe Publishing. (2002).

Hill, A. V. *Living Machinery*. London: G. Bell & Sons. (1945)

Holmer, I. 'Physiology of swimming man'. *Acta Physiologica Scandanavica* 407(Suppl.). (1974)

Howard, H. and Poortmans, J. R. *Metabolic Adaptation to Prolonged Physical Exercise*. Basel: Birkhauser Verlag. (1975)

International Association of Athletics Federations. *Too Thin to Win*. Monaco: IAAF. (1989)

International Olympic Committee. 'Consensus statement on sports nutrition.' *Journal of Sports Science* 29(Suppl. 1): S3–4. (2011)

Jeffries, M. *Know Your Body*. London: BBC Publications. (1976)

Jeukendrup, A. E. 'Nutrition for endurance sports: marathon, triathlon and road cycling'. *Journal of Sports Science* 29(Suppl. 1): S91–9. (2011)

Jones, A. M., Krustrup, P., Wilkerson, D. P., Berger, N. J., Calbet, J. A. and Bangsbo, J. 'Influence of exercise intensity on skeletal muscle blood flow, O2 extraction and O2 uptake on kinetics'. *Journal of Physiology* 1: 4363–76. (2012)

Jones, D. A. and Round, J. *Skeletal Muscle in Health and Disease*. Manchester: Manchester University Press. (1990)

Karlsson, J. 'Lactate and phosphagen concentrations in the working muscle of man'. *Acta Physiologica Scandanavica* 358 (Suppl.). (1971)

Katch, V. L., McArdle, W. D. and Katch, F. I. *Essentials of Exercise Physiology*. 4th edn. Baltimore, MD: Lippincott, Williams & Wilkins. (2010)

King, J. B. *Sports Medicine*. Edinburgh: Churchill Livingstone. (1992)

Komi, P. V. *Strength and Power in Sport*. Oxford: Blackwell Scientific. (1992)

Kelman, G. R., Maughan, R. J. and Williams, C. 'The effects of dietary modifications on blood lactate during exercise'. *Journal of Physiology* 251: 34–5. (1975)

Lee, M. *Coaching Children in Sport: Principles and Practice*. London: E. & F. N. Spon. (1993)

Luce, G. G. *Body Time*. London: Temple Smith. (1972)

McCardle, W. D., Katch, F. I. and Katch, V. L. *Exercise Physiology: Nutrition, Energy and Human Performance*. Baltimore, MD: Lippincott Williams & Wilkins. (2009)

Macleod, D. A. D., Maughan, R. J., Nimmo, M., Reilly, T. and Williams, C. *Exercise: Benefits, Limitations and Adaptations*. London: E. & F. N. Spon. (1991)

Macleod, D. A. D., Maughan, R. J., Williams, C., Madeley, C. R., Sharp, J. C. M. and Nutton, R. W. *Intermittent High Intensity Exercise*. London: E. & F. N. Spon. (1993)

McLintic, J. R. *Basic Anatomy and Physiology of the Human Body*. New York: John Wiley & Sons. (1975)

McNaught, A. B. and Callender, R. *Illustrated Physiology*. Edinburgh: Churchill Livingstone. (1963)

McNeill, A. R. *The Human Machine*. London: Natural History Museum Publications. (1992)

Maffetone, P. *In Fitness and In Health*. Stamford, NY: David Barmore Productions. (2002)

Maffulif, N. *Color Atlas and Text of Sports Medicine in Childhood and Adolescence*. London: Mosby Wolfe. (1993)

Margaria, R. *Biomechanics and Energetics of Muscular Exercise*. Oxford: Clarendon Press. (1976)

Martin, G. E. 'Influence of elevated climatic heat stress on competition in Atlanta 1996'. *HSA* 12(4): 65–78. (1997)

Morehouse, L. E. and Miller, A. T. *Physiology of Exercise*. 5th edn. St Louis, MO: C. V. Mosby. (1967)

Murphy S. *Marathon from Start to Finish*. London: A. & C. Black. (2004)

Pernow, B. and Saltin, B. *Muscle Metabolism During Exercise*. New York: Plenum Press. (1971)

Richardson, R. G. 'Proceedings of the Joint Conference with the British Olympic Committee on Altitude Training'. *BASM* 8(1). (1974)

Robergs, R. A. and Roberts, S. O. *Exercise Physiology.* St Louis, MO: Mosby. (1997)

Robson, H. E. 'Proceedings of the XVIIIth World Congress of Sports Medicine (1970)'. *British Journal of Sports Medicine* 7(1–2). (1973)

Scheuer, J. and Tipton, C. N. 'Cardiovascular adaptation to physical training'. *Annual Review of Physiology* 39: 221–51. (1977)

Sergeant, A. J. and Kernell, D. *Neuromuscular Fatigue.* Amsterdam: North Holland. (1993)

Sharp, N. C. C. 'The Health of the Next Generation: Health through fitness and sport'. *Journal of the Royal Society for Health* 116(1): 48–55. (1995)

Shepherd, R. J. and Astrand, P. O. *Endurance in Sport.* Oxford: Blackwell Scientific. (1992)

Shirreffs, S. M., Casa, D. J. and Carter, R., 3rd 'Fluid needs for training and competition in athletics'. *Journal of Sports Sciences* 25 (Suppl. 1): S83–91. (2007)

Sperryn, P. 'Proceedings of the International Symposium on Anabolic Steroids in Sport'. *BASM* 9(2). (1975)

Stanton, R. *Eating for Peak Performance.* London: Allen & Unwin. (1988)

Sufte, N. K., Gushiken, T. T. and Zarins, B. *The Elite Athlete.* New York: SP Medical and Scientific Books. (1986)

Tanner, R. and Gore, C. *Physiological Tests for Elite Athletes.* Champaign, IL: Human Kinetics, (2013)

Tanner, J. M. and Taylor, G. R. *Growth.* 5th edn. Amsterdam: Time Life International. (1975)

Tipton, K. D. and Wolfe, R. R. (2004) 'Protein and amino acids for athletes'. *Journal of Sports Sciences* 22(1): 65–79.

Weiler, R., Allardyce, S., Whyte, G. P. and Stamatakis, E. 'Is the lack of physical activity strategy for children complicit mass neglect?' *British Journal of Sports Medicine* doi:10.1136/bjsports-2013-093018 (2013)

Wells, C. L. *Women, Sport and Performance: A Physiological Perspective.* Champaign, IL: Human Kinetics. (1985)

Wilki, D. R. 'The relationship Between Sport and Velocity in Human Muscle'. *J Physiol,* 110; 249–280 (1949)

Williams, C. 'Special forms and effects of endurance training'. *5th Coaches' Convention Report.* (1974)

Williams, C., Kelman, G. R., Couper, D. C. and Harris, C. G. 'Changes in plasma FFA concentrations before and after reduction in high intensity exercise' *Journal of Sports Medicine and Physical Fitness* 15: 2–12. (1975)

Wilmore, J. H. and Costill, D. L. *Physiology of Sport and Exercise.* Champaign, IL: Human Kinetics. (1994)

PART 3
MISSION CONTROL

It has been suggested that coaching is 'more an art than a science'. This is, in part, because coaches are working with athletes who are young and multifaceted. It is perhaps also because much of the early research on coaching was about exceptional coaches who had little formal education and spoke of learning from other coaches and from their own experiences. These are certainly effective ways to learn. However, in the current world of competitive sport, coaches who want to thrive and excel are wise to pursue a formal education and begin to see themselves as life-long learners. Competitive sport has simply become far too complex. Coaches must now learn about biomechanics, anatomy, and physiology, as well as become students of human behavior. This knowledge includes how to motivate athletes, how to teach effectively, how to build a cohesive team, how to communicate and effectively manage conflict, and how to enable athletes to manage the anxiety and fears that are inherent in competitive sport. Indeed, coaching is both a science and an art. It is your responsibility as a coach to prepare your athletes physically, technically and psychologically for sport and for life after sport, and do so in an ethical manner. This requires a deep knowledge of the sciences. The art is to take that scientific knowledge and apply it in many different contexts and with many different athletes.

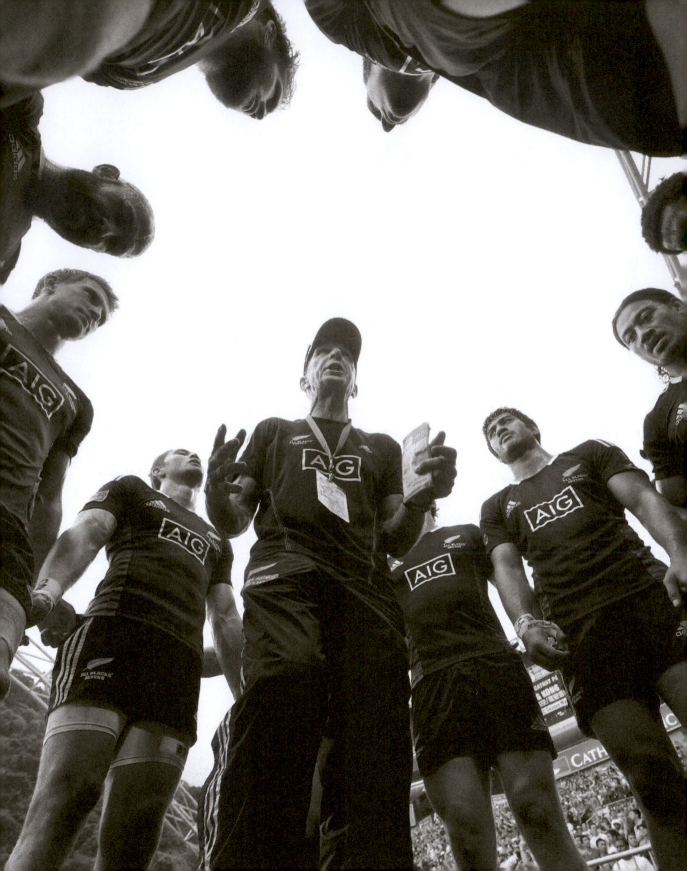

10 SPORT PSYCHOLOGY FOR COACHES

There are a number of pieces of what we might call 'the performance puzzle' that are crucial for success at the high performance sport level. The largest pieces of the performance puzzle are certainly on the physiological side (part 2) and training theory and practice (parts 4 and 5). Another piece of the puzzle encompasses aspects such as socio-culture, family, school, friends, and partners (this chapter and chapter 13). A final piece of the performance puzzle is the psychological side – while the physical side is the most important during the training phase, as the competition phase begins the psychological aspects become more important. Why? The psychological aspect becomes important close to and during competition simply because competition is inherently stressful and athletes need to learn to effectively manage the stress in order to perform optimally in such an environment. Therefore as coaches, you must prepare your athletes both physically and psychologically. We should not deny the inherent stress of competition – we should embrace it and prepare for it!

This chapter looks at psychology for your athletes under three headings to discuss the most relevant aspects of psychology ... your athletes:

1. The art of coaching
2. The skills of psychological preparation
3. Creating the best environment for young developing athletes.

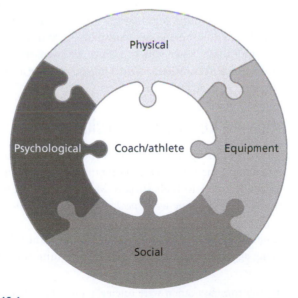

FIGURE 10.1 Components of the 'performance puzzle' impacting the athlete and coach

THE ART OF COACHING

Coaching is about leadership. It is about working with athletes at varying ages and experiences and it can be argued that a coach's goal should be twofold: (a) to create an independent and capable athlete, and (b) to create more skilled performances and ultimately personal best performances when it counts most – at a national championship, at a selection competition, at a world championship, at an Olympic Games.

As a coach you are a leader, and leadership has been defined in many different ways. James Kouzes and Barry Posner, who wrote *The Leadership Challenge* (2002), have defined leadership as the art of mobilising people to want to struggle for shared aspirations. Max DePree, former CEO of the prestigious furniture company, Herman Millar, in his excellent book, *Leadership Jazz*, wrote: 'From a leader's perspective, the most serious betrayal has to do with thwarting human potential, with quenching the spirit, with failing to deal equitably with each other as human beings.' (DePree, 1992: 34)

Kouzes and Posner developed a leadership model based on research with over 75,000 women and men, in a wide range of leadership roles, about the experiences where they were able to accomplish something extraordinary. What they discovered was a recurring pattern of five leadership practices and a set of behaviors that were present when leaders are effective. The five leadership practices are: *model the way, inspire a shared vision, challenge the process, enable others to act,* and *encourage the heart.* For example, when, as a coach when you effectively '*model the way*' you are clear about your core values and your coaching philosophy, you do what you say you will do, and you demonstrate the same behaviors you expect of your athletes. When you '*inspire a shared vision*', you speak clearly about your purpose, talk with energy about your own goals and your athletes' goals, believe in each athlete's ability to succeed, and listen well to any concerns and issues. When you '*challenge the process*' you regularly reflect on your training programme and look for ways to do things differently and better, you question accepted practices, schedule opportunities to continue learning throughout your coaching career, experiment and assess, and look outside your own sport for new ideas. When you '*enable others to act*' you understand that it is crucial you build independent, thinking athletes, who take responsibility for their actions, you develop a relationship of confidence and trust with your athletes, you involve your athletes and others in decision-making, and when appropriate, make it easy for your athletes to ask questions. And finally, when you '*encourage the heart*' you look for the good work and reward that work with a smile and a quick acknowledgement, and you provide a combination of critique and positive feedback on a regular basis.

Effective communication – a key leadership skill[*]

The key skill that underlies effective leadership, and that allows you, as a coach, to execute what Kouzes and Posner (2002) called the five leadership practices, is *effective communication.* Many leading coaches say that their ability to communicate skillfully is key to their success. More specifically, to be an effective communicator you need to develop the skills of *listening well, speaking clearly and concisely, providing constructive feedback,* and *resolving conflict effectively.*

Before addressing the key skills of good communication, it is important to understand the difference between being assertive and being aggressive or passive. Skillful communication is about two individuals,

---

[*] Portions of this section on effective communication were originally published in http://www.coach.ca/women/e/journal/jan2001

or groups, who are engaged in a discussion, being able to remain assertive. The danger, particularly when something contentious or difficult is being discussed, is that one of the individuals – you or your athlete – fall into the trap of becoming either aggressive or passive.

What does it mean to be assertive rather than aggressive or passive? According to Webster's Dictionary *assertive* means 'to state positively, to affirm.' *Aggressive* is defined as 'to undertake an attack, to begin a quarrel' and *passive* is defined as 'being the object of rather than the subject of action; unresisting, submissive.' Being assertive in communicating with your athletes means you value and care for each one of them as an individual. (Over the years, many athletes have said that they wish their coach had treated them as an individual, and not always as just a part of the team.) Being assertive means you treat your athletes with respect, even when you are not in agreement.

Listening well

One of the more difficult and least understood skills of effective communication is the ability to listen well to what is being said. In fact, when you are listening well, you listen to understand what the other person is thinking or feeling, rather than focusing on your response. One of the most powerful ways to enhance understanding is to stop talking! And you have to remember that understanding what someone says does not necessarily mean agreement. To listen effectively, you need to permit yourself to really listen to your athlete – to clearly hear what they are saying before you respond or even begin to think about how to resolve a problem. Kline (2003) argues that 'giving good attention to people makes them more intelligent' (p. 37) and 'to help people think for themselves, first listen' (p. 39).

Why is it so important for a coach to listen well? First of all, so much conflict between individuals results because of incorrect assumptions – and incorrect assumptions often happen because we are eager to respond and solve rather than listen first. 'Oh, I thought the practice was at 3 o'clock.' 'I thought we were practising *this* play.' 'I thought you meant … ' 'I thought my job was to …'

These are examples of what can happen when one does not listen well – whether it is you not listening to your athletes or your athletes not listening to you. When you are able to listen first, there is a lot less misunderstanding and therefore a great deal less conflict. Second, and equally important, when you listen to your athletes, you are better able to understand what they are thinking and feeling and you can then make specific and effective corrections to a training session or create a better plan for a future competition. Third, when you regularly allow your athletes to express their thoughts and concerns, they begin to take responsibility for their actions and think for themselves. Taking personal responsibility and becoming an independent thinker is what they need to be doing, and exactly what you need them to be capable of doing on the field or track, or in the pool, in training, and particularly during competition. After all, it is the athlete who ultimately has to run the race or play the game.

Importantly, allowing yourself to listen to your athletes does not mean that you then allow them to make all the decisions. What it does mean is that when you are able to listen well, you are able to make an informed decision. You can decide if a change is warranted, and if it is not, then you can clearly explain your reasoning.

Speaking clearly and concisely

Two significant aspects of your job as a coach are giving direction and instruction to your athletes during training sessions and competition and dealing with issues or conflicts as they arise. In both situations you want to speak clearly and concisely.

For example, what if one of your athletes is late for training three days in a row and you are beginning to feel quite angry. What is the best way to deal with such behaviour?

Name the behaviour. '**I** want to discuss being late three days in a row.'

Name what *you are feeling*. '***I'm*** quite upset.'

Say what *you need.* 'I need to talk with you about this because we cannot get the practice done effectively when you are a half hour late.'

'I' messages such as the above are clear, concise, and come from what you feel and what you need. Name the issue in an even tone of voice, with no judgment or sarcasm attached. Name the emotion you are experiencing, but stop there. Do not go on with all the concurrent feelings you might be having. And finally, and importantly, state what you need, because only you know what that is.

Providing constructive feedback

Your coaching job, simply stated, is to help each athlete you work with to become increasingly better at executing the speed, skills, or game strategies of your sport. As a result, you are constantly feeding back information to your athletes. What is important to understand, in terms of feedback, is that almost every athlete needs a 'healthy' balance of *critique-to-praise ratio*. What that healthy ratio is will vary from athlete to athlete and vary according to the proximity to a competition.

Giving critical feedback has been cited as one of the least favourite tasks by leaders in the business world, yet in the same breath it is also cited as being essential to success (Lizzio, 2008). The key for coaches is to ensure that their feedback is *constructive*.

Critique-to-praise ratio – generally speaking, the closer to the competition, the more you need to shift your feedback to what the athlete is doing well and away from what is not going well. You do this, first of all, because at some point it is too late to fix the issue. You have to go with what you have until after the competition. Second, and perhaps most importantly, you do this because the athlete's confidence can be fragile and this fragility can increase as competition nears. Most athletes will begin to question their readiness, their skills, their ability. This is a natural reaction to stress. A significant part of your job as a coach is to alleviate that stress and reassure each of your athletes or your team that they are well prepared.

Importantly, shifting your feedback ratio toward 'what we are doing well' does not mean that you do not critique. It means you are doing less critiquing close to a competition. Shifting that ratio and being positive means intentionally observing what your athlete or team is doing well and specifically feeding back that information to them.

Resolving conflict effectively

As a coach you regularly encounter situations that have the potential to escalate into a conflict. Athletes within your training group or on your team may not like each other. An athlete may not like your way of coaching. You may have problems with a member of your sport science team.

The very nature of conflict is an interesting and sometimes misunderstood concept. Conflict is a natural occurrence in our lives and some degree of conflict is often inevitable whenever two or more individuals come together. It is important to recognise and understand conflict and to seek, first of all, to prevent as much conflict as possible and, when it occurs, to work toward resolving conflict effectively.

Indeed, conflict can be *constructive* when it opens up discussion on issues of importance, when it results in solutions to those issues, and when it increases the involvement of individuals in the discussion. But conflict is *destructive* when it begins to take too much energy and diverts focus from more important activities (like training and recovery), destroys an individual's sense of self-confidence, and polarises a team into two groups.

How does conflict occur? One way that conflict begins relates to *information*. There is a misunderstanding, a miscommunication, or a lack of information. A second way conflict occurs is over *how things are to be done* – the methods. If you and your strength coach disagree over the kinds of strength training your team should be doing and the frequency, you have a conflict.

 A third way conflict occurs is over *what is to be done* or achieved, such as goals for your team. You as the coach want to ensure that consensus is built around not only how your athlete will train or practice, but also what the long-term goals are. If you think your athlete has the talent and tenacity to succeed nationally or internationally and his/her parents do not have the willingness or the financial resources to support the travel, you have a potential conflict.

Finally, a fourth way conflict occurs is over *differing values,* and this is probably the most difficult type of conflict to effectively resolve. For example, you may believe that your athlete can compete successfully at the national and international level and still get an education. You might believe that this is a necessary element for a successful life after sport but are faced with your sport governing body that believes if they are providing funding and resources for this athlete then he or she must devote all their time to training. This will be a difficult conflict to resolve.

These are some of the ways that conflict might begin. The good news is that through learning and effectively using all of the skills of effective communication, you will be able to prevent a great deal of conflict within your team and with your athletes. When you listen well, when you speak clearly and concisely, when you provide effective feedback, and when you can share these skills with your athletes, you prevent a great deal of conflict. And when conflict or issues do arise, you will be able to manage them well and resolve the issues effectively, using those same skills.

Finally, within the context of effective communication, you, as a coach, will most likely be coaching both female and male athletes, and it is therefore important to understand there are differences in the way that women and men communicate.

In her book *You Just Don't Understand, Women and Men in Conversation* (1990), and in an article in *Harvard Business Review* entitled 'The Power Of Talk: Who Gets Heard and Why' (1995), Deborah Tannen has written about the influence of linguistic styles on conversations and relationships, particularly in terms of the differences in women and men's communication. What exactly does Tannen mean by *linguistic style*? Everything each of us says, whether we are female or male, is said in a certain way, in a certain tone of voice, at a certain speed, with a certain choice of words, with directness or indirectness, and with a certain degree of quietness or loudness. Each of us has a certain speaking pattern, and Tannen argues that there are fundamental differences between women and men in how those patterns look and sound. 'In other words, linguistic style is a set of culturally learned signals by which we not only communicate what we mean but also interpret others' meaning and evaluate one another as people.' Tannen says that language communicates ideas and, at the same time, negotiates relationships. So how is that relevant for you as a coach?

When you speak with your athletes, you are conveying information and knowledge and you are, in fact, building relationships between you and your athletes and colleagues. Research has shown that the patterns that make up how men and women speak are not the same. According to Tannen, we learn ways of speaking as children, especially from peers, and children tend to play with other children of the same gender. She states that research on North American children has shown that girls tend to play in small groups or with a single friend, spend a lot of time talking, and tend to downplay ways one girl is better than another. Boys tend to play in larger groups. In essence, Tannen argues that boys, growing into young men, use talk to emphasise status and girls, growing into young women, use talk to create connections. (As Tannen importantly notes, not all boys and girls grow up in this way, but it tends to be the way conversational styles are learned.) Often young women athletes are as concerned with being liked by their teammates as they are with being skilled. As a coach working with these young women athletes, you want to help them understand that they can be competitive, excel at their sport, and still be liked and appreciated by the team.

In addition, Tannen argues that in terms of verbal behaviour, women are more likely to downplay their certainty and men are more likely to minimise their doubts.

What does this mean for you, particularly if you coach both female and male athletes? Primarily it means that you need to hone your listening skills. Is the male athlete who appears confident really feeling ready and well prepared? Is the female athlete who is reluctant to state out loud that she is confident and ready really lacking in confidence? Here is where you need to be very careful about making assumptions. You need to step back, ask questions of each of your athletes to find out what they are thinking and feeling, and really listen as they speak. What they say and what they mean may differ. At the same time, as a coach, you need to be aware that while there may be differences between how female and male athletes communicate, there are also a great deal of similarities as they mature. As one coach has said 'Both genders want to know everything – it is more about the readiness and maturity of the athlete than gender.'

Keeping in mind these notions of differing communication styles of women and men, what implications might they have for you? Awareness of how the conversational styles of women and men differ will make it easier for you to ensure that each athlete has a voice and is heard by you. There really is no one best way to communicate, but understanding your own personal communication style and preferences, and then listening for the style and preferences of others, will go a very long way in improving the effectiveness of your coaching and the success of your athletes.

Skilful communication is a flowing, ongoing process. The speaker, the listener, and the message are ever changing. For you as a coach, it is a continuous dialogue. You can't speak one time only with your athletes about an issue and assume that it will never come up again. Inevitably, it will. And new issues, concerns, and ideas will also arise. Be generous in sharing these communication skills with your athletes and your support team. After all, if everyone you work with becomes more effective at communicating, all of you will be much more effective. And you will be 'successful' as a coach – not only in terms of results, but also in developing thinking, independent, responsible athletes.

THE SKILLS OF PSYCHOLOGICAL PREPARATION

There are a group of psychological skills that must be trained to provide an athlete with the opportunity to succeed and become consistent in performance. You as a coach certainly know that physical skills, and technical and tactical components, must be practiced regularly and refined to become competent in a sport. Psychological skills must be practiced in a similar way. The specific psychological skills are: *the ability to develop a deep level of self-awareness, to regularly debrief and analyse training and competition results, to focus on the correct cues, to manage negative distractions, to set effective long and short term goals, to image, to build an effective team, and to manage arousal levels.* Each of these skills will be discussed in detail. It is suggested that many of these skills are also crucial for you as a coach. As a coach, you will often experience stress and developing these skills will help you become a calm and clear thinking coach which will, in turn, help your athletes' performances. As well, if you choose to work on these skills for yourself, you will see that they take time to learn – often a season or two – and this understanding will help as you work with your athletes on these skills (see figure 10.2).

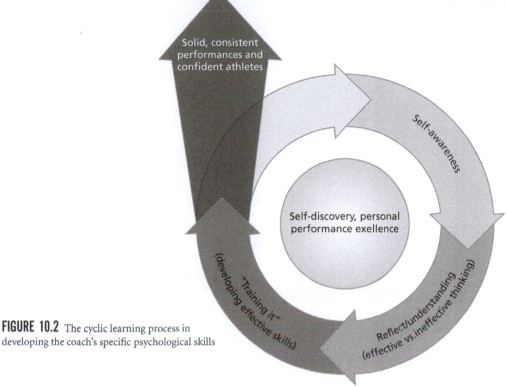

FIGURE 10.2 The cyclic learning process in developing the coach's specific psychological skills

Developing self-awareness

Martens (1987) stated many years ago that sport psychology's motto is 'know thyself'. Helping your athletes, and yourself, develop a good sense of self-awareness is a crucial skill for competitive sport. Knowing what one is good at technically, tactically, strategically, and psychologically, and knowing what one needs to work on, is developed through regular dialogue with your athletes during training sessions, and regular analysis and a debriefing process after competitions. This process builds self-awareness, self-responsibility, creates a level of self-confidence, and ultimately ensures consistently good performances.

Debriefing/analysis of performance

What is debriefing?

Great coaches and athletes *dream* (set goals); *plan* (create a strategy); *do* (execute); and *review* (debrief and learn) (see figure 10.3). Debriefing is a critical learning opportunity for both athletes and coaches and is crucial for excelling at the highest levels. Debriefing is defined as 'an evaluative activity either in training or in competition, with the intended purpose of analyzing existing performance states and determining what might be improved to ensure future performance satisfaction, enjoyment, success, and fulfillment' (Hogg, 2002, p. 182). Effective and regular debriefing encourages continued improvement, fosters clear and honest communication, helps the athlete take responsibility for his performance, and allows him to close the chapter emotionally on past performances – good and poor – in order to move on to the next training block and competition (Kellmann et al., 2006). Debriefing is a tool to promote accountability, objective discussion about progress and results, as well as an integral piece to ongoing learning.

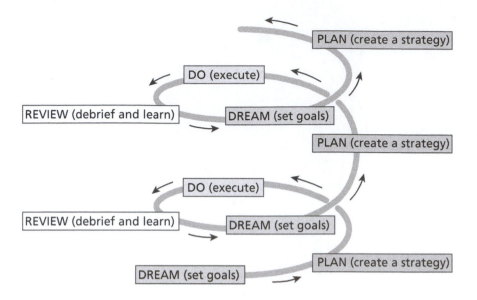

FIGURE 10.3 The approach to setting goals; planning how to achieve them; delivering necessary action, learning from the experiences; then setting the next goal is a continual spiral

Every race or game situation provides an opportunity to help your athlete increase self-awareness and define new actions for improvement. The practice of debriefing involves analysing a performance soon after a competition. Following a debriefing session the athlete should be clear on precisely how they are progressing, where they stand relative to identified performance goals, and what they need to focus on to improve.

Why is debriefing important?

Debriefing at any level of competitive sport is important because it allows meaningful discussion and constructive feedback relating to both the performance process and the outcome. A successful debrief has been shown to increase learning, motivation and confidence, cognitive and emotional recovery and improved self-awareness (Gould et al., 1999; Hogg, 2002; McArdle et al., 2010).

Psychological recovery is also an essential part of effective debriefing. There are often strong mental and emotional responses after a competition and it is important for recovery that the athlete is able to talk about those emotions – to avoid carrying negative emotions (e.g., self-doubt, perceptions of incompetence, feelings of fear, feelings of failure) into the next competition. After a sub-optimal performance, athletes often suffer immense disappointment and yet are more likely to recover well if they can express their emotions, step back and reflect objectively on the whole performance, and learn from any mistakes. And it is important to debrief good performances as well as poor performances. Much can be learned from a great race or game – for example, asking questions such as 'How did that happen?' 'What did I do that resulted in a personal best?' – and then constructing a plan to incorporate that learning into the next competition.

What do I need to know about myself before starting the debriefing process?

Just like athletes, coaches (and support staff) are also accountable for whether or not the athlete is able to perform to expectations. The pressure for performance has the potential to generate strong emotions in coaches and can lead to a rather subjective evaluation of an athlete's performance. External feedback is 'meaningless if it is regarded by athletes as biased and self-serving or if coaches are overly preoccupied with negative outcomes and impose guilty feelings' (Hogg, 2002, p. 183). The goal of debriefing is to look openly and objectively at a performance without judgement, and to collaborate on how learning and performance can be enhanced. A key tenet of the debriefing process is the process of communication between the athlete, coach and identified support staff. One-way performance evaluations that are autocratic in nature limit the athlete's capacity to think and may also promote fear of evaluation and judgement. The athlete must believe that you are there to promote learning and to support their endeavor.

There are various ways you can debrief. First, on a regular basis, you can do an informal debrief with each of your athletes after each competition. This level of debriefing might just be a half-hour conversation, listening well to what the athlete is thinking, and then providing some feedback that will shape the next few weeks of training and the next competition. Another level of debriefing is at the end of the season of competition or after a major competition, such as a World Championship or an Olympic Games. Here, the outcome of the campaign is viewed as the consequence of input from all the individuals who have influenced the consequence. So the debrief with the athlete is simply one part of the overall debrief with all of those individuals involved in the preparation for the campaign. At this level, open and honest *self*-reflection by the coach and sport science support staff involved should be completed prior to engaging in the debriefing process with the athlete. Coaches, athletes, and sport science support staff can reflect individually prior to meeting. Then you, as the coach, bring the group together to discuss and subsequently plan for the following season. A variation of this would be if you, as the coach, did this with your sport science support team, and then just you and the athlete met.

How to prepare your athlete(s) for the debrief process

Initially, athletes do not always have the capacity to self-reflect effectively and objectively. If an athlete is overly self-critical, which is sometimes the case, you risk creating an environment where the athlete becomes discouraged and anxious. It is also possible that the athlete is simply striving to feel comfortable and is not able to critique constructively and that will also not help him or her progress. The balance therefore is in becoming comfortable and open with the debriefing process. (See appendices A and B for examples of a debrief form that can help with the process.)

How to guide the debriefing process effectively
Timing
When scheduling the post-performance debrief it is important to consider the timing. Immediately post-competition, you and/or your athlete may be quite emotional, particularly if the performance is sub-optimal. In this case, it is wise to wait until a good warm down has been completed or perhaps until the next day. Nevertheless, it is important that debriefing occur soon after the event so that vivid detail of the competition can be retained. The athlete and coach should determine the optimal time and place to debrief where they can both be in a productive self-reflective frame of mind. It can be completed the following day, but generally not two weeks later!

Athlete self-reflection
Athletes, if they aspire to a high performance level, must develop the ability to objectively assess performance and determine whether or not they did what was required. A thorough self-reflection on all aspects of performance (technical, physical, tactical, and psychological) will allow for the athlete to learn from his or her experiences. An athlete must be able to openly acknowledge both strengths and weaknesses and be aware

of what she or he must do to ensure optimal recovery and improve future performances. Debriefing allows the athlete to express his or her views about what happened and what could be improved.

Significant others performance analysis

For major debriefs, such as after a Word Championship, an Olympic Games or the year-end reviews, coaches and other sport science staff should also complete a full reflection on the performance before entering the debriefing meeting.

The debrief meeting

Attitude and approach are critical to a successful and productive debriefing process. Positive communication requires all individuals involved to be open, honest, and sincere. Coaches can help create this environment by remaining calm and objective and not overly critical or judgemental. They can also help the athlete manage emotions by encouraging the same calm objective approach for them. Coaches should ask the athlete to speak first. And then listen well to what he or she thinks and feels. You then provide your analysis, and discuss any differences you might see. You create an environment for a healthy analysis and positive solutions by completing the debriefing by focusing on resetting goals and restructuring plans to move forward.

Evaluation of the debriefing process

For the debriefing process to be effective, it must be consistent and regular! It is not a one-time thing and it cannot be ignored especially at the end of the season and after important events. After implementing a debriefing programme with your athlete, reflect on: (a) whether it was helpful for the athlete's learning, (b) if improvements in performance were made or not, (c) if your communication and relationship with the athlete was enhanced or diminished, and (d) if the athlete was able to engage in the process and become more accountable for future performances.

Developing the ability to focus effectively

The skill of focus, or knowing what to 'pay attention to' is a key psychological skill.

Focus can be defined as the 'deliberate investment of conscious mental effort … to focus on the task at hand while ignoring distractions' (Moran, 2009, p. 18–19). An effective focus is when an athlete focuses on 'actions that are specific, relevant to the task at hand and, above all, under his or her own control' (p. 20). Research on the skill of focus has demonstrated that it is a crucial skill for sport performance success (e.g., Bois et al., 2009; Greenleaf et al., 2001; Moran, 2003; Orlick and Partington, 1988; Wulf and Su, 2007), and may differentiate elite from non-elite performers (Meyers et al., 1999).

Nideffer (1976) and Nideffer and Segal (2001) described attentional focus along two dimensions (broad or narrow) and direction (internal or external). An example of a broad attentional focus is a basketball player needing to attend to his play as well as what is going on around him on the court. An example of a narrow attentional focus is a golfer preparing to putt. An example of an external focus is an athlete directing his attention to a ball in field hockey and an internal focus is an athlete is thinking about his thoughts and feelings in a run-up to the triple jump.

The 'correct' focus will be dependent on the sport you are coaching and the individual athlete. For example, from an event perspective, if your athlete competes in an event of short duration – for example, 100 or 200m in athletics – then a clear focus on a couple of technical cues must be maintained for that approximately 10–12 seconds/20–24 seconds. If your athlete competes in the marathon, which will take over 2 hours in duration, focus will be different – an athlete might alternate between a focus on several cues on relaxed running technique and a rather less-focused state of rhythm and enjoyment, particularly early in the race. If you are coaching an athlete in a game sport such as soccer, the athlete must learn to focus when on the field – preferably on aspects related to his position and 'job'/role, and then when on the bench, relax, recover, and then prepare to play again. You must also consider where the athlete is in his career and maturity level. For example, a young, very talented athlete in ice hockey became very frustrated when things did not go well. He would come off the ice after his shift, smash his stick and yell at himself and his teammates. So a plan was developed: first he could not yell or smash his stick. Then, with the two minutes he had on the bench before he went back on the ice, he had 30 seconds to be angry and frustrated and feel all the emotions he might have, 30 seconds to slow down his breathing and relax, and one minute to refocus and plan what he would do differently and better when he got back on the ice. With some practice, it was a strategy that worked well.

So what are other difficulties with understanding and training how to focus effectively? There are a couple of key issues you face as a coach. First, in this age of the iPhone, personal computers, Facebook, Twitter etc., most of your athletes will be more accustomed to multi-tasking rather than maintaining a singular focus. Second, often when athletes become fairly skilled at their sport, they do not 'need' to focus in order to execute the skills in the training environment. However, when we step into the stressful environment of competition, if they have not trained what and how to focus, they often underperform. Third, often athletes who are 'driven' to excel will 'over analyse' and focus too much, for example, on the movement pattern of the skill. And fourth, competition is stressful, and many things can negatively distract an athlete from an effective focus. Negative distractions and how to cope with them will be discussed in a later skill section.

How will you help your athlete improve her or his ability to focus effectively?

1. With your athlete, *set specific daily goals* for each practice/training session, with key technical, strategic or split times to work on. When *committed* to a daily technical or tactical goal, you ensure your athlete is focused in practice – and then in competition, the focus should be the same, not more! For example: in working with a diver who went on to win an Olympic medal in 10m, her objective each day was 100 per cent good dives. So when working on the hurdle, the twist or the entry, as instructed by her coach, the objective was for each dive to be very good. Therefore, to give herself the best chance to accomplish this, she needed to pay attention to what her coach said and try her best to execute. Of course, she did not execute 100 per cent – but her percentage of very good dives increased from 70 per cent to 92 per cent over the course of the year leading up to the Olympic Games. Then, at the Games, the coach joked that all she needed to do was 15 good dives – she dived superbly and won the Olympic silver medal.

2. With your athlete, develop a set of words – *cue words* – that will help him to be calm and focused. It could be reminders such as 'shoulders down', 'breathe', 'explosive', and/or technical cues such as 'left hip down', 'stay forward' and/or words that build confidence, such as 'I have trained hard', 'I am well-prepared'. These words will be successful when the athlete has tried them out in a competition and reflected on what works. Mallett and Hanrahan's (1997) study with sprinters supports the benefit of using cue words for improving focus and performance.

3. With your athlete, develop *pre-competition plans and race/game plans*. Pre-competition plans help an athlete be organised prior to competing, ensures they do not forget equipment, and that they are on time.

All of this helps manage the anxiety that is inevitable in the competitive environment. For example, in a study on golfers, Cohn, Rotella, and Lloyd (1990) detailed the importance of pre-competition plans.

A plan for racing/playing is very much a 'focus plan' – this is what your athlete will focus on when they are playing the game, racing, executing the skill. Many in-depth interviews with elite athletes have confirmed the importance of race or game plans in helping sustain an optimal attentional focus. (i.e. Greenleaf et al., 2001; Orlick and Partington, 1988).

4. You can simulate the competitive setting, by introducing delays, crowd noise, the presence of officials, poor referee calls, training sessions in the heat or cold if that is what the conditions may be. All of these are possible negative distractions for your athletes. This is not always easy to do but it can be quite important in preparation for a World Championship or an Olympic Games.

Managing negative distractions

Negative distractions can pull an athlete out of 'best focus'. Orlick (2007) suggests that the ability to adapt and refocus in the face of distractions is a key psychological skill. Negative distractions come from myriad sources – internally, an athlete's own expectations: 'I need to qualify today' and other thoughts: 'I can't do this move, I always mess it up' and externally: such as other's expectations, winning, losing, teammates, coaches, financial issues, school, partners, family members, fatigue, injuries, etc.

How can you help your athletes manage negative distractions? You can develop, with your athlete, a 'what if' list – a list of all the possible distractions – and then list possible solutions to each 'what if'. For example, what if there is an issue with a parent, what will we do; what if there is a delay in the competition, what can we do in terms of a warm-up plan. The most important aspect to remember is you, as a coach, and your athlete, always have *a choice* to be negatively distracted or not. Learning to effectively focus, and refocus on the correct cues is always a choice – but managing distractions effectively is a skill that needs a lot of practice to be perfected – so that it works for the athlete in the stressful environment of competition. It is also important to remember that when fatigue is present it is harder to focus, refocus, and manage those negative distractions, so sleep is a key component of managing oneself.

Setting effective goals

A goal is an objective standard, or aim of some action. Subjective goals are more general statements of intent such as 'I want to have fun', 'I want to do my best' and objective goals may be more general, such as making a team or more specific such as working to attain a certain proficiency of a skill. Locke and Latham (2002) have said objective goals are about 'attaining a specific standard of proficiency on a task, usually within a specified time' (p. 705).

There are essentially three types of objective goals that you can set with your athletes – *outcomes goals, performance goals and process goals*. An *outcome goal* emphasises a focus on results, achieving a victory in a competitive situation, winning a game or championships, and is dependent on others. A *performance goal* emphasises achieving a standard based on an athlete's previous performance. This is a more internal goal and not quite so focused on other athlete's performances. And finally, a *process goal* emphasises actions an athlete will engage in during a performance to execute or perform well (number of rebounds, making a good pass, being relaxed and doing one's job, stretched out arm, running a certain pace) and is independent of other competitors.

What is important is that you set all three types of goals *with* your athletes – each of your athletes should be part of a dialogue with you, the coach, discussing what can and needs to be accomplished. Write down these goals and regularly revisit the goals you set – sometimes an athlete may surpass what you both believed was possible, and sometimes they get injured, sick, or do not commit to the work needed. When you set realistic and measurable goals, you can assess accurately, and when a goal is met it is incredibly motivating. So set lots of small, measurable, daily process goals, commit to them, and enjoy pursuing them!

It is also crucial that you understand that while all three types of goals are important, outcome goals become a very real stressor for most athletes close to a competition because the outcome is not within one's control. Close to competition and on competition day, process goals are the best because they direct an athlete's attention to what they can control, regardless of what their competitors might be doing. Remember, setting effective goals is not easy and you want to be reassessing and adjusting the goals you set several times during a season.

Imagery

Imagery is actually a form of simulation. Most athletes will 'image' all the time – what you want is that each of your athletes become more *conscious* and more 'in control' of those images.

Images can be visual ('seeing' how it can happen), auditory ('hearing' the sounds of the competition), kinesthetic ('feeling' the movement), olfactory (the 'smell' of the competition site). Each athlete will find what sense or combination of senses will work best for them.

There are two types of imagery – internal (where your athlete images the execution of a skill from his own vantage point) and external (an athlete 'sees' himself executing the skill, as in watching a video). There has been ongoing discussion in the research literature on which perspective is more effective. For example, Hardy and Callow (1999) have argued that an internal perspective is better for closed task sports that depend on perception and anticipation, and an external perspective is better for tasks that depend on form, such as gymnastics. Cumming and Ste-Marie (2001) found that the imagery perspective did not make a difference in relation to the type of task performed. So the research is certainly equivocal at this point. What is most important is that athletes develop an ability to 'see' and 'feel' correct execution of skills, their role on the field, their plan for racing. When imagery is effective, it can help build confidence, enhance motivation, speed up motor learning, and compliment the physical practice of specific skills.

How will you start to teach this skill? You can begin by asking your athlete 'to remember' or *recreate* a positive past performance or technical aspect that he already does well. When an athlete reminds himself about a past good performance – how it felt, what he focused on – it builds confidence. Then when they have developed an ability to image past events, you can ask them to 'image' or *create* something that has not happened yet, such as next week's national championships – what the venue looks like, how they want to race, what they want to focus on. This is about creating a '*blueprint*' for each of your athletes of how they want to perform.

Finally, you can have your athletes visualise potential crises and how they will be solved. For example, an athlete might visualise being called for a third attempt at an opening height in decathlon pole vault. He reaches for the selected pole but the wind picks up and it begins to rain. He must visualise how to make an effective decision with the changing conditions so that he can still deliver a successful performance.

Building an effective team

Great performances happen in sport when an athlete feels a sense of team. As a coach it is important to reflect on how to build an effective team with your group of athletes regardless of whether you coach in an individual sport or in a team sport. So how to move a group of individuals into a well functioning team? And are there different kinds of teams? Before answering those questions let's look first at the difference between a group and a team. A *group* can be defined as two or more people who interact with and exert mutual influence on each other (Aronson et al., 2002). A *team* has been defined as any group of people who must interact with each other to accomplish shared objectives (Carron and Hausenblas, 1998).

A number of models have been developed over the years of research in the area of group and team development and group cohesion, but one model that remains useful in understanding how to move a group of athletes to an effective team is Bruce Tuckman's four stages of team development (Tuckman, 1965). Tuckman proposed that groups progress through four different stages – forming, storming, norming and performing. He argued that if issues are dealt with effectively at each stage the group moves to the next stage. In the first stage, forming, athletes begin to get to know each other and look for where they might fit (Am I the best runner in this group? Am I going to be a starter on this team?). In the second stage, storming, individual athletes/players start to question you as the coach and question where they fit. This is a crucial stage for you to manage. You will need to listen to your athletes' concerns, answer their questions, be clear about the 'how' and 'why' of the training programme and competition schedule, and establish some common goals. When you do this well, the athletes begin to accept how the programme will be run, and therefore move to the third stage, norming. This third stage is when your group begins to become a team. They understand and accept their roles and start to work together to achieve those common goals. The final stage, performing, is when everyone is very much focused on the task at hand, such as winning the team championship or each performing well to accomplish best ever performance by each team member. It is important to understand that each time you bring in a new team member or members, you will likely go back to the storming stage with the group because everyone needs to find their place again. This is normal and again, if you manage it well by listening to each athlete's concerns and questions, and are clear about the direction you are leading the team, you will move the group/team on to the norming and performing stages.

So, are there different kinds of teams? When we think of building a 'team' we often think first about sports such as basketball, football, or hockey. This is not surprising because to play well and succeed in those sports, it is necessary for the athletes to share a common goal, value being part of the team and understand and accept their role on the team. When we think of individual sports such as athletics, swimming, or diving, we do not automatically think of 'team.' But you can build an effective 'team' in these types of sports although it might be done differently. You might think about individual sports from two differing 'team' perspectives. There are sports such as rowing and canoe/kayak where once a team is selected only one athlete competes in each event. Then there are sports such as swimming, speed skating and athletics, where two or more teammates contest each event. An aspect of 'team' that does exist in several individual sports, for example, are the relay teams in athletics and the crew boats in canoe/kayak and rowing.

So, how to build a team in such individual sports? Building an effective team in any sport is a critical factor in ensuring an environment that allows great performances by each athlete on a team. When you are able to move athletes from a group of individuals with a focus on themselves to a team where there is a common goal and an emphasis on helping each other, the chances of succeeding in the competitive arena grow significantly. The nature of team sports requires you, as the coach, to conduct regular team meetings to agree on and revisit team goals, discuss team strategy, resolve issues, plan for and debrief after each game. Individual athlete meetings are very important but will occur less regularly. In individual sports, the shift in emphasis is noticeable. As a coach in an individual sport, you will have training groups, but the majority of your feedback will be with the individual athlete.

Effectively managing arousal

Another key psychological skill for athletic performance is arousal control (e.g., Boiset al., 2009; Jones, 2003; Taylor et al., 2008). While arousal is the key concept, it is necessary to understand the differences between the concepts of arousal, stress, and anxiety. Arousal is a blend of physiological and psychological activity and is not necessarily related to pleasant or unpleasant events. Anxiety is a negative emotional state and has a thought or cognitive component and a somatic component. Stress has been defined as 'the nonspecific response of the body to any demand made upon it' (Selye, 1974: 27). Selye noted that stress is not just nervous tension and it is not always to be avoided. What is important is to accept that competitive sport is inherently stressful and what is crucial is enabling your athletes to learn to manage that stress by managing their arousal and anxiety levels. According to Janelle (2002), expert athletes 'are capable of regulating emotional fluctuations and their physiological manifestations to a greater extent than novices' (p. 245).

Why is understanding and finding that right level of arousal or 'activation' so important for your athlete? It is important because arousal levels affect performance, physically through increased muscle tension, fatigue, movement impairment, and psychologically with an impairment of attention/focus. There have been a number of studies that have demonstrated improvements in athletes' arousal control through a variety of methods including bioneurofeedback (Dupee and Werthner, 2011), relaxation strategies (Fournier et al., 2005) and centering, progressive muscle relaxation, and positive energy (Mamassis and Doganis, 2004). In a later section, bioneurofeedback and its benefits will be discussed in greater detail.

The concept of mental toughness

As your athletes begin to develop the psychological skills listed above, they begin to develop what has been called 'mental toughness.' This is a concept Jones, Hanton and Connaughton (2002, 2007) developed after they interviewed eight Olympic or world champions, three coaches and four sport psychologists. From this body of research they identified four dimensions and 30 attributes. The first dimension, attitude/mindset included attributes such as a strong sense of self-belief and an effective focus. The second dimension, training, included such attributes as loving training and using effective goal setting. The third dimension, competition, included attributes such as loving the pressure of competition and being able to adapt to change and challenges. The fourth and final dimension, post competition, included such attributes as handling failure and success. They concluded with a definition of mental toughness: 'a natural or developed construct that enabled mentally tough performers to cope with the demands of training and competition better than their opponents' (p. 244).

When you train each of the key psychological skills, what you develop is mental toughness with a strong sense of self-confidence. Self-confidence is a direct result of strengthening these psychological skills. When your athletes have developed the ability to know what to focus on when training and competing, know how to manage their activation levels, know how to manage negative distractions, they will also understand they always have a *choice* in what they think and how they react to various situations and they will begin to trust and believe in themselves.

A sense of confidence

At all levels of competitive sport, most athletes' level of self-confidence is quite fragile. The ebb and flow of that self-confidence is linked to their ability to manage themselves physiologically and psychologically and yet is also linked directly to past performances and the relationship with their coach. When competition is going well, many athletes feel quite confident in their abilities. When they are working well alongside their coach, have a trusting and respectful relationship, and have confidence in the training programme, then they also describe themselves as confident. But for many athletes, when one of those components is missing, so is a significant degree of self-confidence.

A psychophysiological orientation

The challenges inherent in competitive sport often produce anxiety (i.e., negative cognitive and somatic activation) in many athletes, which can lead to performance decrements if not managed effectively by building self-awareness and acquiring self-regulatory skills (Gucciardi et al., 2009). Therefore, athletes must learn to effectively self-regulate on multiple levels (i.e., psychological, emotional, and physiological) (e.g. Bar-Eli et al., 2002; Jones, 2003; Taylor et al., 2008). Bioneurofeedback is a training tool that can help athletes learn to self-regulate effectively and consistently. So what is bioneurofeedback and how does it work?

In the last few decades, bioneurofeedback has received increasing research attention as an assessment and training tool for psychophysiological self-regulation in sport (e.g., Bar-Eli et al., 2002; Blumenstein et al., 1997; Dupee and Werthner, 2011; Prapavessis et al., 1992; Werthner et al., 2013). Blumenstein and colleagues (2002) indicated 'a major application for biofeedback is detecting and helping in the management of psychophysiological arousal, especially over arousal' (p. 37).

Bioneurofeedback training or psychophysiological training is a way to examine the physiological processes of the brain on sport performance. Bioneurofeedback targets the development of an athlete's psychological skills of focus, management of anxiety, and recovery/relaxation ability in order to enhance overall sport performance. The training involves the development of self-awareness and self-regulation of both physiological and neurological activity in the body and brain. Focus training provides tools for an athlete to help him develop alertness and concentration and manage emotions, fears and distractions (i.e. negative self-talk, anxiety and doubts) in order to more fully focus on the task at hand, which is primarily training and performance in competition. Anxiety management training ensures the athlete develops the skills to shift into a parasympathetic dominant state at will and regulate, or turn down, the stress response. Training to engage the body in deep relaxation serves to release stress from the nervous system. Bioneurofeedback training is designed to enhance the athlete's awareness of, and ability to influence and control their optimal performance state.

Bioneurofeedback is based on the underlying principle that the nervous system is the command centre of the body. The nervous system can be divided into two parts: the central nervous system and the peripheral nervous system. Information travels within and among the two divisions via neural tissue. The central nervous system includes the brain and spinal cord. Neurofeedback training, also known as EEG bioneurofeedback, is focused on cerebral functions, and more specifically, the brain's electrical activity. The peripheral nervous system has two divisions: somatic (voluntary) and autonomic (involuntary). Bioneurofeedback training targets the autonomic nervous system, which is further divided in two parts: the sympathetic, which activates the fight and flight response in the body (the stress response) and the parasympathetic which deactivates the fight and flight response in the body and allows the body to rest and regenerate (the relaxation response). Ultimately, the controlling source of all systems is universally central and under the control of the central nervous system.

More specifically, the bioneurofeedback training intervention uses instrumentation to assist athletes with self-observation and self-monitoring in order to learn to control physiological and neurological function. During bioneurofeedback training sensors are attached to the body for the purpose of acquiring biological and neurological signals such as those produced by muscles, sweat glands, body temperature, respiration, and heart rhythm (the bioneurofeedback modalities) and brainwaves (the neurofeedback modality). Biological and neurological signals are 'fed back' to the athlete with the goal of gaining mental control over biological and neurological processes. The athlete receives moment by moment information about changes from the sensors. Information is in the form of auditory tones, digital or analogue displays, or computer graphics. The training, which develops the skill of self-regulation through self-awareness, assists athletes and coaches in learning to regulate aspects of their central and autonomic nervous systems.

Bioneurofeedback

Specifically, the bioneurofeedback training (BFK) focuses on developing voluntary control of the autonomic nervous system with the goal of developing conscious regulation of the arousal state and the ability to enter into the state of parasympathetic predominance, which in effect, decreases the stress response. When an athlete experiences anxiety or stress, the sympathetic nervous system becomes dominant. The goal of the bioneurofeedback training is to enable each athlete to improve the balance between sympathetic and parasympathetic nervous system activity, often referred to as autonomic nervous system balance.

The types of bioneurofeedback training used are muscle or electromyograph (EMG), skin conductance/electro dermal activity, heart rate and heart rate variability, respiration rate and peripheral body temperature. During the training, the athletes develop self-awareness and self-regulation of the various feedback modalities. Muscle feedback training enables an athlete to become aware of tension in the muscles and train the muscles to relax and release tension. Skin conductance feedback training allows an athlete to practice decreasing his arousal level (when feeling anxious or overly stressed) and to increase his arousal or activation level (if feeling 'flat' before a competition). Heart rate variability feedback training induces greater parasympathetic nervous system activity and a relaxation response. Respiration feedback training reduces sympathetic arousal, encouraging regeneration, release of tension, and increased physical and mental relaxation. Peripheral temperature feedback training is used to initiate a relaxation response in order to combat competition anxiety and to enhance recovery after a competitive event. A more in-depth explanation follows.

Muscle or electromyograph feedback training

Muscle feedback training provides an athlete with enhanced information about muscle tension in a particular area and facilitates an athlete in learning to control tension in that muscle. Relaxation of excessive and inappropriate tension is the goal. Muscle tension below 1.5mV is considered very relaxed and is the target criteria set. Sensors are attached to the skin on the muscle being targeted for change. Since forehead, jaw and upper shoulder muscles are valid indicators of general arousal and muscle tension, they are commonly targeted during the training. Measurement of muscle activity preceding muscle contraction is called electromyography or EMG. EMG measures, in microvolts, the electrical energy discharged by the motor nerve endings signalling a muscle to contract. These tiny electrical signals emitted by the muscles, proportional to the degree of contraction, are amplified and fed to a visual display or audio signal. The visual display is digits, polygraph-style lines, and changes in colours or patterns.

Skin conductance or electrodermal feedback training

This modality, known as electrodermal activity (EDA), or the more classic term, galvanic skin response (GSR), is related to the electrical activity of the skin. Sweat contains salt that makes it electrically conductive. A skin conductance device applies a very small electrical pressure (voltage) to the skin, typically on the volar surface of the fingers, where there are many sweat glands, and measures the amount of electrical current that the skin will allow to pass. Electrodermal activity (EDA) has been recognised as distinctly sensitive to transitory emotional states and mental events, as well as being closely correlated with sympathetic nervous system activity. Self-calming by physical or cognitive means tends to lower skin conductance and negative emotions such as fear, worry or anger usually raise it. In learning to reliably regulate EDA, an athlete learns to resist distractions which disrupt attention and to maintain a state of mind which is neutral or pleasant. EDA can also be used by an athlete to increase his arousal or activation level before a competition if they feel they are not activated enough. EDA is measured in micro-Siemans and is known to increase during stressful times and decrease during relaxation.

Heart rate and heart rate variability feedback training

Using a photoplethysmyograph monitor on the non-dominant thumb gives an indirect measure of heart rate. Under stress the number of beats per minute (bpm), or heart rate, goes up and should lower after the task. Typically athletes show much lower than average heart rates but genetics and conditioning determine the baseline. Well-trained athletes often have heart rates of 45–60bpm while the average non-conditioned individual is between 72–80bpm. Normally, there are increases of 10–20bpm with activity and a return to baseline within a minute.

Heart rate variability (HRV) refers to the rise and fall of the heart rate synchronised with each breath (i.e. faster on inhalation, slower on exhalation). The magnitude of this systematic variability reflects a healthy alternation between two autonomic influences on the heartbeat, the sympathetic and the parasympathetic. Lack of this variation reflects an imbalance between the two aspects of the autonomic nervous system (ANS), most likely deficient parasympathetic influence. By calming one's emotional state and by making the breathing slower and more regular, the HRV can be increased. This involves an athlete learning to regulate breathing rate and rhythm in order to induce greater parasympathetic nervous system activity and create a relaxation response.

The feedback for HRV involves monitoring heart rate, or heart rate plus respiration. Heart rate is detected from a photoplethysmographic sensor on the finger. A trace reflecting cyclic variations in heart rate is displayed on a video screen. The variability of heart rate is what is of interest. The athlete observes the trace and uses it as feedback for regulating the breath and his emotional state. The heartbeat variability is maximised at a particular resonant frequency, which is breathing rate per minute, and this rate is determined for each individual by observation and experimentation.

Respiration rate feedback training

Respiration pattern, which is depth and frequency of breathing, is highly sensitive to changes of both arousal level and emotional factors. A shallow breathing pattern in athletes has been identified as one of the physiological indicators of stress. The rate of breathing is controlled by the partial pressure of carbon dioxide in the blood stream and can be decreased by blowing out all the carbon dioxide from the bottom of the lungs. Doing this will lower the breathing rate to 5–8 breaths per minute. An ideal rate of breathing for most adults is approximately 6 breaths per minute. Effortless diaphragmatic breathing reduces sympathetic arousal, encouraging regeneration, release of tension, and an increase in physical and mental relaxation.

The instrument used to determine respiration rate is a strain gauge around the abdomen below the ribcage. Smooth continuous expansion of the abdominal region with inhalation is a sign of effortless breathing. Deregulation in breathing often happens during tasks and is usually indicated by one of three variations: a) shallow breathing, with the shoulders doing most of the work rather than the abdominal region, b) breath holding during tasks, and/or c) increasing respiration rate (breaths per minute or brpm). All three of these variations are often associated with poor performance in sport.

Peripheral body temperature feedback training

Skin temperature changes of the fingers provide information about peripheral circulation. The cardio-vascular mechanisms that regulate skin temperature in the hands are closely related to the activity of the sympathetic division of the autonomic nervous system. When this system is activated, the smooth muscles surrounding the blood vessels near the skin surface are likely to contract, resulting in vasoconstriction. This causes a decrease in the flow of blood in the area bringing about a drop in skin temperature. Low peripheral body temperature is a physiological sign of inner tension. Conversely, an increase in hand temperature is accompanied by vasodilation, which is relaxation of the smooth muscles surrounding the peripheral blood vessels in the hands, and results from relaxation of sympathetic activity.

A thermal sensor, called a themistor, is taped to the skin, usually on the palmar surface of one of the fingers. The temperature of the skin changes the resistance of the thermistor, thereby altering the electrical signal in proportion to the temperature. The signal is displayed visually through a tone that changes in response to changes in temperature. The values of peripheral skin temperature range from 18–21°C (i.e. high sympathetic arousal) to 32–35 °C (i.e. low sympathetic arousal). The goal is to maintain peripheral body temperature at or above 32°C during both rest and activity. Temperature training is typically combined with other BFK modalities to initiate a relaxation response in the body in order to combat competition anxiety and to enhance recovery after a competitive event.

Neurofeedback

The neurofeedback training (NFK) focuses on optimising brainwave patterns in specific regions of the brain that influence an athlete's emotional state and cognitive performance. During the NFK training, the athlete trains his or her own brainwaves to function more efficiently. The brain frequencies that are in excess are reduced, and those with a deficit are increased. This technique is used to help improve concentration, deal with distractions and negative thoughts, and help the brain to recharge itself.

The underlying process in neurofeedback involves training and learning self-regulation of brain activity. The brainwaves reflect what a person is doing from moment to moment. Neurofeedback training enhances flexibility in order to access the appropriate state to get a particular job done. In essence, the overall goal of neurofeedback is to improve mental flexibility so that an athlete can produce a mental state appropriate to the situational requirements. During the training, each athlete learns to regulate his brainwaves in order to produce a desired mental state. With the training, NFK helps athletes to be in control of their mental state.

The neurofeedback training technique uses quantitative electroencephalographic (QEEG) feedback. The amount of electrical activity at different brainwave frequencies (i.e. the EEG signal) is amplified from the minute voltages, quantified, and then translated into information that the athlete can learn. The athlete's EEG is actually what they use to operate the displays and games on a computer screen. The feedback from the screen, which may be both visual and auditory, alerts the athlete to what his brain is doing – concentrating, daydreaming, ruminating – and he can then use this information to change brain activity. With training, the athlete learns to use the EEG to control the displays and games on the computer screen. Controlling the computer display teaches the athlete how to produce the brainwaves that are associated with effective focus, staying in the present moment, remaining calm, and quieting the mind. As training progresses, the researcher slowly adjusts the thresholds, shaping the behaviour of the athlete's brain into a more optimal pattern. With practice, the athlete learns how to do this on his own, without the computer feedback.

Neurofeedback for optimal performance is a method for repeatedly exercising the pathways related to attention, and quieting the mind to facilitate their growth and development. With practice the athlete is able to recognise both the state of focus and when they drift off into daydreams, ruminating thoughts, or negative self-talk. The net result is that the athlete becomes better able to self-regulate his mental state, manage distractions, and sustain focus on the task at hand. Analogous to exercise building muscle mass, the utilisation of the brain builds the mass of the brain's dendritic connections. Neurofeedback training can be thought of as 'weight training' for the brain to assist with better utilising one's potential. More specifically, neurofeedback optimises functioning of the brain by enhancing its flexibility, and thus creating the ability to shift mental states at will. Athletes need to develop the ability to focus effectively on task when required (the mental state is beta), to shift into relaxation and recovery when focus is not required (the mental state is alpha), and to recognise and shift out of worry and rumination (the mental state is hi beta).

CREATING THE BEST ENVIRONMENT FOR YOUNG DEVELOPING ATHLETES

When athletes are younger and inexperienced, a more *directive* style of coaching is often appropriate. This means that you as the coach would be setting up the training with little discussion with the athlete, as he will just be beginning to learn about how to train. You may still be starting the process of debriefing, but it will be limited. As the athlete learns and progresses, you may be *facilitating* more and asking for more input from each athlete – their feedback to you will be useful. The athlete may contribute by suggesting warm-up variations and your interactions will entail more discussion. In thinking of this as a continuum, the preferred 'style' becomes *supportive* as the athlete becomes very self aware, has consistently good performances and takes responsibility. Here the coach and athletes work together in a collaborative manner to ensure consistently excellent performance. The coach still provides systematic support and still directs many training sessions, but the athlete is a true partner, providing feedback that allows the coach to make informed choices about training and competing. While describing this as a progression, an athlete may respond better to one 'style' than another, so one of the challenges for a coach is to discover what works best for each athlete and indeed, adapt their way of coaching.

Many articles have been written over the years on the concepts of personality and motivation in sport. Simply put, personality refers to the characteristics that make a person unique and motivation refers to the direction and intention of one's effort.

Understanding the personality of your athletes, particularly as they begin in sport, helps you as a coach. Martens (1975) suggested that personality be divided into three levels – the psychological core, typical responses, and role-related behaviours. The psychological core would include an athlete's values and beliefs about themselves, such as 'I am really good at distance racing' or 'I am not very good at hitting a ball'. The level of typical responses would be how an athlete has learned to respond to the world, such as being loud and brash, reserved and shy, a perfectionist. The third level, role related behaviours refer to the roles we play in our lives, such as being an athlete and a student.

There are many ways that researchers have examined the concept of personality, but what is important for you as a coach to understand is that each athlete will have developed ways of being who they are and some may be helpful or not, and some will be easier to change than others. What is most important is to help your athletes become self-aware and develop an ability to learn and analyse their training and competitive performances without being too critical. While there are questionnaires and tests of trait and state inventories, one of the best ways to help your athletes of all ages develop self-awareness and skills to self-manage is to talk with them, ask questions and create a well-developed analysis/debrief process – all of which helps them to reflect and learn. How to do this effectively is discussed in the section on psychological skills. There is also a great deal of research about the differences between how to coach female and male athletes. Some of those differences are discussed under effective communication.

Motivation is an interesting concept for a coach. It can be viewed from at least three different perspectives: internal and external motivation, motivation as it relates to competitive stress, and achievement motivation. When motivation is discussed in terms of direction of effort it refers to, for example, whether an athlete is motivated to seek out an individual sport such as athletics, or a team sport such as basketball. When it is discussed in terms of intensity of effort it refers to, for example, how much effort an athlete may put into training on a daily basis. What is important for you as a coach is to understand there are a number of variables you must consider in order to motivate young athletes. Here are four key considerations:

- First, you want to be creating an environment that, at least initially, is welcoming and encouraging for all. This certainly means more emphasis on skill development and less on winning games or races. Along with this, you must also consider the inherent personality of each of your athletes, in the sense that you may find yourself with athletes who love to compete, those who can learn to love to compete, and those who eventually will be better doing recreational sports. But often you will not know that initially. You can start by asking questions of your athletes. Gill and Williams (2008) conducted a review of the literature and concluded that children are motivated by skill development, becoming more competent, being challenged and having fun. And remember, there are often cultural and gender differences in motivation. For example, numerous studies have shown that while having fun and developing skills are common across both genders, girls will often cite being motivated by developing skills and the social aspects of sport and boys often emphasise competition and fitness. The key is asking the athletes you coach what they enjoy about sport and understanding that those motives may change over time. What motivates your athlete when he is 15 years old, may be quite different to what motivates him when 25 years old. So you should regularly monitor individual's motives, and when you do, you will be able to create practices and competitive settings that are both challenging and fun.
- Second, you need to regularly adjust the training environment. Some days you might practice hard, another day you might cross-train in a different sport, still developing agility and fitness, but increasing motivation. Provide play and competition.
- Third, do your best, within the group of athletes you coach, to be individualising training. Every athlete wants to feel that you, as the coach, understand what they need and care about them. Again, one of the best ways to do this is to regularly ask them how they are doing, and get their feedback on what they think is working and what might need to change. Whatever they say is great information for you as a coach. If they are incorrect, you certainly correct, but that tells you there are aspects they have not understood in the training. If they are correct, and give you good feedback, they are on their way to becoming more reflective – more of a thinking and responsible athlete. Such an athlete will go a long way in terms of performance.

- Fourth, you want to create a task rather than an outcome orientation for your athletes. When you emphasise a task orientation, you create an environment where work ethic, persistence, and optimal performance can flourish! This creates a focus on personal accomplishment and personal control – how good can I be? An outcome orientation creates an environment where athletes judge their success based on comparison to others, and of course, we have no control over what other teams or athletes do. Competition is inherently about outcome, about winning, about beating others – we cannot ignore that. But as a coach, as you work with young developing athletes, and plan an environment that will encourage them to stay in the sport long term, a task orientation is more productive.
- Fifth, how you deliver feedback as a coach is crucial to increasing levels of motivation. As you downplay outcome goals and emphasise task and personal mastery goals, you want to be thinking of your feedback. You want to be providing a detailed critique so the skill can be improved, and at the same time building confidence – 'you need to move the ball with your left foot and keep your head up as you move down the field – no worries, it will come with more practice'. Be specific with both the critique of a skill and the positive aspects – 'you need to remember to keep your shoulders down as you make the turn, but great work on the 200m split time – excellent.'

These are the key components to creating an environment where young athletes grow into competition in a healthy way and hopefully stay involved for many years to come!

SUMMARY

In a process which is athlete centred, coach led and performance services supported, you as the coach must have a high degree of competence in leading both process and people. Such leadership is strongly value based and goal oriented. Respect and trust in managing relationships of coach–athlete; coach–team; coach–significant others (e.g. parents, performance scientist and managers) are fundamental. This grows not only through what you do but how it is done. So it is as much attitudinal and behavioural as technical. Communications and listening skills are key here as you the coach shifts your style from one of teaching to one of facilitating learning in a climate of constructive candour. Your skills of psychological preparation focus on equipping the athlete to take ownership of personal development and performance; to make considered, responsible decisions; and to deliver effective and excellent performance under pressure. This requires creating the right learning environment at each stage of the athlete development pathway affording non-judgemental feedback for the athlete to develop those techniques which prepare him to focus mental, emotional and physical energies on achieving the task at hand. Bioneurofeedback is a valuable resource in this. Building effective teams leans heavily on your competence in harmonising diversity and conflict resolution. There is a delicate balance in this to address psychological preparation for each team member's role; for team cohesion, cooperation and collaboration; and for leveraging individual team member's unique personal strengths.

REFLECTIVE QUESTIONS

1. What would you want your athlete(s)/each of your team players to be focused on during a race/performance/game situation? What would help you feel confident in helping athletes/players practice the correct focus?

2. How often should you debrief/analyse your athletes' performances? Would you do it by yourself or would you include your athlete(s)? Design a review strategy to build into an athlete's/team's year plan. What would you need to make that feasible?

3. How would you gain accurate intelligence of the right range of physiological activation for team/athlete(s) in order to perform optimally?

4. How well do you feel you are equipped to create an effective high functioning team?

5. Do you know how to help athletes recover psychologically – and not be 'thinking about' competing all the time?

If you are already coaching athletes/teams, please respond to these questions on the basis of your experience and practice.

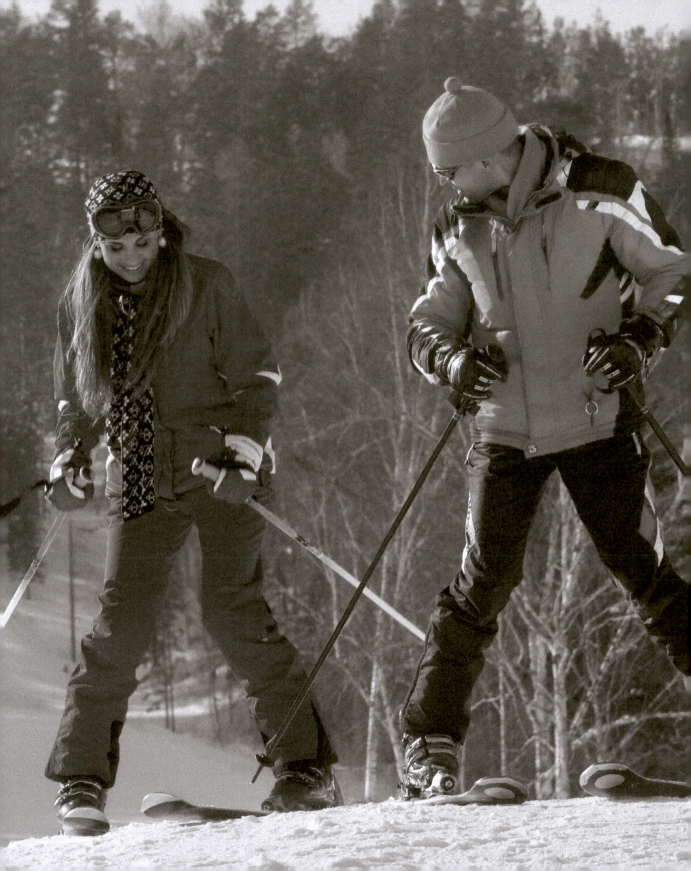

11 PERCEPTUAL-MOTOR LEARNING

In most Western countries, knowledge about the acquisition of skill is frequently neglected. This may be due to the nature versus nurture emphasis of recent years, with controversial statements such as 'winners are born not made!', or to the fact that new information on the perceptual and decision-making aspects of sport has not been effectively disseminated through coach education programmes.

Regardless of the reasons for this oversight, every individual has a need of movement, whether this is the fundamental requirement of the movement of inner organs, or the muscles. Movements can be described in the context of patterns and skills. A motor pattern is the movement involved in the carrying out of a particular task. This is different from a motor skill, which places emphasis on the accuracy, precision, and economy of performance of the task execution. One of the most fundamental tasks of early childhood is the development of the dominant movement patterns and motor skills through variety, increasing experimentation, and progressive learning. A major aim of motor development in the first two years of life, for example, is walking. Once initiated, proficiency in this basic motor skill develops at an exponential rate (Malina and Bouchard, 1991).

Education aims, through physical activities, to promote the understanding of regular systematic movement as a part and philosophy of life, with the idea that sport is a school for life. More specific movement, as required in sports performance, requires motor skill training to cultivate and refine highly skilled performance. Perceptual-motor skill training reflects the enhancement of those characteristics required for skilled performance. While the capabilities of a skilled athlete are numerous and sport-determined, there are identifiable aspects to expert performance, relating to economy of effort and precision of movement:

'A complex, intentional action involving a whole chain of sensory, central and motor mechanisms which, through the process of learning, have come to be organised and co-ordinated in such a way as to achieve predetermined objectives with maximum certainty.'

(Whiting, 1975, p. 6)

Defining skilled performance is important for the coach attempting to balance the amount of time dedicated to the various components of training. The practice of movement elements in open skill sports such as ball sports (particularly drill practice of basic skills) often takes up a disproportionate amount of time, despite the fact that perceptual and decision-making skills are regarded as highly influential in determining success (Abernethy et al., 1999). The perceptual-motor skill is context-determined. With few exceptions, the expert performer in one sport will not demonstrate the same level of skill in another sport. There is virtually zero transfer from one sport to another (Lotter, 1960), although the learning process is transferable. Some sports, such as soccer, rely upon perceptual and decision-making abilities, with the uncertainty of opposition play, tactics, and timing. Other sports define expert performance by control and movement precision, for example artistic gymnastics, where actions can be planned in advance and performance conditions are predictable.

The characteristics of each respective high-level performer differ enormously, yet each stands to gain perceptual-motor skills training.

PERCEPTUAL-MOTOR SKILLS TRAINING

An ability is a stable characteristic or trait, inborn and unaffected by practice and rehearsal. A skill is distinct – it can be developed or lost. Given this, the coach can assist the athlete through the development of skills central to movement technique, and ultimately performance. To do so using perceptual-motor learning theory in practical technique training, the coach emphasises first the sensory part of reactions or responses and, second, complete awareness and control over what is going on.

Sensory perception is a multi-dimensional construct blending external events with an accompanying interpretation of internal activity. Perceptual information is obtained via a collective process. An individual's ability to identify what is going on in the external environment, such as where a competitor is during a race; to interpret what is occurring internally, such as loss of concentration; to understand body positioning, such as trail-leg angle in hurdling; and to establish the actual relationship between the body and the environment, are accounted for by sensory perception. Perception is more than the body's reception of information by its various sensory systems. Associated sub-processes potentially limit performance. These are identified as detection, comparison, recognition, and selective attention. Whether a signal is present or not can be determined through detection. Comparison assesses whether two stimuli are the same or whether they differ. The identification of stimuli, objects and patterns known previously occurs by recognition, and selective attention ensures the appropriate allocation of processing resources where deemed relevant or ignoring distracting or less relevant information (Abernethy et al., 1999).

Every sport has sensory aspects. Where a hierarchy of sensory dominance is suggested, perceptual priority is afforded to vision. The dominant means of controlling skilled movement for the sighted athlete is via the visual system. Kinaesthesis, audition and the remaining senses follow thereafter. Different sensory information is made available to facilitate 'reading' performance. The advantages of training perceptual-motor skills are varied. Fatigue-induced distortion can be minimised, or the athlete can learn to anticipate requirements. Feed-forward – information sent ahead in time to prepare for the following sensory feedback – has been shown through research on visual perception to be of an advantage to the performer (Gallistel, 1980). A copy of the motor (efferent) command sent to the eye muscles is, in addition, sent to a location in the brain; the visual perception system is in this way informed about the imminent movement of the eye. This 'efference copy' mechanism may indeed exert similar parallel control over the movement of the limbs as well (Schmidt, 1988). Neurological evidence has indicated that sensory information to be received by the muscles is also sent to locations in the brain (Evarts, 1973). Thus the aim of such activities may be to inform the sensory system and to prepare it for reception of feedback.

Fundamental to training are the sources of non-visual information and how they interact with vision. To develop sensory perception and necessary awareness, modified activities and games can be used to create a rich reservoir for understanding and perfecting techniques. The ballet dancer rehearsing movements before a mirror is educating the body in an entire movement range, teaching it through predetermined sequences and acquiring more knowledge of what is involved. The athlete must consciously make himself aware of responses and reactions, thereby accumulating movement information.

It is evident that this movement must be harmoniously controlled, a function carried out by the pyramid and extra-pyramid cells coming from the sub-cortex and connecting every part of the brain responsible for movement. Cooperation between pyramid and extra-pyramid nerves is very subjective where potential influences include feelings and emotions. A lack of coordination results in a certain mental state, expressed by a movement error during performance. Each small, uncoordinated activity contributes to failure. Thus the aspect of self-control under a range of conditions faced by the athlete should be rehearsed where the athlete is to maintain a performance-facilitating equilibrium. The ultimate aim of perceptual-motor skills training is to ensure that the decoding of information being picked up by the sensory systems is attenuated and enhanced by accompanying learning.

Feedback and knowledge of results

The coach regularly provides the performer with feedback regarding athletic movement. Feedback is information from the environment that informs the athlete about performance efficiency during and/or following the movement. Feedback can be further classified into intrinsic feedback, which provides a basis for movement evaluation, and extrinsic feedback, information produced to augment intrinsic feedback. Both are of great importance to the athlete wishing to develop his performance. The value of feedback, however, would be severely limited without a dimension of external feedback known as knowledge of results (KR). A verbal form of feedback, KR provides the performer with information comparing the actual performance with the intended goal. The athlete can use this information to improve performance. Another function of KR is that of motivation. The athlete's knowledge of results can motivate further performance improvement. Goals must be established for KR to be effective and meaningful to the athlete. A result without a predetermined goal offers little value.

As discussed in chapter 10, feedback is not about one way traffic. The athlete will constantly be providing feedback to the coach, for example, in terms of movement perceptions and understanding of information and advice to ensure quality communication.

THE LEARNING CONCEPT

A more complex model of events supersedes the concept of learning as a process of conditioned responses. This model might be represented as a type of self-regulating system (Bernstein, 1957, figure 11.1a). Although the terminology differs from that used in Bernstein's (1957) picture of things, Anochin (1967) and associates explained the underlying theory of learning a technique along similar lines (figure 11.1b). This popular theory purports that two types of afferent supply incoming information.

1. The situation afferent embraces all environmental stimuli and consequently includes stimuli that are both relevant and irrelevant via the sensory organs (proprioceptors). Recollected stimuli may also be included. This area of afference causes an integration of the nervous processes that precede the causal afferent.

2. The causal afferent is the 'reading' of the situation afferent and selection of the relevant from the irrelevant.

This collective afference is referred to as the afferent synthesis and it concludes with the intention to act. Such intention is given expression by the effector apparatus. When afferent synthesis ends and action is affected, a specific afferent apparatus – the action acceptor – is formed. This compares the afferent synthesis (intended action, I) with the completed action (performed action, P) on which information is brought back

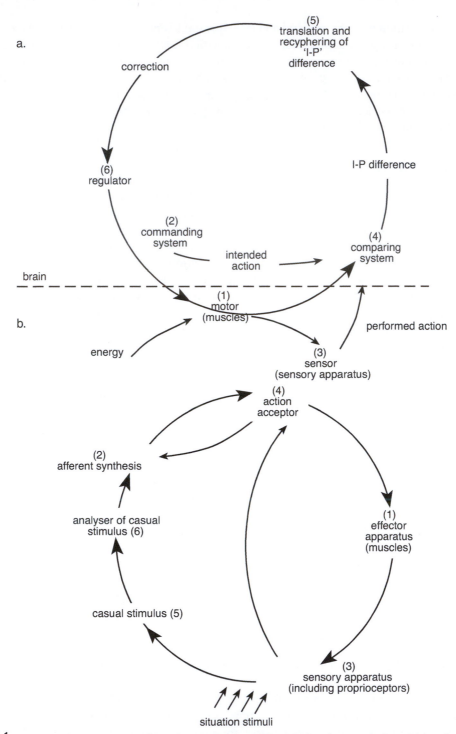

FIGURE 11.1 Events in the learning process (a) based on Bernstein's model and (b) based on Anochin's model (numbered to help comparison)

via situation and causal afferents. If there is agreement (i.e. no I–P difference), the cycle is complete. If not, new reactions are formed as the I–P difference is assessed and corrections made as the effector apparatus modifies the original action until agreement is reached. In cybernetics, this concept of reafference is referred to as back-coupling or feedback. Principal types of reafferent may be classified as follows.

1. Kinaesthetic afferents, which are represented by proprioception.

2. Resultant afferents, which comprise all afferent characteristics which relate to the result of the performed action. All new actions, however, arise from previous actions, and those new actions will, in turn, form the basis for future actions. Hence Anochin's (1967) subdivision of resultant afferents:

   - episodic reafferent, which provides information on intermediate actions;
   - final reafferent, which provides information on the final execution of the original plan of action.

The suggested existence of an afferent synthesis confirms the importance of factors such as training environment, motivation and a comprehensive understanding of a given technique by the coach, while the action acceptor emphasises the importance of previous experience and a complete appreciation of a given technique by the athlete. It rests with the coach to ensure that such factors are carefully assessed if technical training is to be efficient.

Senses and the afferent syntheses

Although we traditionally recognise five senses: vision, audition, taste, smell, and kinaesthesis, a hierarchy of sensory dominance exists. The major sensory system utilised by humans is vision, where visual information is dominant over other received information (Posner et al., 1976). Where a discrepancy may arise between visual information received and that offered by other sensory systems, the brain and nervous system resolve it by regarding the visual information as correct (Smyth and Marriot, 1982).

Internal and external proprioceptors register signals that form a complex support system often under-utilised by the performer in sport. While visual stimuli often lead the sensory complex, followed by kinaesthesis, other sensations affect the performer, such as the feel of the weight and size of the ball used by the footballer or basketball player, or the smell of the chalk on asymmetric bars. Established Russian and Czech coaching methodologies have long made successful use of sport-specific leading senses within the sensory complex. This is known as the afferent synthesis, providing the performer with permanent information prior to, during, and following performance. The motor learning of an activity includes an appropriate breakdown of the skill, identifying and reinforcing the afferent synthesis. For example, a breakdown of high jump technique (Dick, 1993) can easily include the appropriate development of the leading analyser which will be athlete-determined (table 11.1).

During the movement series the leading senses are dynamically changed according to the demands of the movements of the body. If, for instance, the high jumper fails to clear the bar, knocking it off with the lower leg, then the afferent synthesis will automatically facilitate greater attention to the awareness of the activity of the lower leg in the next attempt. The performer is informed through this mechanism at every moment.

FOSBURY FLOP	PHASE	REFERENCE	CRITERION	LEADING ANALYSER SENSORY REINFORCEMENT	ASSESSMENT
	I Approach PENULTI-MATE STRIDE	A 1 foot plant 2 body/trunk 3 arms B 4 front supp. BC 5 supp. knee B 6 rear arm C 7 arms	ball contact/curved path inclination/slight forward lean counter arm swing heel lead yielding held back parallel/behind trunk	*Visual* as look for spot above the bar; *Kinaesthetic* as feel high knees to penultimate stride.	
	II Approach LAST STRIDE	D 8 trunk 9 supp. leg DF 10 take-off leg E 11 arms F 12 body/trunk F 13 foot plant EF 14 free leg	upright horizontal pushing action fast & active plant/pre-tension/'long' starting double swing inclination/backward lean 'through' the bar/optimal take-off pos. bending/forward-upward movement	*Kinaesthetic* as feel tall; *Auditory* as hear foot plant; signal then to initiate upward push; *Kinaesthetic* as feel arms then lean.	
	III TAKE-OFF	FG 15 take-off leg FH 16 arms FH 17 free leg GH 18 free knee H 19 arms H 20 shoulders H 21 body	minimal & passive yielding active double arm swing active knee drive 'opening'/block in horizontal pos. blocked/bent lifted/horizontal vertical/parallel to upright	*Kinaesthetic* as feel arm swing & knee drive.	
	IV RISING OPENING	I 22 head I 23 outside arm IK 24 body IK 25 arms IK 26 free leg K 27 back K 28 head	view; along the bar 'leading' longitudinal axis rotation 'opening' lowering parallel to bar backward movement	*Visual* as spot over the bar; *Kinaesthetic* as feel body opening; feel rising.	
	V LAYOUT	KL 29 arms L 30 hips L 31 legs L 32 back L 33 head L 34 longit. axis	extended/'diving action' hyperextended/elevated bent/directed downwards 'arched' thrown back rectangular to bar	*Kinaesthetic* awareness of back & hips; exaggerate arched feeling.	
	VI RECOVERY	LM 35 pelvis M 36 head/trunk M 37 hips M 38 legs M 39 arms	active lowering 're-active' countermovement active bending synchronous active knee extension bending	*Kinaesthetic* acknow-ledgement of lowering of pelvis; *Visual* as see clearance of legs.	
	VII PREPARA-TION FOR LANDING	NO 40 head NO 41 hips NO 42 arms NO 43 body NO 44 legs	raised bent/blocked spreading in 'L-position' extended/directed upwards	*Kinaesthetic* with raised head; maintain 'L' shape feeling.	

TABLE 11.1 Guiding technical adjustment using visual or kinaesthetic leading analysers as coaching points

Technical feedback

As discussed in chapter 10, feedback is fundamental to the value of the coach-athlete relationship and is central to the learning process which the coach leads. The importance of technical feedback in learning and developing sports techniques was probably the earliest to be recognised. This affords a constructive environment where technical models may be established, refined and rendered robust and where error is readily eliminated. It enables the athlete to analyse the afferent synthesis so that he can read the appropriate sense and use it for anticipatory purposes. Beginners do not have this sense and so may find themselves stretched. For example, a young soccer player may pass the ball behind an oncoming teammate. Anticipation together with the process of cognition gives the prediction and prognosis of events. It is sensible, then, for the coach to include this type of training within the planning of competitive conditions.

An operational understanding of the benefits of various data collection techniques will enhance the value of specialised input in coaching/training. Irrespective of the analysis method undertaken, it is fundamental that a systematic approach is used in the analysis of sports movement (Marshall and Elliot, 1999). Predictive analysis methods use computer simulation to explore 'what if' scenarios. A model of a person or apparatus is created to predict changes occurring as a result of varying input parameters. Motion and image capture and analysis technology coupled with relevant software allows sophisticated notational analysis which is now an essential element for coach and athlete in high performance sport (Hughes and Franks, 2004).

The importance of imagery was discussed in chapter 10. Intelligent application of notational analysis in technique training at once enriches both internal and external imagery, given that the coach has already introduced internal and external imagery skills in the athlete's learning programme.

The kinaesthetic sense is the focus of internal imagery. It is often regarded as the 'dark' sense as it is difficult to know what the muscular apparatus senses! Appropriate skill breakdown where the sensory complex is managed and reinforced will enable the performer to exert control over this automatic process. In this way, the leading sensory channel and the dynamic change of leading channels are developed. The actual breakdown with an integrated series of practices helps the athlete learn control at a conscious level.

This type of sensory training shadows the athlete through his skill development. At the initial stages of games learning, activities for children involving throwing a variety of suitable objects such as soft miniature implements and balls will introduce sensory awareness. Likewise an elite javelin thrower can benefit from increased kinaesthetic awareness of the hand by changing the throwing implement with emphasis on good technical form. Where every activity has a specific complexity of afferent synthesis, both coach and athlete can explore training opportunities to reinforce appropriate sensory perception. Approaching the hanging ball from different directions will assist the footballer with the skill of heading; the tennis player maintaining a bouncing tennis ball on the racket while keeping a balloon off the ground with his foot couples sensory awareness with the attention required for a specific activity. Patience is required as motor learning is not directly observable.

Learning

Learning is a process involving the acquiring of increased skill capability. A series of internal processes associated with practice or experience will influence this capability for skilled behaviour, resulting in relatively permanent change. An individual will learn from participation itself within an appropriate situation, and from the breakdown of skill. Whole and part approaches should be combined. To optimise later skill automaticity, part-skill practices may shape initial learning conditions. A learning ceiling is presumed when some success is experienced by a performer, yet there is evidence to suggest that further practice brings about continued skill enhancement due to 'over-learning' (Schmidt, 1988), as opposed to learning beyond the original learning goal. Given the possibility of further improvements in performance, the learning design should facilitate adequate opportunity: part skill – whole/modified; part skill – whole/less modified; part skill – whole/realistic situation; part skill – whole/game situation. The approach is not prescriptive but tailored to the individual's response.

Unfortunately, simply accumulating time in the game does not eradicate sufficient bad habits and patterns acquired due to lack of a stable learning base. Basic skills should be mastered sequentially to arrive at precise task performance. At every competitive level, fundamental errors are apparent, particularly when the performer has to mobilise reserves in order to cope with changing conditions in a game or event. If an athlete succumbs to externally induced or self-perceived factors such as the opposition scoring and panic resulting, or celebrating a point and losing concentration as a result, the least established skill patterns are more vulnerable.

Associated with this notion is that of effort. As an athlete learns a motor skill, the subsequent execution of that skill requires less effort (Kahneman, 1973), leaving the athlete more freedom to attend to game/event-specific information. Learning should allow the athlete processing and movement efficiency. Every life activity is directed by a high level of automisation of the basic elements of sensory and motor control. Given that the athlete must be able to concentrate on a range of game/event-induced aspects if performance is to be successful, information processing should not be overloaded. Automaticity implies that skills do indeed become automatic, thereby interfering less with other tasks. Learning taking place in the over-learning phase reduces attentional load and allows more accurate secondary task performance (Schneider and Fisk, 1983). Such improvement can perhaps be attributed to less interference from the main task.

Standard situation learning

Given the need for sports literacy – the ability to read performance-related internal and external cues – practice variation is vital. Both athlete and coach will be aware of performance hot spots, regular incidents, most frequently used moves, techniques, or skill patterns. Statistical analysis reveals how such standard situations impact upon performance and thereafter can influence the content of the learning to be automated by the athlete. This does not mean that outlying possibilities are not considered when dedicating time to technical training, but that the athlete has a ready library response from which he can select what is required. The established learning process gives greater room to manoeuvre, freeing up space more easily for the allocation of reserves in the event of unexpected contingencies, or by helping facilitate more economic (saving time) and efficient (preserving energy) learning.

AIMS OF TECHNICAL TRAINING

The general aims of technical training are as follows:

1. To direct the athlete's learning, and to perfect the most efficient technique(s) relative to a given sport. This demands that the coach has a complete understanding of the sport and its particular technical demands; of the athlete's present capabilities and his potential development; of techniques used by other athletes who are enjoying success; of teaching and developmental methods. In short, the coach

must establish a sound technical or biomechanical model, based on athlete and sport, towards which he must direct the athlete.

2. To direct the athlete towards a stable performance of the learned technique. This implies a progressive 'opening' of the situation, in which the athlete must perform the given technique. One might visualise an initial stage in the process where all conditions for learning are perfect and totally without distraction. A final stage might also be visualised where, irrespective of the bombardment of distracting factors and within biological limits, the performance of a given technique is as perfectly reproduced as if the situation was without interference. Environmental interference may come from wind and weather, apparatus, altitude, spectators or other athletes.

3. A further aim might be considered for sports where the athlete is forced to make a rapid selection of correct technique from a reservoir of many. To solve a situational problem the coach must direct the learning of this capacity. Thus, it is not only the techniques themselves that separate the weightlifter from the football player, but also the total nature of the competitions in which their techniques are executed.

Classification of technique

Attempts have been made to classify technique. The three classifications are determined by the nature of technique: single or multiple; and the performance/competition situation: constant or variable.

1. Sports in which a single technique determines the performance, and which are based on a constant technical model, where the structure of competition is relatively constant. This includes most track and field events, swimming, bowling, shooting and archery. Any variation within the structure of competition is restricted to factors such as weather, competition surfaces, facilities and equipment.

2. Sports in which a multiplicity of techniques determines the total performance, and where the structure of competition is relatively constant. Within each sport there exists a similarity of technical model between certain techniques, but each technique is distinct. Constancy of technical performance is made possible by the structure of competition and the conscious differentiation of techniques. Into this category will come artistic gymnastics, dance, figure skating and diving.

3. Sports in which a multiplicity of techniques may be demanded of a rapidly changing competition structure. Athletes here must select appropriate techniques to meet the changing demands of competition, but must also master each technique in the 'pool' at the athlete's disposal. Into this category come all team sports, combat sports, sports in which there are exchanges with an opponent (such as racket games) and sports in which environmental demands other than the opponent (e.g. weather, terrain), necessitate rapid and/or accurate selection of the most expedient technique (sailing, climbing, golf or canoeing).

The development of technical training must follow a different course for each classification.

Class 1

- Develop the technique in a closed situation (e.g. without environmental or competitive interference) as a 'performance'.

- Introduce a progressively open situation (e.g. more variables) while maintaining the 'performance' approach.
- Introduce a progressive intensity of competition.
- The general progression is from performing a technique to applying the technique in competition. In some cases the latter demands greater application of strength, or speed, (e.g. long jump), while in others, accuracy of performance is essential (e.g. shooting).

Class 2

- Develop each technique separately and in an order which permits the learning of each to proceed without the interference of the other.
- Again, the situation for learning each technique must be closed.
- The situation is now opened through the use of other equipment or different facilities. It may also be opened through a combination of techniques in movement sequences.
- This progression may be pursued throughout the athlete's future development as new techniques are introduced and new permutations and combinations of these techniques are advanced.
- Introduce a progressive intensity of competition.
- Here the progression develops accuracy of reproduction in the performance of techniques.

Class 3

- Develop each technique separately in a closed situation and in an order which permits no mutual interference.
- The situation is opened primarily by applying the technique in a changing situation (e.g. active opposition, varying climbs, sets).
- The athlete must also be exposed to technical adjustments necessitated by varying playing conditions. A more complex opening is where the athlete in the face of active opposition or varying terrain may choose one of several techniques.
- Introduce a progressive intensity of competition or environmental stressor.
- From here the progress is from learning, developing and making robust each technique, to reading the game situation; deciding how to deal with it; selecting the right technique; and effectively and excellently executing that technique under pressure of reducing timescales.

Technique may also be classified by considering the aim of each technique. On this basis, Dyatchkov (1967) offered the following classifications:

1. Sports in which the aim of the technique is to express intensive strength of brief duration within the ideal technical model, such as sprints, jumps, throws, or weightlifting.

2. Sports in which the aim is endurance development with an optimal expression of strength. This embraces middle and long-distance running, skiing, rowing, swimming and cycling.

3. Sports in which the aim of technique is development of those physical abilities permitting accuracy of performance of movements within a prescribed programme. This includes gymnastics, trampolining, figure skating and diving.

4. Sports in which the aim is the solution of those complex problems associated with interplay of athletes and/or environment, i.e. team games, combat sports, racket games.

Despite these attempts to classify technique, certain activities may fall within several categories. The aim of classification, however, is primarily to establish the planned technical development of an athlete. Consequently, it is sufficient that the coach identifies the specific aim of technique for an athlete in a given sport. Having done so, it rests with the coach's knowledge of anatomy, biomechanics, physiology, rules of the given sport, experience within that sport, and the performance status of the athlete, to formulate a plan of technical development.

Learning technique

In general terms, it would appear that the learning process can be shown to display a discernible pattern (table 11.2). These stages or phases fit closely with an extension of the 'conscious competence learning model'. Origination of the model has been variously attributed to Noel Burch of Gordon Training International ('Four Stages for Learning Any New Skill'); Martin M. Broadwell ('Teaching for Learning', *The Gospel Guardian*, 20 Feb 1969); and Abraham Maslow. The stages may be described as:

- Unconscious incompetence
- Conscious incompetence
- Conscious competence
- Unconscious competence
- Reflective competence*
  (*This fifth level was coined by David Baume in 2004.)

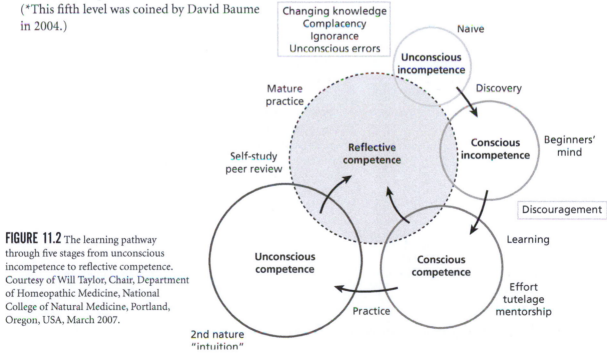

FIGURE 11.2 The learning pathway through five stages from unconscious incompetence to reflective competence. Courtesy of Will Taylor, Chair, Department of Homeopathic Medicine, National College of Natural Medicine, Portland, Oregon, USA, March 2007.

Stage or phase	Morphological/ functional	Regulative/neural	Teaching/coaching methods and conditions
1. Irradiation of stimulation	First concept of movement is learned, followed by an attitude to its learning.		Previously acquired related knowledge plus general total concept of action influence this stage.
2. Irradiation of stimulation processes	First ability to perform action and first acquisition of the action i.e. the basic form of the action is performed.	There is a generalisation of motor reactions together with muscle tensions and unnecessary movement, brought about by irradiation of stimuli to neighbouring areas of the cerebral cortex.	Teaching objective is to produce an accurate basic action and eliminate unnecessary movements, etc. Demonstration and video accompanied by verbal instruction (simple) is indicated.
3. Concentration through development of inhibitory processes	Correction, refinement of differentiation. Finer coordination of movement.	Concentration of focus of cerebral cortex processes. Movement is accepted more fully into the consciousness and in greater detail. Individual phases of movement become stabilised. Proprioceptors begin to take leading role.	Training must be concentrated but too frequent repetition within a training unit will fatigue the beginner and impede learning. Detailed learning of the movement is now worked on. Methods based on kinaesthesis (the feel of the movement) are used.
4. Stabilisation and automisation	High degree of precision in performing the action in a closed situation.	Complete harmony of neural processes where proprioceptors and cerebral cortex eliminate interference due to unnecessary movement; and rapid adjustment to changing conditions allows performance of a perfect action.	Intervals between training units can now be increased, as can the number of repetitions within each unit. Stabilise action and perfect technical detail. Training is designed to eliminate variables and give opportunity for 'perfect' execution of the action.
5. Stabilisation and automisation	Precision in performing the action in an open (more variable) situation.		Progressive development of physical capacities (e.g. strength, elastic strength, speed, etc.) necessary for long-term development in performance.

TABLE 11.2 Outline of learning stages in the acquisition of techniques

This process has been illustrated by Will Taylor, Chair of the Department of Homeopathic Medicine at the National College of Natural Medicine (Portland, Oregon), in figure 11.2.

'We revisit conscious incompetence, making discoveries in the holes in our knowledge and skills, becoming discouraged, which fuels incentive to proceed (when it does not defeat). We perpetually learn, inviting ongoing tutelage, mentoring and self-study (ongoing conscious competence). We continually challenge our 'unconscious competence' in the face of complacency, areas of ignorance, unconscious errors, and the changing world and knowledge base: We challenge our unconscious competence when we recognise that a return to unconscious incompetence would be inevitable. We do this in part by self-study and use of peer review – such that mature practice encompasses the entire "conscious competence" model, rather than supercedes it as the hierarchical model might suggest.'

It is recognised that the well-conditioned athlete arriving at stage 1, equipped with many (if not all) of the basic components of the total technique to be learned, is better prepared to advance through the stages than the athlete with little experience or conditioning to call upon.

Returning to the concept of the learning process, one might suggest that it is in the interest of the athlete to experience a wide range of motor coordinations in the shape of multiple sport skills in pursuit of establishing a more sophisticated action acceptor. Physical education appears to have focused emphasis on increasing the scope of a child's 'movement experience'. If such experience moves from the general and extends along a specific avenue of activity, it seems logical to anticipate the natural evolution of 'fundamental components'. From these fundamental components, highly specialised techniques may develop (figure 11.3). The concept of fundamental components, and the development of exercises based on them, has been successfully applied to sport, with the former German Democratic Republic (GDR) particularly benefiting from this methodology.

Establishing exercises based on components, demands a detailed knowledge of the original technique used. Each of these exercises must have the greatest possible range of application in techniques within its sphere, yet the essence of the component must not be destroyed by further breakdown or modification of parts. This suggests the possibility of derivatives. Derivatives of the first degree coincide with the essential parts of the component, while derivatives of the second degree are characterised by comprising only some of the essential parts of the component. The role of these components in the former GDR research was in two parts.

1. The integrating role (establishing the complete technical model from the components).

2. The differentiating role (establishing stability of the technical model by ensuring an ability to clearly separate one technique from another, correct movement from wrong movement). From this, and similar work, some important points emerge:

- When the first component learned is one that unites as many parts as possible of the final technique, learning time is reduced.
- Learning time for differentiation is also reduced by this approach.
- The use of first degree derivatives does not demand stability of the component, but second degree derivatives must not be introduced until the component is stable, otherwise there will be negative interference.

Each component must be constantly related to the whole technique. This is most important where the derivative is of the second degree, or where the derivative of the first degree contains a limited range of essential parts. Harre (1986) noted that athletes who learned derivatives of the first and second degree, by conscious acquisition of fundamental exercise, and who were made to differentiate consciously, proved, when learning

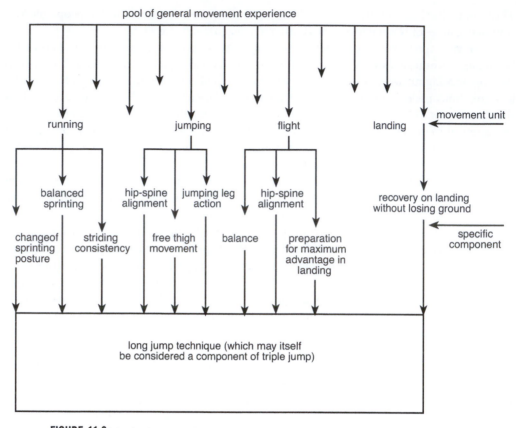

FIGURE 11.3 The development of specific technique via fundamental components

new movements, to be more capable of distinguishing the details of the movement and performing them with accuracy. A progressive development in ability was noted with the increasing mastery of varying exercises. The athlete must be offered the benefit of expert guidance during the learning of technique. Consequently, the practice of providing instruction for beginner athletes via novice coaches might be the basis of a poor technical education which will make itself evident at a later date in faulty technique.

Faults and corrections

Without the assistance of sophisticated equipment, the coach offers instruction based upon the comparison of a 'mental' technical model and what may be readily perceived. There are very obvious limitations to what can be perceived at any one time, so the coach relies mainly on experience of cause and effect. The immediately apparent problems are that coaches have varying amounts of experience and, even with experience, cause and effect are not always easily identifiable. It is nevertheless essential to the athlete's development that accurate information be readily available when kinaesthetic impression and concept of movement are fresh in the athlete's mind. If there is no immediate feedback for the athlete, there is considerable risk of stabilisation of faults. The use of photosequence cameras, videotape, kinographs, videographics, print-outs on force components, velocities, photo-electric apparatus, notational analysis, virtual reality, software packages which allow real time technique comparison, or computerised segmental analysis can provide such feedback. Even if some of this equipment is not readily available for showing the athlete's own performance (e.g. video), it should still be possible to show the correct technique where the athlete is not matching the technical model. The efficiency of technique might be evaluated in one or several of the following broad categories of method.

1. As implied above, evaluating the athlete's technique against the technical model. This approach is used in many so-called 'skill tests', with the athlete 'scored' against norms. It is also used in comparative analysis of the athlete with another athlete known to be technically proficient, or of the athlete with a video of himself performing a technically proficient jump at some previous date. Video techniques, photo-sequence techniques, light-track photography techniques, dedicated software packages, or standard testing processes may be applied to this type of evaluation.

2. Another method is the comparison of actual performance with theoretical performance. For example, a comparison of the height through which the athlete raises his centre of gravity with the height actually jumped in a high jump competition. This method may be extended to include comparison of performance with related criteria in standard tests. Thus, the long jumper may compare competition long jump performance with, on the one hand, standing long jump, sargent jump, 30m sprinting speed; or on the other hand, the horizontal velocity and parabola of flight of the athlete's centre of gravity. Again, video techniques, dedicated software packages, and a knowledge of related standard tests may be applied to the evaluation.

3. A third class of method evaluates a particular technique relative to its success or failure against opposition. Technique is evaluated on the basis of gaining advantage in attack over defence or, conversely, in gaining advantage in defence over attack. It could be argued that tactical input rather than technique is being evaluated in, for instance, team games. Video techniques and notational analysis are essential to this class of evaluation for it to be more effective.

Despite detailed and expert planning, it is nevertheless possible for faults to arise. Before any attempt is made to correct such faults, the exact cause or causes must be determined. This is emphasised due to the fact that 'effect' is more readily recognised; the coach may occasionally reduce the effect of a fault rather than eliminate the cause. It is also important to assess how well established the fault has become. Faults that come to light during the early stages of learning are less difficult to correct than those which have become stabilised to such an extent that they are almost a part of the athlete's technique.

Correction should always ensure the athlete understands the technical model, the fault and the correction. This is vital because frequently athletes who are technically lacking in proficiency may produce superior performances and the novice may seek to follow that technique because it produces favourable results.

Faults must be discovered and corrected early. To delay will stabilise the fault and possibly cause stagnation in performance. Moreover, should the athlete 'grow with the fault' then any attempt at correction becomes more difficult. This is due to the basic inertia of an entrenched pattern and also because performance in general will fall below that recorded when the 'wrong' technique is used, thereby causing a loss of confidence in the process of developing a correct technique. Finally, the additional time required to correct a well-established fault is hard to justify when the time should be directed towards improving an athlete's performance. Getting it right will always prove less expensive than putting it right!

Correction may be pursued by contrasting a faulty and correct technique component. Arranging that faulty performance is impossible so it might prove a useful exercise to practise the movement with, for example, the other leg or arm. The progressive replacement of a faulty technique with a correct technique appears to advance in the same four stages as in learning a new skill. The time span involved varies with the stability and nature of the fault.

Stage 1: the faulty technique asserts itself whenever concentration is lost. The correct technique is occasionally reproduced.

Stage 2: neither the faulty nor the correct techniques are strong enough to dominate, so there is frequently a confusing or mixing of techniques. The correct technique is reproduced more frequently.

Stage 3: there is a conscious differentiation, with the correct technique only occasionally lost, in fatigue or stress.

Stage 4: complete stability of correct technique.

Opinions differ on the relative merits of massed and distributed practice as the athlete learns technique. Personal experience, in the absence of conclusive evidence, suggests an initial massing of practice until the whole activity can be put together, then a gradual separation of practice units. Even when well established, time must be taken to regularly realign technical models and in the first mesocycle of the annual cycle there should be a thorough review of the technical models and careful assessment of the physical competencies related to those models.

General points on technique training units

There must be flexibility in determining exact durations for technique training units because individual athletes vary not only in their capacity for concentration, but also in their status of physical abilities. Several points might be made, however, as a basis for establishing suitable unit construction in technique training.

1. Concentrated technique work should not go beyond 20 minutes without a break.

2. The prospect of a long unit of technique work prepares the athlete for an extended distribution of effort. Consequently, a prolonged unit must be divided into subsections, possibly with each section having a separate emphasis.

3. Reduction of fatigue improves motivation, not only within the session, but also from day to day. Thus, within a training workout, a technique-training unit must come before a conditioning unit and a heavy 'conditioning day' should not precede a 'technical day'.

4. A compromise must be effected between maintaining the excited state of the neuromuscular system and allowing recovery from a previous effort. This will be individually arrived at. It would appear that during recovery from technical training there is a perseveration of neural processes. This may be because when intense external stimulation ceases, internal consolidation occurs. It has also been suggested that organisms are refractory to (resist) early repetition of an act.

5. During recovery there may be a tendency for incorrect associations to be 'forgotten' faster than correct ones. This could be due to the non-existence of positive reinforcements.

6. In technical development, unit construction should be so arranged that all practices are related to the given technique, unless the objective of the unit is to develop the ability to differentiate techniques, select appropriate techniques, or put together a sequence of techniques. Practices may be related by similarity of content, technique, principles, etc. It should be appreciated that these practices are techniques or sports in themselves and are not to be confused with components.

7. Only one technical point should be considered at any one time.

8. Adapt the sport to the athlete before adapting the athlete to the sport. This principle should be followed unless adapting the sport creates a wrong basis for development. For example, hurdles should be reduced in height and spacing, and 'mini' ball games developed for early learning.

9. For sighted athletes, approximately 80 per cent of what is learned is from visual stimuli, so a correct demonstration or a well-explained video is more appropriate than words alone. Auditory and kinaesthetic stimuli are the key learning conduits for blind athletes.

10. It is important to note that the novice athlete must be given expert technical instruction when being introduced to a sport. Conversely, the novice coach must not be used as teacher of the novice athlete unless under the supervision of an experienced coach.

11. 'Repetition is the mother of learning.' The athlete must know the correct technique(s) to repeat and have an appropriate physical competency profile completed to perform sufficient repetitions without fatigue-induced compensations creeping in.

12. The progressions of adding endurance, resistance or speed to development of technique can only be introduced within the limits of keeping the technical model intact. To continue technique work without an intact technical model can lead to 'chronic' (persistent, embedded and very difficult to correct) rather than 'acute' (recent and impactful, cause and effect clear and more readily corrected) technical errors.

13. When technique breaks down, it is essential that 'rebuilding' be done at a slower overall speed. The speed should be such that the athlete can feel the correct sequence of individual body segments' contribution to the technique.

14. Conditions must be favourable, as concentration and freedom of movement are fundamental to learning technique. A warm, windless environment without interfering variables such as noise or distracting movements must be available. Once the technical model is well established, the athlete must learn to keep technique intact in a climate where hostile variables increase in number and degree.

15. There appears to be little difference in the methods used in teaching techniques to men and women. However, due note should be taken of the communication differences suggested in chapter 10. There can be variance in the techniques of men and women, however, even in the same discipline.

16. Children may not be equipped to learn techniques used by mature elite performers. It is the basic technical model that the young athlete learns, and not some sophisticated elaboration of that model.

17. When working to correct a technical fault, the best advice is to go back one or even two steps before the appropriateness of the exercises selected to effect correction. For example, if selecting specific drills for foot movement in tennis, work first on strength exercises to develop those muscles on which efficient performance of those drills depends.

18. Maintain constructive dialogue with the athlete throughout the technical training process and build in time for reflective learning for the athlete and for you at conclusion of the technical training unit.

SUMMARY

Fundamental to the athlete's long-term development is the learning of sound technique. The coach directs such learning and works towards stability of technique through technical training. The classification of technique determines its course of development but, broadly speaking, coaching methodology is geared to various learning stages. An interpretation of cybernetic theory affords an explanation of the concept of learning. Within the framework of this concept the coach will identify the role of fundamental components; the need for accurate identification and speedy correction of faults; the best relevant technology; and the importance of providing the beginner athlete with the best available technical expertise.

REFLECTIVE QUESTIONS

1. You have been asked to design an exercise programme for a tennis player who struggles to make the small footwork adjustments necessary for quick movement about the court. Following study of the player's footwork, you create exercises to develop footwork speed. Unfortunately the athlete cannot coordinate his foot movement. List possible strength, mobility or motor coordination reasons and why they may be causing the coordination difficulties. What would you do to effect correction in each of these reasons?

2. Discuss the statement, 'It is not the faulty technique you see that you must address but the learning stage that preceded it.'

3. An athlete is selected for the national hockey team based on his excellent performances for his club. In the national team, however, he struggles to deliver the same level of technical performance. He is the only player from his club in the national team. Discuss possible explanations for such difference and what would you suggest is done to remedy things.

4. With a faulty technique, your athlete achieves more success than with the corrected model you are coaching the athlete to perfect. Discuss how you will reconcile this with the athlete. If the situation continues and the coach–athlete relationship is becoming fragile, how might you look to resolving the situation and reaffirm the strength of the relationship?

5. Technological advance has brought a proliferation of aids for coaches and athletes. They range from technical feedback apps to remote monitoring and analysis of movement. They also make it possible to compare an athlete's technique with a top performer's and to access technical advice remotely from other technical specialists. Conduct a search for such technology and design a programme for what you discover where it may be used to enhance your technical skills coaching.

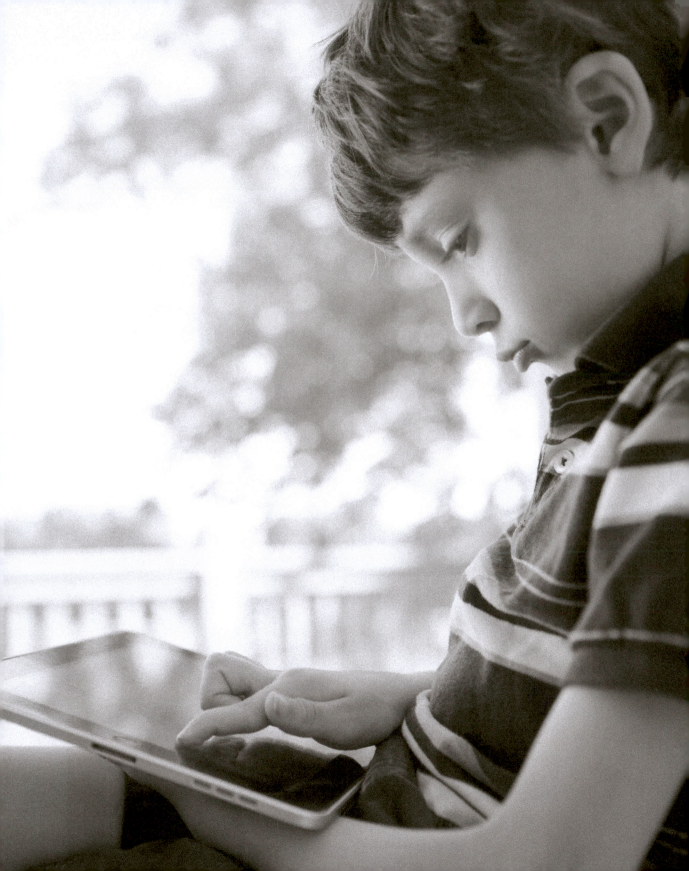

12 PSYCHOLOGICAL CHANGES AND THE GROWING CHILD

Perceptual skills impact upon performance. Given that simple kinaesthetic skills – body movement sensations arising from musculoskeletal sensors – develop during childhood, the coach should be aware of the various stages of development through which the child is required to progress towards adulthood. The trainability of a range of performance-influencing factors is age-determined. The following age divisions are offered as guidelines. Their appropriateness will vary according to many factors, including individual rates of development, male/female differences, and cultural variables.

GENERAL PATTERNS
Early primary school (5–7 years old)

By the age of five the child has developed a wide range of abilities and skills, and individual differences are already apparent. While heredity plays a major role in this individuality, the seeds from which many psychological functions and characteristics of the developing personality have grown (and will grow) are to be found in the many forms of play which constitute the major activity of the child through the early primary school years. He is emotional, thinks graphically, seems to live in a world of half fantasy and half reality, has mastered a wide vocabulary and its use, and thinks rapidly in short, intense bursts which is a mark of mental agility rather than a lack of ability to concentrate. The roles he adopts in play are drawn most accurately from his immediate social environment and, towards the end of this period in primary school, relationships with other children become more stable.

During these formative years, the importance of play must be stressed in the introduction of sport because it is through play that the child develops. His imagination must be stimulated, with success attainable. Above all, activities must be intrinsically enjoyable. Award schemes (and variations) are extremely valuable at this stage for they offer a framework within which it is possible to shape the pupil's behaviour. Finally, it is worth noting that psychological characteristics developed by the age of five may be dampened by the imposition of school discipline at that age. In most other cultures, school is postponed by at least one year. It becomes clear then that the play concept must be the key to maintaining the impetus of developing in a broadening social world, as represented by the school. A guided play approach achieves better results when learning motor skills than free play does. The teacher plays an important part in the child's life at this time. Possibly the coach could come to fulfil a parallel role in terms of an early introduction of the child to coaching in certain sports (e.g. gymnastics).

Primary–secondary school bridge (8–11/13 years old)

This period may be described as a gentle shift from naive realism to critical realism. At the beginning of this period, the child is acquiring knowledge of the world without understanding relationships or trying to see what lies behind reality. Nevertheless, he concentrates on the detail of his environment and can be analytical in perception, memory and thought. His power of concentration is still unstable, so the teacher or coach should avoid lengthy explanations. Variety both in content and method are prerequisites to successful instruction. Throughout this period, the child often requires guidance in the stabilising of social relationships and experimentation in group situations should be encouraged and observed.

As the period progresses, the child becomes capable of concentrating on specific tasks for longer periods of time and begins to seek logical connections and generalisations. As intellectual development progresses, so does his play. Early play experiences (before five years of age) are to gain mastery over his environment and, having achieved this, past successes are re-enacted in a symbolic manner as play develops towards the formality of the game situation. The trend, then, is away from imagination and towards logical thinking. Also worth noting is that towards the end of this period children will have a well-developed ability to memorise. This period also marks the separation of the sexes, in that acceleration towards maturity is greater in girls. One consequence of this is that interests become extremely varied between the sexes. Emotions, while well-balanced and optimistic early in this period, can begin to shift towards a less carefree profile. Consequently, at the end of this period the child has completely altered physically, intellectually, socially and emotionally. Most children will already have entered the period of adolescence.

Mid-/post-secondary (11/13–16 years old)

The start of this period is a whirlwind of change in every characteristic mentioned earlier. Learning becomes an intellectual exercise and productive activity assumes a major role. More social opportunity is now available and relationships within the family unit assume a different form. Social and physiological changes result in emotional imbalance and instability of mood. The young person's uncritical self-assurance is replaced by a fluctuation between esteem and doubt as he gradually pieces together a concept of himself from the collective impression he has of how others see him. This situation is a crucial factor in the information of attitudes that the young athlete in this age range will have towards participation in sport. How he sees himself in the eyes of his peers may influence whether or not he will continue his commitment to pursuit of competitive advantage.

This phase over, the adolescent moves to the final phase in this period. The agitation and disharmony of the first phase gives way to inner assurance that is linked with a visible increase in social capacity. Hopefully, the society in which he grows will not only make high demands of him, but will grant him the right to, and every possibility for, an all-round development of personality and, in particular, progressive situations demanding responsibility. Intellectual development reaches a near-adult level and his attitudes are consciously critical and searching in pursuit of independence of opinion and judgement. A continual awareness of this developmental continuum is important if the child is to grow within the social framework of the 'club' in particular, and the sport of his choice, in general.

Throughout his development, the sport should be adapted to the child before the child is taught how to adapt to the sport. The spirit, not the letter, of both constitutive and regulative rules and regulations should be applied to afford an attractive and flexible framework within which the child will be attracted to express himself. Gradually, by careful planning of his programme of sports education, the official rules will replace this flexible framework without prejudicing his interest, enthusiasm or enjoyment. As the adolescent moves towards the 17–22 year age group, the personality fills out around those basic characteristics evolved up to this period. More and more, however, that personality will seek to stamp itself upon the society about it, and our society (i.e. sport) must learn to accommodate rather than contain it.

MOTOR LEARNING CHARACTERISTICS
Early primary school (5–7 years old)

The period of development probably begins around 3–4 years of age, when a few basic forms of motor patterns are at his disposal. He can crawl, walk, pull, swing, climb, clamber, jump down, run, throw from standing, jump low heights and short distances, and can both catch and kick a ball. These actions represent each of the three forms of movement: locomotor, in which the body is moved through space – walking, running, jumping; non-locomotor, where specific body parts are moved via pushing, pulling, twisting; and manipulative, through which objects are moved – catching, throwing, striking. Already a preference to left or right is evident. In the course of development, all these forms of movement are improved in quality and their repetition seems endless. The first combined movements (rather than movements in sequence) can be seen, i.e. running and jumping, high throwing and catching, running and throwing, running and slinging, running over low barriers in balance, jumping onto objects, running to swing on a rope. Consequently, by the end of this period it is possible to carry out all-round exercise with plenty of variety and intensity of movement.

For many reasons, little is known of the development of physical abilities (e.g. strength) in this age group. It has been shown, however, that speed of movement is only very slightly developed and does not reach more significant values until 9–10 years of age (e.g. up to eight years of age, reaction time is in excess of 0.5 seconds). Also, as far as can be assessed, strength and agility are not well developed at this stage. On the other hand, mobility and aerobic endurance are well developed towards the end of this period. The explanation of the former lies in the elasticity of the movement apparatus and the looseness of joints, while the latter is well developed due to the varied and active play activity. At this stage, a general approach serves to improve strength by using bodyweight and apparatus together with light resistances such as medicine balls and sling balls, as well as to improve the coordination of movement at speed. The introduction of many skills is quite practicable and the following may be borne in mind. These youngsters:

- have a powerful but uncontrolled and non-directed joy in movement
- concentrate for very short spells
- remain undeveloped in their direction of effort
- are limited in their capacity for motor learning
- display a weak retention for what has been learned
- exhibit a limited group consciousness – exercising individually or in very small groups is recommended.

Primary–secondary school bridge (8–11/13 years old)

This is without doubt the most important period in the progress of motor ability. It is that phase of development in which already familiar forms of movement are vastly improved and many new ones learned and stabilised, often without instruction, as demonstrated in activities such as roller skating, ice skating, skateboarding and cycling. New movement patterns are frequently mastered at the first attempt, following suitable demonstrations, concise explanation and one or two trials and accurate corrections. This period has been termed 'the age of specific achievement' or 'the child's best age for learning'. Almost all measures of physical achievement have their greatest rate of improvement at this stage, with speed, agility and aerobic endurance showing the most outstanding rises. Mobility, however, will decline shortly after this period begins and considerable work must be done to improve upon, or even maintain, the levels already acquired.

During these years, the youngster may develop a keen interest in sport, an enthusiasm for learning sport skills, a love of activity, an uninhibited attitude in the learning situation, and an increasing ability to embrace the value of learning athletic skills. The educator is in a favourable position as the youngster wants and has the ability to learn, and enjoys an activity and its related practices. There is a longing for achievement and for challenge. Consequently, training loads can already be quite high, provided the principle of gradual progression to sub-maximal loading (80–90%) has been strictly followed. Particular caution is urged in speed endurance and strength training. The former is known to be among the most severe stresses of athlete training and would certainly seem inadvisable at this stage. In addition, it is debatable whether the youngster is well equipped to tolerate lacticanaerobic stressors. Maximal strength training is not advisable on the grounds of an unconsolidated skeletal structure to which only sub-maximal work should be offered as a load. With initiative and intelligent use of equipment and apparatus, the youngster should find sufficient resistance in the handling of his bodyweight. Certainly there is no justification at this stage for loading the spine by taking weights on the shoulders. Legwork is best done by other means and time would be better spent exercising the spine's own muscular apparatus.

Mid-/post-secondary (11/13–16 years old)

The majority of physical ability statistics continue to show improvement through the traumatic phase of puberty (figure 12.1). The neuromotor system should now have achieved full capacity and be able to offer a store of movement from which more and more complex permutations and combinations can be produced. The increased trainability of the strength components of speed is a consequence of the augmentation in muscle mass resulting from naturally increasing levels of testosterone or oestrogen during puberty.

From now on, development will mean the increasing sophistication of technique, despite interference of environmental variables. The athlete learns by instruction and experience to reproduce perfect movement despite wind, rain, temperature, or opposition tactics. Problems may arise in the shifting relationships of limb proportions in the early years of this period. Such problems, should they occur, will affect coordinative ability, harmony of movement, ability to learn new skills, and motor adaptability. Agility suffers under these circumstances. The problems will manifest themselves in a temporary lack of performance stability, particularly where movement patterns were not learned in the 8–11/13-year-old stage. This emphasises the importance of that stage, and it is suggested that when such problems arise, no new skills be introduced but that work be done on the improvement and consolidation of known skills. It would be ill-advised, for example, to start working on hitch-kick, but right to spend time on stride-jump, in long jump, if this flight technique had been used up to this point.

Gradually the youngster concludes the period of pubescence and slides gently into adolescence, which takes him towards adulthood and the relatively conclusive appearance of all physical and motor characteristics. A second opportunity exists here to introduce new patterns of movements, and progress towards the sophistication mentioned earlier begins. Harre (1986) summarises this period as one of 'harmonisation, increased individualisation, relative stabilisation, and sex differentiation'.

With the relative conclusion of physical growth, untrained youngsters gradually reach their individual best achievements. Girls mature at 15–16 years of age, in contrast with boys at 18–20 years of age. Strength, elastic strength and endurance capacities are all highly trainable during this period and will continue to be so for several years. However, speed improvements become more difficult unless speed has been temporarily stagnated due to habitually low levels of stimulus (e.g. running with slower athletes, running solo, or running on slow tracks).

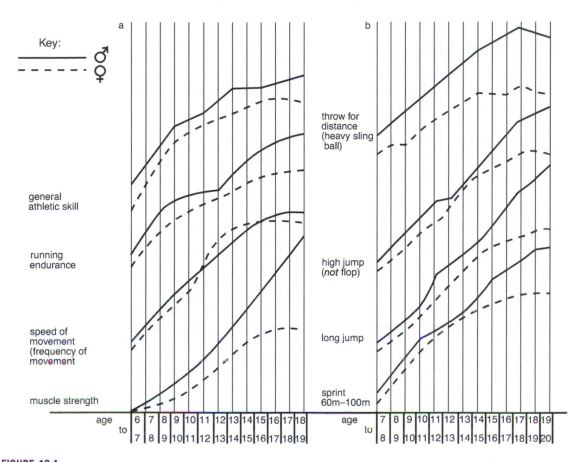

FIGURE 12.1 (a) Non-parametric representation of development, specific to age, of some physical characteristics, 1959); (b) non-parametric representation of development, specific to age, of some basic athletic events (from Harre D., 1973)

SUMMARY

The coach clearly has a role to play in contributing to the education of the growing child. This brief outline of psychological and motor learning characteristics provides a basis for planning this contribution. Development of play constitutes an essential vehicle of total development and the concept of a progression from informal individual play through group games to the formality of organised sport, serves as a framework within which the coach will develop the child's ability to express himself. The most critical period of technical development is suggested as 8–11 years of age (girls) and 8–13 years of age (boys). Sound technical expertise interpreted through play must be available in these years. As coaching does not occur in a vacuum, more than technical efficiency is required. This more holistic approach ensures that the coaching exchange is much more than mere skill acquisition.

REFLECTIVE QUESTIONS

1. Several sports have created modified versions of the sport for young athletes. Select a sport with which you have an interest and experience and design a programme of technique development to take the young athlete from the modified version to the real version.

2. Discuss the advantages and disadvantages in a multi-skill sport of your choice of:
   a. teaching one technique and not moving to another until a robust effective model is established, thus building techniques in sequence, versus
   b. introducing a wide range of techniques simultaneously and building the models in parallel.

3. Discuss the following statement from the point of view of (a) female athletes and (b) male athletes in the age group 14–16. 'The problem we have in retaining young athletes is less about how to motivate them as how to avoid demotivating them.'

4. 'Mobile phone and iPad technology has changed not only how young people communicate, but how they think, how they behave and how they make decisions.' Discuss this statement as a basis for a communications strategy to be more effective as a coach in working with athletes through their teenage years.

5. The tidal wave of physiological, physical, mental and emotional change impacting both male and female athletes through the growing years can be as difficult for them to handle as exciting. Outline your personal continuous professional development plan over the next two years to build relevant competencies in understanding this area. Set out a strategy for developing your skills in helping athletes through these years, indicating conditions under which you would refer the athletes directly to the sport psychologist you will work with. Outline your approach to giving athletes ownership of effectively managing such changes.

SUMMARY OF PART 3

The coach works to improve the efficiency of energy production and of energy expression. At a simplistic level, this means getting the right fuel to the engine and making sure the engine can use it. But athletes are adaptable and creative and, unlike engines, become involved in their own development. The coach must understand and be able to apply not just the 'technical business' but the 'people business'. Both are essential for the coach to be effective. Consequently, the coach requires a sound working knowledge of education and self-education when developing the athlete towards an independence in delivering a quality performance, whether in an individual sport or a team sport and whether in a contributory role or a cooperative role within a team. The coach should understand the learning process, from the specific components which are moulded into a whole in developing an athlete's particular technique(s), through to the climate of emotional arousal, motivational environment, tentative maps of personality, and psycho-regulative phenomena which make every coach-athlete contact period far more unique than generic.

CHAPTER 10 REFERENCES

Aronson, E., Wilson, T. and Akert, R. *Social Psychology*. 4th edn. Upper Saddle River, NJ: Prentice Hall. (2002)

Bar-Eli, M., Dreshman, R., Blumenstein, B. and Weinstein, Y. 'The effect of mental training with biofeedback on the performance of young swimmers'. *Applied Psychology: An International Review* 51(4): 567–81. (2002)

Blumenstein, B., Bar-Eli, M. and Tenenbaum, G. 'A five-step approach to mental training incorporating biofeedback'. *The Sport Psychologist* 11(4): 440–53. (1997)

Blumenstein, B., Bar-Eli, M. and Tenenbaum, G. *Brain and Body in Sport and Exercise: Biofeedback Applications in Performance Enhancement*. New York: John Wiley & Sons. (2002)

Bois, J., Sarrazin, P., Southon, J. and Boiché, J. 'Psychological characteristics and their relation to performance in professional golfers'. *The Sport Psychologist* 23(2): 252–70. (2009)

Carron, A. V. and Hausenblas, H.A. *Group Dynamics in Sport*. 2nd edn. Morgantown, WV: Fitness Information Technology. (1998)

Cohn, P. J., Rotella, R. J. and Lloyd, J. W. 'Effects of a cognitive-behavioral intervention on the preshot routine and performance in golf '. *The Sport Psychologist* 4: 33–47. (1990)

Cumming, J. L. and Ste-Marie, D. M. 'The cognitive and motivational effects of imagery training: A matter of perspective'. *The Sport Psychologist* 15: 276–88. (2001)

DePree, M. *Leadership Jazz*. New York: Dell Publishing. (1992)

Dupee, M. and Werthner, P. 'Managing the stress response: The use of biofeedback and neurofeedback with Olympic athletes'. *Biofeedback* 39(3). (2011)

Doidge, N. *The Brain that Changes Itself*. New York: Viking (2007)

Dick, F.W. *Winning Matters*. London: Abingdon. (2010)

Fournier, J., Calmels, C., Durand-Bush, N. and Salmela, J. 'Effects of a season-long PST program on gymnastic performance and on psychological skill development'. *International Journal of Sport and Exercise Psychology* 3(1): 59–77. (2005)

Gill, D. and Williams, L. *Psychological Dynamics of Sport and Exercise*. 3rd edn. Champaign, IL: Human Kinetics. (2008)

Gould, D., Guinan, D., Greenleaf, C., Medbery, R. and Peterson, K. 'Factors affecting Olympic performance: Perceptions of athletes and coaches from more and less successful teams'. *The Sport Psychologist* 13: 371–94. (1999).

Greenleaf, C., Gould, D. and Dieffenbach, K. 'Factors influencing Olympic performance: Interviews with Atlanta and Nagano U.S. Olympians'. *Journal of Applied Sport Psychology* 13(2): 154–84. (2001)

Gucciardi, D., Gordon, S. and Dimmock, J. 'Evaluation of a mental toughness training program for youth-aged Australian footballers: II. A qualitative analysis'. *Journal of Applied Sport Psychology* 21(3): 324–39. (2009)

Hardy, L. and Callow, N. 'Efficacy of external and internal visual imagery perspectives for the enhancement of performance on tasks in which form is important'. *Journal of Sport and Exercise Psychology* 21: 95–112. (1999)

Hogg, J. 'Debriefing: A means to increasing recovery and subsequent Performance'. In M. Kellmann (ed.), *Enhancing Recovery: Preventing Underperformance in Athletes*, 181–198. Champaign, IL: Human Kinetics. (2002)

Hughes, M. D. and Franks, I. M. *Notational Analysis of Sport: Better Systems for Improving Perfomance and Coaching*. 2nd edn. London: Routledge. (2004)

Janelle, C. 'Anxiety, arousal, and visual attention: A mechanistic account of performance variability'. *Journal of Sports Sciences* 20(3): 237–51. (2002)

Jones, G., Hanton, S. and Connaughton, D. 'What is this thing called mental toughness? An investigation of elite sport performers'. *Journal of Applied Sport Psychology* 14: 205–18. (2002)

Jones, G., Hanton, S. and Connaughton, D. 'A framework of mental toughness in the world's best performers'. *The Sport Psychologist* 21: 243–64. (2007)

Jones, M. 'Controlling emotions in sport'. *The Sport Psychologist* 17(4): 471–86. (2003)

Kellmann, M., Bußmann, G., Anders, D. and Schulte, S. 'Psychological aspects of rowing'. In J. Dosil (ed.), *Sport Psychologist's Handbook: A Guide for Sport-Specific Performance Enhancement*, 479–501. Hoboken, NJ: John Wiley & Sons. (2006)

Kline, N. *Time to Think: Listening to Ignite the Human Mind*. London: Ward Lock. (2003)

Kouzes, J. and Posner, B. *The Leadership Challenge*. San Francisco, CA: Jossey-Bass. (2002)

Lizzio, A., Wilson, K. and MacKay, L. 'Managers' and subordinates' evaluations of feedback strategies: The critical contribution of voice'. *Journal of Applied Social Psychology* 38(4): 919–46. (2008)

Locke, E. A. and Latham, G. P. 'Building a practically useful theory of goal setting and task motivation: A 35-year odyssey'. *American Psychologist* 57: 705–17. (2002)

Mallett, C. and Hanrahan, S. 'Race modeling: An effective cognitive strategy for the 100m sprinter?' *The Sport Psychologist* 11(1): 72–85. (1997)

Mamassis, G. and Doganis, G. 'The effects of a mental training program on juniors' pre-competitive anxiety, self-confidence, and tennis performance'. *Journal of Applied Sport Psychology* 16(2): 118–37. (2004)

Martens, R. *The Social Psychology of Sport*. New York: Harper & Row. (1975)

Martens, R. *Coaches Guide to Sport Psychology*. Champaign, IL: Human Kinetics. (1987)

McArdle, S., Martin, D., Lennon, A. and Moore, P. 'Exploring debriefing in sports: A qualitative perspective'. *Journal of Applied Sport Psychology* 22(3): 320–32. (2010)

Moran, A. 'Improving concentration skills in team-sport performers: Focusing techniques for soccer players'. In R. Lidor and K. Henschen (eds), *The Psychology of Team Sports*, 161–89. Morgantown, WV: Fitness Information Technology. (2003)

Moran, A. 'Attention, concentration and thought management'. In B. Brewer (ed.), *Sport Psychology*, 18–29. Oxford: Blackwell Publishing. (2009)

Moss Kanter, R. *Confidence: How Winning Streaks and Losing Streaks Begin and End*. New York: Three Rivers Press. (2004)

Nideffer, R. M. *The Inner Athlete*. New York: Crowell. (1976)

Nideffer, R. M. and Segal, M. 'Concentration and attention control training'. In J. M. Williams (ed.), *Applied Sport Psychology: Personal Growth to Peak Performance*, 4th edn, 312–32. Mountain View, CA: Mayfield. (2001)

Orlick, T. *In Pursuit of Excellence*. 4th edn. Champaign, IL: Human Kinetics. (2007)

Orlick, T. and Partington, J. 'Mental links to excellence'. *The Sport Psychologist* 2(2): 105–30. (1988)

Posner, M. I., Nissen, M. J. and Klein, R. M. 'Visual dominance: An information-processing account of its origins and significance'. *Psychological Review* 83: 157–70. (1976)

Prapavessis, H., Grove, J., McNair, P. and Cable, N. 'Self-regulation training, state anxiety, and sport performance: A psychophysiological case study'. *The Sport Psychologist* 6(3): 213–29. (1992)

Robazza, C., Pellizzari, M. and Hanin, Y. 'Emotion self-regulation and athletic performance: An application of the IZOF model'. *Psychology of Sport and Exercise* 5(4): 379–404. (2004)

Tannen, D. *You Just Don't Understand: Women and Men in Conversation*. New York: Ballantine Books. (1990)

Tannen, D. 'The power of talk: Who gets heard and why'. *Harvard Business Review* 73: 138–48. (1995)

Taylor, M., Gould, D. and Rolo, C. 'Performance strategies of US Olympians in practice and competition'. *High Ability Studies* 19(1): 19–36. (2008)

Tuckman, B. W. 'Developmental sequence in small groups'. *Psychological Bulletin* 63: 384–99. (1965)

Werthner, P., Christie, S. and Dupee, M. 'Neurofeedback and biofeedback training with Olympic athletes'. *NeuroConnections* Summer: 32–7. (2013)

Wulf, G. and Su, J. 'An external focus of attention enhances golf shot accuracy in beginners and experts'. *Research Quarterly for Exercise and Sport* 78(4): 384–9. (2007)

CHAPTERS 11 AND 12 REFERENCES

Abernethy, B., Wann, J. and Parks, S. 'Training perceptual-motor skills for sport'. In B. Elliot (ed.), *Training in Sport*. Chichester: John Wiley. (1999)

Anochin, D. K. *Das Funktionelle System Ais Grundlage Der Physiologischen Architektur Des Verhaltensakte*s. Jena: Veb Gustav Fischer Verlag. (1967)

Baume, D. A., 'A Dynamic Theory of Organizational Knowledge Creation', Organization Science 5: 14–37, (2004)

Bernstein, N. A. *The Coordination and Regulation of Movements*. London: Pergamon Press. (1957)

Broadwell, M., 'Teaching for Learning (XVI)', The Gospel Guardian, vol. 20 (41), pp. 1–3 (1969)

Burch, N., 'Four Stages of Learning Any New Skill' in Learning a New Skill is Easier Said Than Done, Adams, L. Solana Beach, CA: Gordon Training International (2011)

Dick, F. W. *High Jump*. Birmingham: British Athletic Federation. (1993)

Dyatchkov, N. V. *Soversenstsvovanie Techniceskogo Masterstva Sportsmenov*. Moscow: Fiskultura i Sport. (1967)

Evarts, E. V. 'Motor cortex reflexes associated with learned movement'. *Science* 179: 501–3. (1973)

Gallistel, C. R. *The Organisation of Action*. Hillsdale, NJ: Erlbaum. (1980)

Harre, D. *Principles of Sport Training*. Berlin: Sportverlag. (1986)

Harre, D. *Trainingslehre*. Berlin: Sportverlag. (1973)

Kahneman, D., *Attention and Effort*. Englewood Cliffs, NJ: Prentice Hall (1973)

Lotter, W. S. 'Interrelationships among reaction times and speeds of movement in different limbs'. *Research Quarterly* 38: 202–7. (1960)

Maslow, A. H. and Lower, R. (ed.), *Towards a Psychology of Being*, 3rd edition. New York: Wiley & Sons (1988)

Malina, R. M. and Bouchard, C. *Growth, Maturation, and Physical Activity*. Champaign, IL: Human Kinetics. (1991)

Marshall, R. N. and Elliot, B. C. 'The analysis and development of technique in sport'. In B. Elliot (ed.), *Training in Sport*. Chichester: John Wiley. (1999)

Meyers, M. C., Bourgeois, A. E., LeUnes, A. D. and Murray, N. A. 'Mood and psychological skills of elite and sub-elite equestrian athletes'. *Journal of Sport Behavior* 23(3): 399–409. (1999)

Schneider, W. and Fisk, A. D., 'Attentional theory of mechanisms for skilled performance' in Magill, R. A., (ed), Memory and Control of Action. Holland: Elsevier (1983)

Schmidt, R. A., *Motor Control and Learning: A behavioural emphasis*, 2nd edition. Champaign, IL: Human Kinetics, (1988)

Selye, Hans. *Stress without Distress*. Philadelphia, PA: Lippincott Williams & Wilkins (1974)

Smyth, M. M. and Marriot, A. M. 'Vision proprioception in simple catching'. *Journal of Motor Behavior* 14: 143–52. (1982)

Whiting, H. T. A. *Concepts in Skill Learning*. London: Lepus Books. (1975)

CHAPTERS 11 AND 12 BIBLIOGRAPHY

Allport, G. W. *Personality*. New York: Holt, Rinehart & Winston. (1937)

Allport, G. W. *Pattern and Growth in Personality*. New York: Holt, Rinehart & Winston (1961)

Allport, G. W, Vernon, P. E. and Lindzey, G. *A Study of Value: A Scale for Measuring the Dominant Interests in Personality*. Boston, MA: Houghton & Mifflin. (1951)

Amrose, A. and Horn, T. S. 'Relationship between perceived coaching behaviours and motivational climate in college athletes'. *Journal of Sport and Exercise Psychology* 9. (1997)

Apitzsch, E. and Berggren, B. *The Personality of the Elite Soccer Player*. Lund: Lund University. (1993)

Apter, M. J. *The Experience of Motivation: The Theory of Psychological Reversals*. London: Academic Press. (1982)

Arkes, H. R. and Garske, J. P. *Psychological Theories of Motivation*. 2nd edn. Monterey, CA: Brooks/Cole Publishing Company. (1982)

Balson, P. D., Elcblom, B., Soderlund, K., Sjodin, B. and Hulfan, G. 'Creative supplementation and dynamic high intensity intermittent exercise'. *Scandinavian Journal of Medicine and Science in Sports* 3: 143–9. (1993)

Bandura, A. 'Self-efficacy: Toward a unifying theory of behavioural change'. *Psychological Review* 84: 191–215. (1977)

Bangsbo, J. 'The physiology of soccer with special reference to intense, intermittent exercise'. *Acta Physiologica Scandinavica* 151(Suppl. 619): 1–115. (1994)

Bar-Eli, M., Hartman, I. and Levy-Kolker, N. 'Using goal-setting to improve physical performance of adolescents with behaviour disorders: The effect of goal proximity'. *Adapted Physical Activity Quarterly* 11: 86–97. (1994)

Bauersfeld, M. and Voss, G. *Neve Wege im Schnellgkeitstraining*. Munster: Philippka. (1992)

Beggs, A. W. D. 'Goal setting in sport'. In G. J. Jones and L. Hardy (eds), *Stress and Performance in Sport*. Chichester: John Wiley. (1993)

Biddle, S. J. H. 'Exercise motivation across the life span'. In S. J. H. Biddle (ed.), *European Perspectives on Exercise and Sport Psychology*. Champaign, IL: Human Kinetics. (1995)

Blanchard, K. and Johnson, S. 'The one minute manager'. In K. Blanchard, P. Zigarmi and D.Zigarmi (eds), *Leadership and the One Minute Manager*. London: Willow Books. (1983)

Blanchard, K. and Schula, D. *Everyone's a Coach*. New York: Harper Business. (1995)

Bloomfield, J., Ackland, J. and Elliott, B. *Applied Anatomy and Biomechanics in Sport*. Melbourne: Blackwell Scientific Publications. (1994)

Boutcher, S. H. 'The role of performance routines in sport'. In G. J. Jones and L. Hardy (eds), *Stress and Performance in Sport*. Chichester: John Wiley. (1993)

Burton, D. 'Multimodal stress management in sport: current status and future directions'. In G. J. Jones and L. Hardy (eds), *Stress and Performance in Sport*. Chichester: John Wiley. (1993)

Carbonaro, G. *Motor Coordination in Sport and Exercise*. Rome: Fidal. (2001)

Carron. A. V. and Ball, J. R. 'Cause and effect characteristics of cohesiveness and participation motivation in intercollegiate ice hockey'. *International Review of Sport Sociology* 12: 49–60. (1977)

Carron, A. V., Widmeyer, W. N. and Brawley, L. R. 'The development of an instrument to assess cohesion in sport teams: the Group Environment Questionnaire'. *Journal of Sport Psychology* 7: 244–67. (1985)

Cattell, R. B. *The Scientific Analysis of Personality.* Harmondsworth: Penguin. (1965)

Cohen, F. and Lazarus, R. S. 'Coping with serious illness'. In G. S. Stone, F. Cohen and N. E. Adler (eds), *Health Psychology.* San Francisco, CA: Freeman. (1979)

Côté, L., Salmela, J., Trudel, P., Baria, A. and Russell, S. 'The coaching model: A grounded theory assessment of expert gymnastic coaches' knowledge'. *Journal of Sport and Exercise Psychology* 17(1): 1–17. (1995)

Covey, S. R. *Principle-Centred Leadership.* New York: Simon & Schuster. (1992)

Cox, R. H. *Sport Psychology. Concepts and Applications.* 4th edn. New York: WCB/McGraw-Hill. (1998)

Counsilman, J. E. *Competitive Swimming.* Englewood Cliffs, NJ: Prentice Hall. (1977)

Dainty, D. A. and Norman, R. W. *Standardising Biomechanical Testing in Sport.* Champaign, IL: Human Kinetics. (1987)

Davidson, R. J. and Schwartz, G. E. 'The psychobiology of relaxation and related states: a multiprocess theory'. In D. Mostofsky (ed), *Behavioral Control and Modification of Physiological Activity.* Englewood Cliffs, NJ: Prentice Hall. (1976)

Dick, F. W. *Winning: Motivation for Business, Sport and Life.* London: Abingdon. (1992)

Dick, F. W. *Players Guide.* Hartlepool: West Hartlepool Rugby Football Club. (1995)

Doherty, J. K. *Modern Track and Field: Promotion, History and Methods.* London: Bailey & Swinfen. (1963)

Donnellon, A. *Team Talk: The Power of Language in Team Dynamics.* Cambridge, MA: Harvard Business School. (1996)

Eysenck, H. J. and Eysenck, S. B. G. *Eysenck Personality Inventory Manual.* London: University of London Press. (1968)

Fredenburgh, F. A. *The Psychology of Personality and Adjustment.* Menlo Park, CA: Benjamin Cummings. (1971)

Freud, S. 'Libidinal types'. In S. Freud, *Collected Papers, Vol 5*, ed. Strachey, J. London: Hogarth Press. (1931)

Frankel, L. P. *Overcoming Your Strengths.* New York: Harmony Books. (1997)

Fromm, E. *Escape from Freedom.* New York: Holt, Rinehart & Winston. (1941)

Fromm, E. *Man For Himself.* New York: Holt, Rinehart & Winston. (1947)

Fuoss, D. E. and Troppman, R. J. *Effective Coaching: A Psychological Approach.* New York: John Wiley. (1991)

Galtanus, G. C., Williams, C., Boobls, L. H. and Brooks, S. 'Human muscle metabolism during intermittent maximal exercise'. *Journal of Applied Physiology* 75: 712–19. (1993)

Galvin, P. 'Applying an organisational developmental model to a sports setting'. In R. J. Butler (ed.), *Sport Psychology in Performance.* Oxford: Butterworth Heinemann. (1997)

Geese, R. and Hillebrecht, M. *Schnelligkeitstraining.* Aacheon: Meyer and Meyer. (1995)

Gollnick, P. D. and Hermanisen, L. *Biomechanical Adaptations to Exercise: Anaerobic Metabolism Exercise and Sport Science Reviews* (ed. Wilmorg, J. H.) Vol. 1, New York: Academic Press. (1973)

Gould, D. and Krane, V. 'The arousal athletic performance relationship: Current status and future directions'. In T. Horn (ed.), *Advances in Sport Psychology*, 119–41. Champaign, IL: Human Kinetics. (1992)

Gould, D. and Udry, E. 'Psychological skills for enhancing performance: Arousal regulation strategies'. *Medicine and Science in Sport and Exercise* 26(4): 478–85. (1994)

Gruber, J. J. and Gray, G. R. 'Factor patterns of variables influencing cohesiveness at various levels of basketball competition'. *Research Quarterly for Exercise and Sport* 52: 19–30. (1981)

Gruber, J. J. and Gray, G. R. 'Responses to forces influencing cohesion as a function of player status and level of male varsity basketball competition'. *Research Quarterly for Exercise and Sport* 53: 27–36. (1982)

Harris, D. V. and Harris, B. L. *The Athlete's Guide to Sport Psychology: Mental skills for physical people.* New York: Leisure Press. (1984)

Hendy, H. M. and Bower, B. J. 'Gender differences in attribution for triathlon performance'. *Sex Roles* 29: 527–42. (1993)

Hickson, R. C. 'Interference of strength development by simultaneously training for strength and endurance'. *European Journal of Applied Physiology* 42: 372–6. (1980)

Hill, K. L. *Framework for Sport Psychologists.* Champaign, IL: Human Kinetics. (2001)

Hollander, E. P. *Principles and Methods of Social Psychology.* New York: Oxford University Press. (1971)

Horne, T. and Carron, A. V. 'Compatibility in coach-athlete relationships' *Journal of Sport Psychology* 7: 137–49. (1985)

Huber, V. L. 'Effects of task difficulty goal setting, and strategy on performance of a heuristic task'. *Journal of Applied Psychology* 70: 492–504. (1985)

Ickes, W. J. and Layden, M. A. 'Attributional styles'. In J. H. Harvey, W. J. Ickes and R. Kidd (eds), *New Directions in Attribution Research*, vol. 2. Hillsdale, NJ: Erlbaum. (1978)

Ingjer, F. and Myhre, K. 'Physiological effects of altitude training on elite male cross-country skiers'. *Journal of Sports Sciences* 10: 49–63. (1992)

Iso-Ahola, S. E. and Hatfield, B. *Psychology of Sports: A Social Psychological Approach.* Dubuque, IA: Wm. C. Brown. (1986)

Jacobson, E. *Progressive Relaxation.* Chicago, IL: University of Chicago Press. (1929)

Jones G. J. 'A cognitive perspective on the process underlying the relationship between stress and performance in sport'. In G. J. Jones and L. Hardy (eds), *Stress and Performance in Sport.* Chichester: John Wiley. (1993)

Jones, R. L. 'Toward a sociology of coaching'. In R. L. Jones and K. M. Armour (eds), *Sociology of Sport.* Harlow: Longman. (2000)

Katzenbach, J. R. *Real Change Leaders: How you can Create Growth and High Performance at your Company.* New York: McKinsey & Company. (1995)

Kinlaw, D. C. *Coaching for Commitment: Managerial Strategies for Obtaining Superior Performance.* Oxford: Pfeiffer & Company. (1993)

Komi, P. V. 'Measurement of the force–velocity relationship in human muscle under concentric and eccentric contraction'. *Medicine of Sport* 8 (Biomechanics III): 224–9. (1973)

Komi, P. V. and Bosco, C. 'Utilisation of stored elastic energy in leg extensor muscles by men and women'. *Medicine and Science in Sport and Exercise* 10: 261–5. (1978)

Kozlov, I. and Muraveyev, I. 'Muscles and the sprint'. *Fitness and Sport Review* 6: 192. (1992)

Krech, D. and Crutchfield, R. S. *Elements of Psychology.* New York: Alfred A. Knopf. (1962)

Kyllo, L. B. and Landers, D. M. 'Goalsetting in sport and exercise: A research synthesis to resolve the controversy'. *Journal of Sport and Exercise Psychology* 17: 117–37. (1995)

Landers, D. and Leuschen, G. 'Team performance outcome and cohesiveness of competitive coaching groups'. *International Review of Sport Sociology* 2: 57–69. (1974)

Legs, A. and Arthur, S. 'An investigation into anaerobic performance of wheelchair'. *Ergonomics* 31: 1529–37. (1988)

Lenk, N. 'Top performance despite internal conflicts: An antithesis to a functionalistic proposition'. In J. W. Loy and G. S. Kenyon (eds), *Sport, Culture and Society: A Reader on the Sociology of Sport*, 393–7. New York: Macmillan. (1969)

Lopez, V. 'An approach to strength training for sprinters'. *Track Technique* 115: 3668–95. (1991)

McAtee, R. *Facilitated Stretching.* Champaign, IL: Human Kinetics. (1993)

Mahoney, M. J. and Avener, M. 'Psychology of the elite athlete: An exploratory study'. *Cognitive Therapy and Research* 1: 135–41. (1977)

Martens, R. *Coaches' Guide to Sport Psychology*. Champaign, IL: Human Kinetics. (1987)

Massimo, J. 'The gymnast's perception of the coach: Performance competence and coaching style'. In R. M. Suinn (ed.), *Psychology in Sports: Methods and Applications*, 229–37. New York: Macmillan. (1980)

Miller, T. W. 'Assertiveness training for coaches: The issue of healthy communication between coaches and players'. *Journal of Sport Psychology* 4: 107–41. (1982)

Moritani, J. 'Time course of adaptations during strength and power training'. In P. V. Korni (ed.), *Strength and Power in Sport*, 266–78. Oxford: Blackwell Scientific Publications. (1992)

Murray, P. E. *IS4: Integrated Sport Science Support Strategy*. Victoria, BC: International Coaching School of Canada. (1994)

Murray, P. E. *Cohesion: A Perspective from Operationalised Coaching Styles in Coaching and Interacting Sports*. Working Papers in Education. Wolverhampton: Educational Research Unit, University of Wolverhampton. (1996)

Murray, P. E. *The Construction and Validation of the Facilitating Coaching Styles Questionnaire*. Wolverhampton: University of Wolverhampton Press. (1999)

Murray, P. F. and Krastev, A. M. *La ejecucion élite y el comportamiento del entrenador. Estudios del Entrenador; apoyo academico para la maestria en las ciencias del deporte*. Chihuahua: Universidad Autonoma de Chihuahua. (1992)

Nolan, T. 'A walk on the wild'. *Coach and Athletic Director* April: 51–8. (1997)

Ozolin, E. S. 'The sprint'. *Soviet Sports Review* 2: 57–60; 3: 142–4; 4: 195–9. (1990)

Pollard, A. 'Sociology and teaching: A new challenge for the sociology of education'. In P. Woods and A. Pollard (eds), *Reflective Teaching: The Sociological Contribution*. London: Croom Helm. (1998)

Pope, W. 'Emile Durkheim'. In R. Stones (ed.), *Key Sociological Thinkers*. Basingstoke: Macmillan. (1998)

Pousson, M., Van Hogeke, J. and Goubel, F. 'Changes in elastic characteristics of human muscle induced by eccentric exercise'. *Journal of Biomechanics* 23: 343–8. (1990)

Steiner, C. *Achieving Emotional Literacy*. London: Bloomsbury. (1999)

Sternberg, R. J. *Thinking Styles*. Cambridge: Cambridge University Press. (1999)

Tellez, T. in D. Hemery, *Sporting Excellence: What Makes a Champion?* London: HarperCollins. (1991)

Verhoshansky, Y. V. and Lazarev, V. V. 'Principles of planning speed and strength; speed endurance training in sport'. *Journal of National Strength and Conditioning* 2: 58–61. (1989)

Wadler, G. R. and Haimling, B. *Drugs and the Athlete*. Philadelphia, PA: F. A. Davis. (1989)

Westre, K. R. and Weiss, M. R. 'The relationship between perceived coaching behaviours and group cohesion in high school football teams'. *Sport Psychologist* 5(1): 41–54. (1991)

Wilke K. 'Analysis of sprint swimming: The 50m freestyle'. *Swimming Science* 6: 33–46. (1996)

Wilson, G., Elliott, B. and Wood, G. 'Stretch shorten cycle performance enhancement through flexibility training'. *Medicine and Science – Sports and Exercise* 24: 116–23. (1992)

Zimmerman, B. J. and Kitsantus, A. 'Self-regulated learning of a motoric skill: The role of goal setting and self-monitoring'. *Journal of Applied Sport Psychology* 8: 60–75. (1996)

PART 4
THE LANGUAGE OF TRAINING THEORY

In parts 1, 2 and 3, relevant aspects of the sports-related sciences have been reviewed. Parts 4 and 5 seek to draw together the practical implications of this review and, by considering these against a backcloth of experience, to apply them to the development of the athlete.

One of the greatest problems in studying training theory is the diversity of terminology. The most obvious examples of this are in the area of fitness and its components. In part 4, a framework of definition and explanation is set out to establish a sound basis in this aspect of training theory. The concept of fitness is examined as it applies to all lifestyles. The major components of fitness, seen here as strength, speed, endurance, mobility, and their derivatives, are brought into focus in separate chapters. The technical component is covered in chapter 11. An understanding of these components is fundamental to the construction of training programmes specific to the athlete and the discipline. The final chapter of part 4 deals with evaluation, a process critical to the ordered progression of training and, consequently, of fitness.

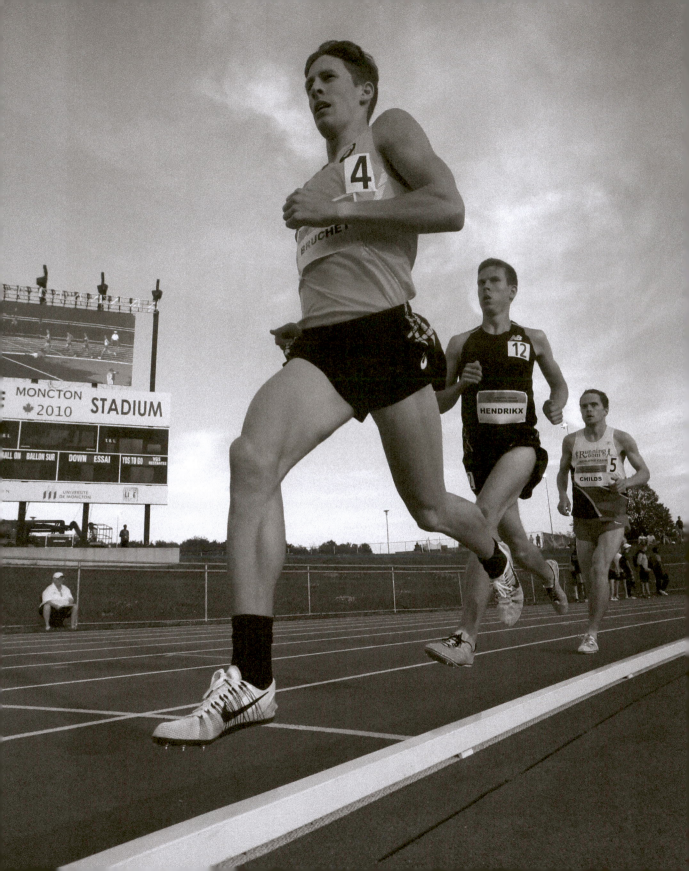

13 FITNESS

Fitness may be defined as the level of adaptation to the stressors of a given lifestyle. It is an essential component in the concept of 'wellness', which might be defined as a persistent endeavour to achieve the highest probability for total wellbeing (figure 13.1). A scientifically based and systematic training programme is fundamental to the athlete's fitness. Training provides the athlete with the basic means to adapt to his particular stressors through controlled exercise. Training theory may supplement the coach's practical knowledge to help him formulate a balanced training programme. The principles of training which apply in designing fitness programmes apply equally to elite performers, recreational performers, developing performers and those whose lives are not oriented towards sport or physical recreation.

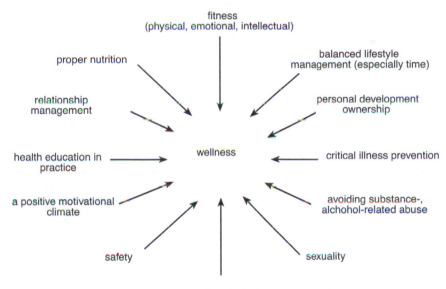

FIGURE 13.1 Critical components of 'wellness'

THE GENERAL PICTURE

If a fitness programme is to be relevant, three questions must be answered. What is the lifestyle of the person involved? Is that person fit for that lifestyle? How can that person become fitter, or maintain present fitness levels?

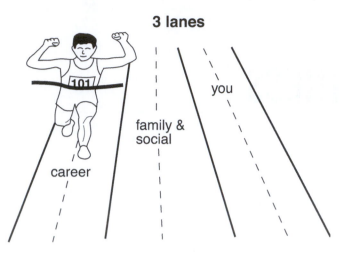

3 lanes

you

family &
social

career

FIGURE 13.2 A balanced approach to personal development requires planning to achieve goals in all three lanes

To answer the first question one must review the stressors of the lifestyle: work, social, family, leisure pursuits, and so on. The review becomes more complex when such factors as ambition and anxiety are taken into account. Without a detailed answer to the first question, it is impossible to consider the second. The review is seldom easy, because not all stressors are obvious. Issues become confused as there is temptation to focus only on those factors which can readily produce the effects of stress-related problems. The fact that a person appears to have the measure of his cumulative stressor climate, as determined, say, by a favourable testosterone/cortisol ratio, should not be interpreted as meaning that one may dismiss the relevance of any component stressor within that climate. Each stressor must be considered – and the athlete's status relative to that stressor evaluated – before addressing the final question of how to ensure that the athlete remains in control, or can regain control.

One's lifestyle might be thought of as a three-lane motorway along which a person travels through life (figure 13.2). The 'Highway Code' is one's values framework – there is overall purpose for the journey variously determined by religious beliefs or philosophies of life. Each lane represents a broad avenue of progression: one's occupation or means of earning (career); one's social and family responsibilities (family and social); and the avenue of one's personal expression or creativity (you). Each person is continually on the move along the 'motorway', meeting the demands of pursuing objectives in any, or all, of the lanes at any time. There are many possible stressors in pursuit of these objectives.

Career

Most careers have their own in-built set of stressors. On starting a new career, one is more aware of what they are. The majority are soon accommodated as routine is established and they consequently represent a low-level package of stressors. However, crises have to be managed, personal emotions must be suppressed despite provocation, and routine must be pursued despite peaks and troughs of general health and instability in the non-working environment.

For the committed athlete, whether professional or amateur, full-time or part-time, 'career' embraces the 'career' that is outside sport, such as study and business, plus the 'career' that is sport. Because performance

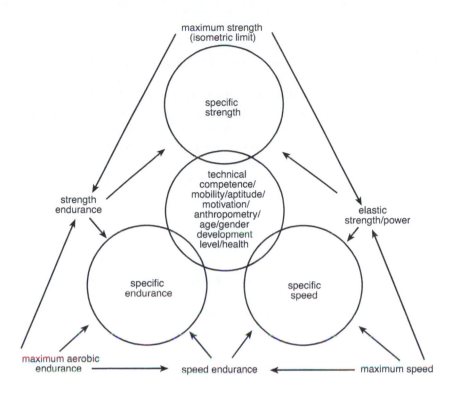

FIGURE 13.3 Schematic representation of the relationship of basic fitness characteristics and their involvement in the specific fitness required of individual disciplines/sports.

is competitive, sport is a total expression of an athlete's complex profile of competence and motivation, and pursuit of achievement represents a considerable range of stressors. They include the physical demands on the organism when training to develop those conditioning characteristics relevant to a given sport. These are represented in figure 13.3. As the athlete progresses through a year plan, the effects of physical stressors vary according to how the athlete's conditioning status matches the specific demands of cumulative training loads. The range of stressors also includes those associated with varied fortunes in pursuit of high ambition, especially when sport is 'career'!

Family and social

Home and social situations also have their own stressor profile. Family bereavement not only represents an immense immediate stressor of emotional trauma, but also the shock waves can last months, or even years, putting health at risk. Moving house is also a most stressful experience as the disorientation can drain reserves of physical and emotional energy. Other states of transition can have high potential as stressors. They include shifting from school to university, or school to employment; from childhood through adolescence; from a stable to an unstable relationship; from employment to unemployment; from having children at home to having them leave; and from a comfortable economic scenario to one where there is seldom enough to meet the next round of bills.

You

Most people seldom attend to addressing those stressors that impact on personal life. Personal development can too readily be considered relative to 'career' rather than the 'real you'. In the interest of emotional, intellectual and physical health/fitness/wellbeing, there should be a strategy for coping with the total environment of stressors and for delivering on personal development. The key to achieving the right strategy is understanding that there is only one pool of adaptation energy available to cope with cumulative stressors (figure 13.4).

Running across these three broad areas of stressor is a person's profile relative to the impact of their personal interpretations and delivery of other 'wellness' components in practice. The total complex of the stressor environment is, then, substantial and unique to a given person. Each person is located somewhere on a lifelong fitness continuum – what fitness means in personal terms reflects where someone is on that continuum, which might be thought of as a progression of roughly decade long stages.

Age

5–14	Learning skills, developing conditioning base and forming attitudes to use over the next 20 years to development advantage.
15–24	Fitness relates to pursuit of development/competitive advantage.
25–34	Cosmetic fitness; weight control; peak competitive years (in sport).
35–44	Wellness focus to protect from coronary disease.
45–54	Balancing lifestyle to avoid stress-related illness.
55–64	Maintaining energy levels to keep pace with 35–54-year-olds.
65 →	Living that pace of life which lets you enjoy it.

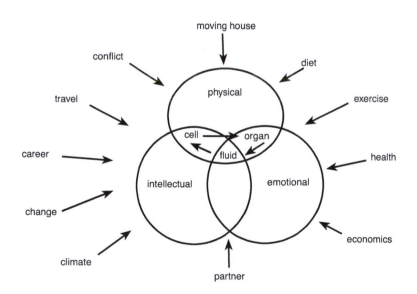

FIGURE 13.4 Stressors persistently bombard us. Our response is stress-increased agitation in the cycle of interdependence between cells, organ and fluids. Because the pool of general adaptation energy required for that response is finite, the stressor effect is cumulative. The total stressor 'package' must then, be identified and managed.

5–14 years old

Family, school, local authorities and activity-focused clubs build on the personal talents/abilities one is born with, plus early life experience, motivational climate and early attitude framework. These years, which bridge the primary and secondary school years, are more development-centred than achievement-centred. They are critical preparation for the next 20 years and, therefore, for life. They prepare young people for what they will do and how they will do it in the challenging and competitive years to come. They are the fitness foundation years for life. It is essential then, that in these years behaviour patterns for regular activity and healthful nutrition and lifestyle discipline are taught and learned. This applies whether these years are the first in the high performance athlete pathway or simply the building blocks for a healthy, active and productive life.

15–24 years old

Even if one is not committed to becoming a 'sports star', these years could be vital in establishing a pattern of physical recreation. Sports centres, sports clubs, sports councils and governing bodies of sport will be able to advise on where and when one may participate in sport and recreation at one's own level. These years see significant and substantial lifestyle situations from school to higher education; making occupation and career choices; changing domestic circumstances etc. Consequently new routines must build upon well-being related behaviour patterns developed in the previous decade. This is not only a matter for thoughtful time management but for a conscious attention to all that constitutes a healthy active lifestyle and the balance between addressing the challenges of these years and regeneration. Regular exercise and balanced diet are the best form of preventive medicine against fitness and health problems in subsequent decades. For those now on the high performance athlete pathway, these are the most critical development years. Coaches leading the process of such development should be specialists in taking athletes through the relevant development stages.

25–34 years old

Problems in this age group find their origins in the previous decade. Difficulties in weight control are derived from indiscriminate eating habits and lack of exercise. By reducing the daily calorific intake, weight will be lost but muscle tone will not improve. Only exercise will improve muscle tone, but it must be aimed at the appropriate muscles. Exercises fall mainly in the strength endurance, heart endurance and mobility areas. However, if one is pursuing continued involvement in sport, all the characteristics mentioned for the previous decade will be developed, and to an appropriate level. Regular aerobic exercise is a vital form of preventive medicine for this age group. Although professional sports may already have some high potential athletes under contract from the late teens, for most sports the 'peak performance years' are within this age range. Early thought should be given to those adjustments in activity and diet in the years following an athlete's competitive years in sport.

35–44 years old

If the years leading into this period have not seen the stressors of lifestyle well managed, their accumulation may lead to cardiovascular and other health-related problems (figure 5.2, p. 90). For example, if people in this age group have done very little exercise, there is high potential for the following:

- Being overweight or even obese, which puts an extra load on the heart and increases risk of diabetes.
- Poor muscle tone, which endangers joints in sudden exertion (especially the back) and leads to postural problems.
- Joint stiffness, which limits movement in the joints and consequently discourages exercise.
- Poor condition of the oxygen transporting system – this leads to breathlessness in even slight exertion, is related to coronary problems, and generally discourages active recreation.

Twenty years or so of inactivity will make it very difficult and even dangerous to launch into vigorous exercise now! The best policy is first to review diet – specifically reducing carbohydrate intake as part of a weight loss strategy. Advice should be sought in this from a GP or nutrition expert. By attacking the weight situation early, exercise will be less uncomfortable. Next, improve joint mobility, then the oxygen transporting system, and then move on to muscle tone. Low impact exercise will help avoid the demotivation which comes with muscle and joint aches. So instead of jogging, try mountain biking, roller blading, langlauf, etc. This, combined with dietary control, will reduce weight. As a result new life will be put into these years with the physical, social and mental benefits of physical recreation.

For the athlete who is into post competitive years, a strategy should be designed and delivered to cope with the wear and tear of the high performance training and competition years while establishing a routine which balances activity, regeneration and diet. Some athletes may of course continue to compete under specialist coaching supervision in 'masters' competition.

45–54 years old

If a momentum to activity, regeneration and diet has not already been established, it is vital that early in this decade it is effectively addressed. Exercise and activity programmes should be undertaken following a general medical check. National and local authority campaigns provide advice on this. That will also be available via gyms, health clubs, spas etc. Twice per week aerobic workouts through walking, jogging, swimming, cycling, etc.; mobility workouts in the shape of daily stretches; and once per week general strength workout from bodyweight circuits to supervised strength workouts in a gym will serve most person's needs as a basic programme. Annual health checks are recommended, for example to monitor cholesterol, blood pressure, sugar, etc., and also gender related health hot spots via appropriate screening procedures. It is also sensible to review stressor climate and stress management effectiveness at least annually. Again, an increasing number of athletes will continue to pursue 'masters' competition preparation and performance under specialist coach supervision.

55–64 years old

Attention to balanced nutrition and other things such as weekly intake of alcohol units remain a matter of sensible self-discipline. Regular activity/exercise along the lines of suggestion for the previous decade should remain, although heavy strength work is not generally recommended except for those who may be continuing in 'masters' weightlifting or strength related 'masters' sports. Again, management of the stressor climate and its impact is essential. Annual health checks as per previous decade, if not continued should now be routine. If not already done, it is time for broadening those fields of personal interest and aptitude which will enrich not only the regeneration process in a world of challenges, but life as a whole. Such things may combine substantial physical activity blended with the therapeutic values of, for example, working in the garden. On the other hand they may afford opportunity for personal skills to be made available to club or community organisations as a leader, manager, coach, mentor, etc. This of course brings value to the club or organisation but also a sense of fulfilment and being valued to the person concerned. Athletes may continue in 'masters' preparation and competition, again given appropriate specialist coaching.

65+ years old

In France, these years are identified as '*le troisième age*' (the third age). This seems more appropriate than 'retirement'! Just as each stage of the high performance athlete pathway builds as preparation for the next, so also with the age stages of life's journey set out here. What's gone before should be preparation for a healthy, active, enjoyable quality of life through the 'third age'. Broadening of personal interests and doing something with them has been prepared for in the previous 10 years. Now it's time to live them and enjoy them to the full by being fit to do so. All the better if, in doing so, there is a real sense of continued personal value within the family, the community and/or other 'teams'. When self-awareness affords any suggestion that personal value is reducing, self-belief ebbs and that constitutes a big negative stressor. On the other hand, when there is a strong sense of personal value and worth, this constitutes a very positive health benefit. For those athletes who travelled the high performance athlete pathway, whether they ceased competition when their peak performance years were over or continue in 'masters' competition, fitness, hopefully, has been approached as a lifelong process.

Where competitive sport is the focus of personal development, fitness must be approached as a process commencing early and continuing through and beyond peak performance years. Of course, the peak performance years vary between sports. The fact is, however, that the components of each development phase must be addressed if athletes are to deliver their true potential in those peak performance years. Forcing the pace of development cannot be considered as reflecting a sense of responsibility for a young person's preparation for a healthy life. Emotional, social and even intellectual development can be compromised. This said, commercial aspects of top-level sport may alter perspective. The ethical issues here must be thought through.

BASIC PRINCIPLES OF TRAINING

The principles, or 'laws of training', of specificity, overload and reversibility are basic to the theory and practice of physical development, but will be more fully appreciated when related to the basic physical characteristics (see p. 224 and figure 13.3 on p. 219).

Specificity

Adaptation is specific to a stressor and the effect of a stressor is specific to an individual athlete. The importance of this should become apparent if we consider two athletes (a), and a training unit (b).

(a) John: best 200m = 22.0 seconds; Angus: best 200m = 23.0 seconds
(b) Unit = 6 x 200m in 24.0 seconds with 90 seconds recovery

This unit cannot have the same effect on each athlete because it represents a different percentage maximum intensity for each.

Overload

Progressing the adaptation status of a physical characteristic requires progressive challenge to status. Such progression is in raising the training stimulus of resistance, duration or speed that defines the stimulus, or a combination of these through the overcompensation cycle (see figures 21.2 and 21.3, p.333).

Reversibility

When intensity, extent or density is reduced, the degree of adaptation brought about by the training loads will gradually weaken. Strength losses are faster than mobility losses. Status improvements brought about by special methods over a short term are lost more quickly than those brought about by 'slower' methods over a long term. Yet there are occasions when loads are reduced deliberately in special preparation for a major competition. The coach must decide the extent to which such training should be cut back and for how long.

EFFECT OF TRAINING

Training might be considered as having three levels of effect.

1. Immediate: the immediate effect of training is the body's reactions to the stressor of the training stimulus. They include increased heart rate, perspiration, increased blood lactate, heightened endocrine system involvement and fatigue. This is the catabolic effect of training.

2. Residual: the residual effect of training is what might be considered as the body's recovery and preparation response. The recovery response is seen in a raised general metabolism for some time after exercise is concluded. During this time the body's resting state is restored with the waste products of energy expenditure removed, and other stressor-related effects gradually eliminated. The preparation response is seen in the heightened level of adaptation to future training stimuli. Having been stressed by a training stimulus, the body organises itself to ensure that next time it will not be 'stressed' so much by the same stimulus! Put another way, this effect of training ensures that the body is prepared for a greater training stimulus next time. This is the anabolic effect of training.

3. Cumulative: the cumulative effect of training is the body's progressive adaptation through the preparation response. This is what is measured in fitness monitoring tests over a period of months or even years. The effect of training will be considered again in chapter 21.

BASIC PHYSICAL CHARACTERISTICS

The interpretation of specificity is clear when one considers the type of fitness required for a given lifestyle. Whereas the athlete works to increase fitness towards some level of excellence, the non-athlete may work to compensate for the damage his lifestyle is causing. Thus, the lorry driver slumped at his wheel uses few abdominal or back muscles and should therefore attempt to improve muscle tone in these areas.

The definition of overload chosen by the coach depends upon the particular physical characteristics that need to be developed.

- **Strength:** overload is increasing the resistance in terms of kg, etc.
- **Strength endurance:** overload is increasing repetitions of an activity with a resistance ranging from the athlete's own bodyweight, to adding weighted belts, etc. to the athlete, to light and sub-maximal loads. The lactic anaerobic energy pathway has high involvement.
- **Aerobic/heart endurance:** overload is increasing the amount of time that the person can continue a low strength demand in a steady state of work of low-intensity repetitions. The aerobic energy pathway is involved exclusively.
- **Speed endurance:** overload is increasing the number of high-quality repetitions of an exercise per unit of time; or increasing the quality of repetition while keeping the number at or above a fixed threshold; although this may take place in a climate of cumulative lactic anaerobic pathway by-products, the alactic energy pathway has critical high involvement.
- **Speed:** overload is performing (and or selecting) a given task faster.
- **Elastic strength/power:** overload is increasing the resistance without loss of speed; or increasing speed of moving a fixed sub-max → max resistance.
- **Mobility:** overload is taking effective joint action beyond its present limit.

Clearly there are several subdivisions and variants of these broad areas of characteristic. Reversibility interpreted for the non-athlete or athlete will give an indication of how much exercise is required each week to maintain a reasonable degree of fitness. It is believed that a minimum of 2–3 units per week is necessary for the non-athlete, while the athlete is often involved in 2–3 units of training per day. The minimum will be used by the majority of non-athletes, e.g. day 1: jogging and mobility exercises, day 2: circuit training and jogging, day 3: some form of physical recreation. On the other hand, it would be ideal if some form of physical activity and regeneration training became part of daily routine.

POINTS ON FITNESS AND TRAINING

The following are some general points on fitness and training for both the athlete and non-athlete:

1. Before beginning any exercise programme, both athlete and non-athlete should have a full medical check-up. It is good practice to make this the start of regular annual or biannual check-ups. Some medical conditions may suggest a modified programme.

2. Children will not damage a healthy heart by exercising – quite the opposite. When children are tired they stop!

3. There is no upper age limit for exercise. The right exercise programme supported by relevant medical advice will keep the heart, muscles, joints, vascular and support systems healthy to provide and use energy required to enjoy one's lifestyle.

4. The starting focus of all exercise programmes is low intensity training – general all-round aerobic activity to prepare a foundation for developing a programme. General activity in terms of strength

should focus from the outset on postural muscles – spine (core strength) and those responsible for balance, stability, etc.

5. Stiffness following exercise is natural – and not serious. Sharp pain rather than discomfort during the next bout of exercise may be cause for alarm. It might be due to slight muscle strain and so rest followed by low-intensity exercise and gentle stretching – or a prescribed rehabilitation programme – should return things to normal. If the pain persists, a physiotherapist must be consulted. If exercise is being commenced after a long period of inactivity, it should be low impact (e.g. aqua-jog) and gentle mobility.

6. Too much training does not shorten life, but too little may. It cannot be said that training will necessarily lengthen life, but it will help make one's 'allotted span' more enjoyable.

7. There is no such thing as 'overtraining'. Physical, mental or emotional 'burnout' is due to the cumulative effect of all the stressors in one's life. Rather than compromise the training programme, the overall picture must be reviewed with the various objectives and tasks prioritised to create 'space' for adaptation to take place.

8. Women are able to train as hard as men. Following pregnancy, women's training load capacity increases and competitive performance in most cases improves above that of the accepted normal progression curve. Women may train hard throughout the menstrual cycle. However, in the 2–3 days prior to menstruation high intensity elastic strength work (i.e. jumping routines) which focus sudden high loads on the hips/lower-back should not take the athlete towards fatigue because the sacroiliac joint is less stable at this point in the cycle and can be strained.

9. People do not 'go to fat' when they finish serious training. The fact is that their appetites often stay high while their energy expenditure is now lower, and, consequently, weight increases. Such athletes should maintain a programme of lighter training as part of their personal fitness programme and review eating habits. This approach will also help maintain general muscle tone.

10. Training does not make people 'muscle-bound'. This is an obscure expression which reflects the fact that certain types of strength training will considerably increase the size of muscles – for example in bodybuilding. This will only happen if this is the objective of training and specific diets or exercise are pursued to this end. Normal exercise programmes do not have this effect. In fact, by reducing fat around the muscle, and improving muscle tone, a clearer definition of the limb musculature will result.

11. Exercise machines are safe for non-athletes to use provided their use is properly explained by a qualified instructor. There are, however, advantages and disadvantages to be considered (see p. 247).

12. For personal safety, neither athlete nor non-athlete should work alone with loose weights or exercise machines.

13. Isometrics should not be used indiscriminately, especially by those aged 35 and over as they may overload the heart.

14. Because fitness is specific, so also are fitness programmes. The objectives of each phase of a training programme should be clearly defined and the programme planned to meet those objectives.

15. Personal fitness programmes, whether for athlete or non-athlete, must on the one hand set out details of physical activity and regeneration and, on the other, afford advice from fitness-related areas such as nutrition, sports psychology and sports medicine – relevant to the individual's needs.

16. No fitness programme can be seriously considered without a definite time commitment on the part of the person for whom the programme is designed.

17. Because exercise programmes are designed to address the specific development needs of an athlete, it is not appropriate to swap programmes between athletes without agreeing with the coach that this is appropriate.

18. Once a regular routine of training is established, there should be a balanced mixture of exercise machines and free weights exercises in the programme. This should be a well-planned programme, to ensure that those muscles acting as synergists in controlling movements are not neglected.

19. Because habitual posture and activity patterns can lead to imbalances and compensatory stress in the joint complexes, it is sensible to consult a chiropractor or osteopath or have a comprehensive all joint movement analysis by a physiotherapist at least once a year for monitoring and corrective treatment.

SUMMARY

The purpose and meaning of fitness is specific to the individual, whether or not an athlete. In general it relates not only to coping with the stressors of a given lifestyle at each stage of life's journey, but enjoying a desired quality of life in the process. Effective fitness through each stage is not only measured against achieving immediate goals but in preparing for the stages to come – it's a lifelong process. Against the background of fitness to tolerate the stressors of day-to-day living, the athlete seeks to develop a fitness specific to the demands of his sport. It must be borne in mind that just as the demands of each sport are diverse, so are the day-to-day lives of the athletes. If the athlete becomes 'unfit' for life outside sport, due to an inability to adapt to its stressors, then there will certainly be an overlap into sport, and his capacity for developing fitness for his sport will be impaired. The coach must view the development of fitness as unique to athlete and situation, and consequently the totality of the athlete's life must be taken into account in identifying his 'uniqueness'.

REFLECTIVE QUESTIONS

1. Taking the three lanes of figure 13.2, outline two personal goals for the next year in each lane in terms of:
   a. a performance or achievement goal
   b. a development goal.
   Then outline your plan for achieving these goals.

2. For a sport of your choice, prepare a profile of the specific fitness the sport requires for high performance athletes using figure 13.3 as a reference framework. Explain your reasoning for this profile.

3. Eight weeks before the Olympic Games, a key athlete selected for the volleyball squad has a metatarsal fracture. Medical opinion is that the fracture will be healed in four to six weeks max. What are the possible fitness issues involved? Outline your plan to address these issues including exercise/activity examples. On paper the team is predicted to make the semi-finals at least.

4. One of your athletes has left home for university studies. In the first year he has added 5kg to his bodyweight, mainly due to fast foods and his social life. You visit him to try and address the situation. Outline the topics you will discuss and the plan of action you would propose to re-establish fitness for sport and as a building block for personal wellness in his life.

5. Discuss how you would apply the 'laws of training' to an upper body strength workout of three exercises over six weeks for:
   a. A 12-year-old female squash player
   b. A 25-year-old paralympian (T54) 1500m male track athlete
   c. A 30-year-old female rock climber.
   (Note: exercises may or may not be the same for each and may or may not be the same throughout the six weeks.)

14 THEORY AND PRACTICE OF STRENGTH TRAINING

Of all the biomotor qualities strength may the most all-encompassing. There is no form of motion that does not require some expression of force; therefore all sports will derive benefit from sport appropriate strength training. The physical quality of strength is the underpinning for the optimum development of the other biomotor qualities.

Because of its importance and ease of measurement it is tempting to try to train strength as an independent motor quality, but as we will see strength is a highly interdependent motor quality that profoundly interacts with and affects all the other biomotor qualities. It must be trained accordingly and this interaction must be accounted for in the whole training programme. The benefits of a sound strength-training programme are:

- improved ability to reduce and produce force
- increased ability to express explosive power
- increased joint stability
- significant contribution to injury prevention and rehabilitation.

Training methods from a variety of other sport disciplines have heavily influenced strength training. The most prominent have been Olympic weightlifting, power lifting and bodybuilding all of which are also competitive sports. In addition, gymnastics and wrestling have had profound effect on what we do in strength training.

Strength is an umbrella term that incorporates a spectrum of activities and training methods designed to enhance the force requirements of the sport trained for. Strength is the ability to exert force with no time constraints – it is simply how much force can be applied. The role of strength training is to condition the bones, tendon, ligaments and muscles to withstand and overcome the high forces placed on them in competition and training.

Power is the ability to express force in the shortest amount of time. Power can be broken down into speed dominated or strength-dominated power. Strength dominated power is characterised by the expression of high force against external resistance. Shot-put and discus, and the several football codes, are activities that demand strength-dominated power. Speed dominated power is the production of high force expressed at high speed with restricted resistance. Throwing a baseball, swinging a golf club or a tennis racket characterise speed dominated power.

Strength is important because it plays a role in all movements. In muscle action, strength functions to move a body part, to help resist movement of a body part and to stabilise or fixate a body part. The traditional emphasis in strength training has been on its role as the mover of a body part. Resisting moving a body part, which is the eccentric component of muscle action is equally, if not more important because it is during this force reduction phase where most injuries occur. Strength also plays a prominent role in stabilising or fixating a body part – this isometric action is also an important performance factor. A good sound strength development programme will carefully direct training to address all three functions of muscle actions in an integrated manner.

Strength acquisition is governed by neuromuscular, muscular, biochemical, structural and biomechanical factors. They are highly interdependent. It is the nervous system, in response to the demands of a specific task, that governs recruitment order and sequence. The brain does not recognise individual muscles; rather it recognises patterns of movement. The clear implication of this is that it is movement rather than individual muscles that we are training. The initial adaptation to strength training is neural through increased firing rate, motor unit recruitment and improved motor unit synchronisation. The body essentially learns to engage the appropriate muscles producing the desired movement and the stabilisers to effectively reduce and produce force.

FACTORS IN STRENGTH GAIN

- A major factor in gaining strength is the cross sectional area of muscle (hypertrophy). Muscles with greater cross sectional area have the capacity to produce more force, taking into consideration that the longer the muscle the greater its potential shortening or lengthening capability. The architecture of the muscle (see page 108) has a profound influence on the force producing capabilities of muscle. Research has shown that muscle architecture can change and adapt to a strength training stimulus in a relatively short period of time.
- Intramuscular coordination refers to the capacity to recruit motor units within a muscle. Intermuscular coordination is the ability of the agonists, antagonists, stabilisers, and neutralisers to work synergistically in an integrated environment. This is dependent on the following: (1) less Golgi tendon organ (GTO) inhibition; (2) decreased antagonistic inhibition; (3) increased dynamic joint stability; (4) increased neuromuscular control.
- The role that the endocrine hormonal system plays in strength training is significant. A properly designed strength training programme can take advantage of the body's natural hormone production to optimise strength gains and gains in lean mass. The endocrine hormonal system serves to maintain homeostasis as well as play a significant role in training adaptations. This requires manipulation of sets, reps, diet and rest to take advantage of the body's natural desire to maintain homeostasis.
- The types of muscle activity have been explained in chapter 6.

Anthropometry (the scientific study of the measurement and proportions of the human body) is clearly as significant a factor in designing a strength training programme as in selecting athletes for certain sports. These factors are largely genetic – successful competitive weightlifters are built that way and are developed accordingly because they have a lever complex advantage. They neither resemble physically nor are developed as would be appropriate for a basketball player.

Notwithstanding the importance of understanding which muscles are agonists, antagonists etc. in a given movement, muscle actions should be viewed in terms of actual function. In movement, the role of a muscle is not determined simply by its anatomical location, the function of the muscle changes during a single movement, in fact it is possible to have all types of muscle action occur during a single movement. Therefore it is necessary to think beyond labelling a muscle as an agonist or antagonist. So it is appropriate to use the terms originated by Logan and McKinney for the reason they articulate below:

'Historically, anatomists and kinesiologists have used the terms "agonists," "antagonists," "synergists," and "fixators" to describe muscular action. These terms are lacking as descriptive terms for muscle actions because they have been used in a context which has not taken into consideration the effects of gravity as well as other external forces acting upon and within the body.'

(Logan and McKinney, 1970, p. 68)

Logan and McKinney go on to explain their theory of muscles most involved (MMI): 'The muscles which overcome resistance and move a joint through a specified plane of motion are called muscles MOST involved' (Logan and McKinney, 1970, p. 67). The contralateral muscle works together with MMI. The guiding muscles help rule out desired action and ensure efficiency. The stabilising muscles fixate a joint or body part to enable other body parts or joints to move. This does not argue against understanding agonist function, antagonist function, and so on; rather it affords context.

Chapter 3 explained Newton's laws of motion and also lever systems. Because both intra and inter individual structural differences can contribute to large differences in mechanical advantage, it is imperative to take this into consideration when designing a strength training programme.

Current thinking demands that we look at strength differently. Contemporary thought is that strength training is *coordination training with appropriate resistance to handle bodyweight, project an implement, move or resist movement of another body, resist gravity and optimise ground reaction forces*. Let's look at the elements of the definition in detail.

- **Coordination training** is that aspect of strength training that incorporates both intramuscular and intermuscular coordination. The key to efficient movement and effective force application ultimately is intermuscular coordination, which is training muscles synergies to apply force at the correct time, in the correct plane and the correct direction.
- **Appropriate resistance** is determined for each of the following demands:
  - » **Handle bodyweight** – If the sport demands handling bodyweight then the emphasis is on relative strength working in various percentages of bodyweight resistances.
  - » **Project an implement** – The weight of the implement will determine the necessary resistance to develop strength to move that implement at the required speed.
  - » **Move or resist movement of another body** – This will determine the type of resistance, duration and direction of force application.
  - » **Resist gravity** – Sports that demand work against gravity necessitate more eccentric and isometric emphasis to express the necessary force.
  - » **Optimise ground reaction forces** – Sport with high ground reaction forces demands realistic reactive strength.

This definition directs the training and incorporates a spectrum of training methods to address the varying strength/power demands of different sports. Remember the goal is to develop strength that the athlete can use. Some is measurable and some is not.

Classification of strength training

General strength – exercises that develop the force component. They are characterised by slower speed, higher force movements. Traditional weight training exercises and other resistance methods that do not seek to imitate any aspect of a specific sport skill. Speed of movement is of little or no concern. This is all about force, not speed.

Special (transitional) strength (also related strength) – The purpose of these exercises is to convert general strength into specific strength. These exercises are similar but not the same as specific sport movements – they incorporate movement with resistance that incorporates the joint dynamics of the skill. Olympic style weightlifting, medicine ball work, stretch cord work and plyometric training fit into this category. A significant force component is present, but there is a much higher speed component. The exercises are more specific.

Specific strength consists of exercises that are characterised by movement with resistance that imitates the joint action of the sport skill. Rather than similar it is very much the same. There is a high degree of specificity in terms of mechanics, skill and above all, speed of movement. This obviously will have the highest degree of transfer to specific sport skill.

Strength training principles

These are the 'laws of training' (see chapter 13) as applied to strength training. **Specificity** might be defined by the acronym SAID – specific adaptation to imposed demands. It is important to understand that except for practicing the specific task or sport itself, no conditioning activity has 100 per cent carry-over. Some strength activities have a more direct carry-over than others because of similarities in neuromuscular recruitment patterns, energy systems and biomechanical characteristics. In most instances the overload in the sport or activity is not a sufficient stimulus on the neuromuscular system to achieve any significant strength adaptation. Essentially it is not as much about specificity as it is preparation for more specific work.

Within specificity is the individualisation concept that the strength training programme must fit the individual athlete. It must match the athlete's developmental age and training age as well as take into consideration injury history, body proportions and recoverability.

In the quest to be more 'functional' we have become overly concerned with making strength specific to the sport and to the movements of the sports at the expense of developing strength as a general quality to improve performance. It is important to remember that specificity is not trying to strictly imitate the sport movement; instead it is an evaluation of the physiological biomechanical and biochemical demands of the activity and then designing a programme to progressively overload the movements that make up the skill in order to enhance the activity. To evaluate specificity of strength training with regard to transfer to specific movements carefully consider the following factors (Kraemer and Häkkinen, 2002):

- Muscle groups involved in the exercise. Strength improves in the muscle groups that are stressed in training.
- Movement pattern – the movement must be similar to the desired movement in order to have carry-over. This relates to posture, the timing of joint movement and the range of movement.
- Joint ranges of movement – strength will increase specific to the joint angle at which one performs the exercise.
- Velocity of contraction – adaptations are specific to the velocity where training occurs.
- Type of muscle action – adaptation is specific to the type of action.

The starting point to ensure transfer of strength training to the sport being trained is to objectively evaluate current strength and power levels relative to the strength demands of the sport, position or event. What are the limitations? What type of strength is needed? How much training time is available? What equipment and facilities are necessary and what is available?

Overload is the foundation for strength gains. In order to achieve an adaptation it is necessary to stress the body to a level beyond which it is normally functioning. Overload is achieved though increasing volume – the amount of work done; by increasing intensity – the quality of work per unit of time or; by increasing frequency – how often the stimulus is applied (see chapter 22).

Reversibility. When strength training is reduced or arrested, previous gains are lost (see chapter 13). Such loss can be dramatic as, for example, when joints are immobilised following injury. Continuous lack of exercise in the shape of strength related work will result in muscle atrophy.

Constructive application of the overload principle is based on the concept of progression. Progression is essential to ensure continued increase of strength capacity and adaptation to the strength-training stimulus. In its simplest form progression will move from simple to complex; easy to hard; and general to specific work. These simple steps in progression give way to complex interactions. All training variables do not progress at the same rate nor do all individuals progress at the same rate.

To ensure proper progression we must clearly define each step and articulate specific goals and objectives for each step. It is important to develop evaluative criteria, to assess the achievement of each of the goals and objectives for each step.

Progression is not linear, therefore do not design programmes in a linear fashion. Start with a clear picture of what the athlete needs to achieve or look like at the end of a training programme, but remember that progression toward that ultimate objective will in all probability proceed in a staircase like progression. Constant progress should be made toward the goal, but some of the incremental steps along the way will be smaller than others. Factor into the plan that there will be plateaus and occasional regression – there is an ebb and flow to this (see chapter 21).

In addition to the principles, strength training must reflect clear understanding of recovery and variation.

Recovery (see chapter 23) – The ability to recover both short and long term from a workload is crucial to positive adaptation to the strength training stimulus. If the athlete is unable to recover from the training stress then it is not an appropriate load. No two athletes are the same in ability, nor are they the same in the ability to recover, different athletes have different recovery abilities.

Variation – Training volume, intensity, frequency and sometimes exercise selection must be constantly varied in a systematic manner to ensure continual adaptation. Because the body adapts to training stressors so quickly it is important to vary training. This variation should not be random or haphazard, but systematically planned in order to measure the effect of the variation. If training is not varied the body will adapt quite quickly and the training effect will be dulled. If no variation is incorporated there is a significant risk of staleness and eventual overtraining.

THE FOLLOWING ARE SOME OF THE VARIABLES THAT CAN BE CHANGED OR MODIFIED TO ENSURE CONTINUED ADAPTIVE RESPONSE:

- Increase volume – in many ways it is the easiest and simplest variable to manipulate.
- Increase intensity – change the quality of work. This alternative is more viable in speed and power sports.
- Change frequency – add or reduce the number of training sessions. Also consider multiple sessions in a training day to address different components.
- Change the actual composition of the workouts – sometimes it can be as simple as a change in rest intervals; it may also be a change in the sequence of exercises. Monotony in workouts can serve to dull the adaptive response. Be sure to make sure the variations have a specific purpose, not just haphazard changes to make things look different.
- Increase the difficulty of training.
- Any logical sensible combination of the above will also ensure continued adaptive response (see chapter 24).

Functional strength training concepts

Train movements not muscles – The central nervous system (CNS) is the command station that controls and directs all movement. The CNS calls for pre-programmed patterns of movement that can be modified in countless ways to react appropriately to gravity, ground reaction forces and momentum. Each activity is subjected to further refinements and adjustments by feedback from the body's proprioceptors. This process ensures optimal neuromuscular control and efficiency of function. Isolation of specific muscles does not appropriately emphasise dynamic, multi-dimensional strength development. Movement does not occur in the anatomical position. Movement occurs in reaction to gravity, ground reaction forces and momentum. Movement is not an isolated event that occurs in one plane of motion; it is a complex event that involves synergists, stabilisers, agonists and antagonists all working together to reproduce efficient triplanar movements.

Train postural (core) before extremity strength – The core – the hips, abdomen and the spine – is the relay centre of the body. Without a strong and stable core to act as a transmission to transfer force produced off the ground or from above by the upper extremities it is virtually impossible to produce efficient movement.

Train bodyweight before external resistance – This is putting the concept of training movement (above) into practice. The athlete must be able to effectively handle bodyweight in a variety of movements and specific exercises before progressing any significant external loading. The basic bodyweight exercises are pull-ups, push-ups, dips, rope climb, crawling, bodyweight squats, lunges and step-ups. Coaches should use creativity and imagination to design exercises and routines that incorporate the following fundamental movements: swinging, pulling, pushing, reaching, extending, bending, jumping, hopping and bounding. Work against gravity, with the bodyweight as resistance, will strengthen the bones, tendons, ligaments and muscles in preparation for further external loading work to follow. It is a small upfront investment for a large backend return. Every exercise should incorporate multi-joint and multi-plane exercises. It is from this foundation that progression can be made to equipment ranging from medicine balls, weighted vests and gymnasium equipment through to formal weight training.

Train strength before strength endurance – Initial strength gains are neural; essentially the initial strength gains come from learning the movements. A quality that has not been developed cannot be endured. There is plenty of time to incorporate strength endurance once a good foundation of strength has been established. The primary means of developing strength endurance is through circuit training.

A sound strength training programme must include the following movements:

- pulling
- pushing
- squatting and squat derivative movements like lunge and step-up
- rotation
- bracing.

In a balanced programme all of those movements should be incorporated into the exercises selected and applied in a microcycle. Consider the following criteria for exercise selection:

- Multi-joint. Use as many joints as possible to produce force, conversely use as many joints as possible to reduce force.
- Isolation exercises that put unusual stress on one joint should be avoided. They cause neural confusion because the muscle is asked to something different in strength training than it must do in movement in performance. Consequently exercises like leg extension, leg curl, concentration curls and 'pec deck flyes' have no place in a functional strength training programme. This is fine for bodybuilding but has little or no transfer to the sport performance.
- Close the chain to utilise gravity and ground reaction forces. Wherever possible exercises should be performed standing.
- Tri-plane motion. Movement occurs in all three planes, sagittal, frontal, and transverse. Therefore it is imperative to select exercises and modes of strength training that allow movement in all three planes of motion.
- Amplitude. Work over the greatest range of motion that is possible to control.
- Speed. Incorporate speed of movement that is safe and the athlete can control.
- Proprioceptive demand. Challenge the joint and muscle receptors to provide feedback regarding joint and limb position and reposition accordingly. The proprioceptors assist the system to generate movement in a form that it is appropriate to the demands placed upon the system. This will ensure that the strength will transfer to the performance.

As a step toward designing the optimum programme consider the following questions:

- What are the strength requirements of the sport?
- What muscle groups are used in the sport?
- What are the movement requirements?
- What is the direction of the application of force?
- What is the range of motion over which force will be produced and reduced?
- What are the common injuries in the sport? (Our purpose is prevention.)

Once those questions have been answered then focus on the qualities of the individual athlete. Carefully consider growth and development factors – has the athlete gone through puberty? Gender must be taken into consideration, the female athlete needs to strength train more often and continue the strength training through to peak competitions. Biological and chronological age are often quite different. Is the athlete an early or a late developer? Cognitive and emotional development should also be considered, as they are quite important in the ability to learn exercises and routines as well as to accept coaching.

Strength training programme design

The exercises must be safe but sufficiently challenging to elicit an adaptive response. They must be appropriate for the developmental as well as the training age of the athletes. Where necessary the exercises should be sport or movement specific.

> Start by developing an extensive exercise menu and from this menu select specific exercises for the programme. Then divide the exercises into logical categories to organise the training:
>
> - Balance and stability
> - Elastic-reactive (plyometric exercises)
> - Postural strength/core exercise
> - Total body exercise/combination movements
> - Lower extremity
> - Upper extremity
> - Multiple throw exercises (ballistic throwing exercises)

Number of exercises – it is best to carefully choose and limit the number of exercises. Keep a focus to the workout. Determine the essential need to do exercises, too many exercises will dilute the training effect.

Sets/reps – for bodyweight exercises a range of 10 to 20 reps is necessary to force adaptation. For weight training the traditional paradigm of sets and reps is still very valid. Higher reps for hypertrophy development, lower reps with multiple sets are good for neural development.

Mode of resistance – depending on the objective and the phase of the programme, choose a resistance mode that is appropriate for the objectives. Each mode has its advantage or disadvantage depending on the specific objectives of the training programme. It is advisable to mix the modes of training on a regular basis.

Progression – progress from bodyweight exercises to external resistance exercises both within the workout and through the training year. Also within each workout perform balance/stability work and core work first before moving to heavy loads. Start with simple easy to perform exercises and then progress to more complex movements. The key to progression is mastery. Do not allow the athlete to proceed further into the programme until the basic exercises have been mastered, if this is not done then there is a higher risk of injury.

Frequency – there are several alternatives, all of which work quite well depending on the objective. The alternatives are:

- Total body – alternate days, for example Mon/Wed/Fri or Tue/Thu/Sat
- Split routine – training on consecutive days, for example Mon/Thu: legs and total body and Tues/Fri: upper body

Duration – generally it is best to keep the entire strength training session in the time range of 1 hour to 90 minutes. The closer to one hour the more optimal the results.

Time of the training year – obviously the greatest emphasis on strength training should be in the preparation macrocycle and in the bridge from preparation to competition. But it is important to develop a manageable programme that can be continued throughout the season or the strength gains acquired in preparation macrocyle will be rapidly lost.

Testing strength – in beginning a programme it is probably best to utilise projected maximums or base weight selection on percentage of bodyweight. This allows the ability to constantly project and assess progress. For the inexperienced, testing for one rep maximum can be unsafe and is unnecessary.

Evaluating results – the traditional evaluation of a strength training programme has been the ability to lift more weight on weight training exercises or more repetitions on bodyweight exercise. In an absolute sense that is still valid, but we need to go beyond that and carefully observe the carryover to the sport. This is much more subjective, but this is the ultimate goal of any strength training programme. Closely observe if the athlete's ability to start and stop has improved. Has there been a reduction in injuries?

TYPES OF STRENGTH

- **Maximal strength** – the most force the muscles can produce voluntarily in a single muscle action, regardless of the time element.
- **Absolute strength** – the most force an athlete can produce, regardless of bodyweight and time of force development.
- **Relative strength** – the maximum force an athlete can generate per unit of bodyweight, regardless of time of force development.
- **Speed strength** – the ability of the neuromuscular system to produce the greatest possible force in the shortest possible time.
- **Starting strength** – initial rate of force development characterised by the ability to produce high levels of force at the beginning of functional movements.
- **Explosive strength** – the capacity to develop a sharp rise in force once movement has been initiated. It is characterised by an increase in force per unit of time.
- **Elastic reactive strength** – the ability to rapidly switch from an eccentric contraction to a concentric contraction.
- **Strength endurance** – the ability to produce and maintain force in a climate of fatigue.
- **Stabilisation strength** – the ability of the neuromuscular system to provide dynamic reflex joint stabilisation during functional movements.
- **Power endurance** – the ability to produce and maintain power in a climate of fatigue.
- **Core strength** – the ability of the lumbar-hip complex musculature to maintain control and dynamic stability during movement.

Postural (core strength)

The core is an integrated functional unit consisting of the lumbar spine and hip complex, the thoracic and cervical spine. It is a muscular corset that lends integrity and support to the body. The core is the centre of the body, the thickest part of the body. In all movement the core musculature must be active to allow for efficient movement. The core works as an integrated functional unit that accelerates, decelerates, and dynamically stabilises the body during movement. All movement is relayed through the core. The core is in effect a swivel joint between the hips and the shoulders, which (1) allows the entire body to accelerate the limbs, (2) allows the entire body to decelerate the limbs and (3) Allows the entire body to support a limb.

Choose exercises that work the core in all planes of motion:

- trunk flexion and extension (sagittal plane)
- lateral flexion (frontal plane)
- trunk rotation (transverse plane)
- combinations (tri-plane)
- throwing and catching (dynamic stabilisation in all three planes).

For the purposes of effective programme design and efficiency the core exercise classifications are as follows:

- stabilisation
- flexion/extension
- rotation
- throwing/catching

The system of classification then allows us to distribute exercises based on classification to ensure adequate recovery and effective coverage of all aspects of core movement (see table 14.1).

Monday/Thursday

DB Complex

DB High Pull x 6	5 Complexes
DB Alternate Press x 6	1:1 work:rest
DB Squat x 6	Pair off with partner
DB Row x 6	

Mini Leg Circuit

Squat x 3	
Lunge x 3 each Leg	Start with 3 circuits, progress to 6,
Step-up x 3 each leg	No rest between exercises
Jump Squat x 3	

TABLE 14.1 Translating the core exercise classification system to designing a balanced programme

Plyometric (elastic/reactive strength)

It is training the stretch shortening cycle of muscle action to enhance the subsequent concentric action. The utilisation of the stretch shortening is essential for efficient human movement. It is a quality of the muscle action that is highly trainable and adaptable.

The goals of plyometric training are threefold: (1) To raise explosive power. (2) To learn to better attenuate ground forces regardless of the event or sport. (3) To learn to tolerate and use greater stretch loads, in essence to increase muscle stiffness.

The last point demands a bit more explanation. Musculotendinous stiffness is the key to elastic/reactive training. It is highly related to the body's ability to store and reuse elastic energy from running and jumping. The concept of stiffness is sometimes confusing because we tend to equate stiffness with a lack of flexibility, for explosive movements this is not the case. Essentially a stiff muscle will develop a high degree of tension as it is stretched. This is very desirable to raise explosiveness. Conversely a non-stiff muscle will collapse and absorb elastic energy; it does not react, as actively to the ground, therefore it will produce significantly less explosiveness. A simple analogy to help to understand stiffness is to compare a soft rubber playground ball and a golf ball. If both balls were dropped onto a hard concrete surface the golf ball would react rapidly and the playground ball would react slowly to the ground. In plyometric training in order to optimise ground reaction forces we want the golf ball type reaction. A stiff muscle is able to produce optimum amounts of reactive force in a short period of time.

Plyometric training is not a stand-alone training method; it is highly compatible with and significantly enhanced by strength training. It is also closely related to speed development. Most importantly it is *not* a conditioning tool! Because of the explosive nature of the work it is of high neural demand, therefore it should not be used for conditioning. It should almost never be trained in a climate of fatigue, with a few notable exceptions. Those exceptions are sports that demand power endurance like soccer, rugby, basketball, 400m or 400m hurdles. In those sports the fatigue element is only introduced after the technical component of the exercise is mastered – this will minimise the risk of injury. The stimulus for adaptation is not volume, it is intensity, and nothing should ever compromise the intensity of the movements. A high volume session is in the range of 90–120 contacts with a range of 250–400 contacts for a microcycle. More is definitely not better. If used properly it is a highly effective tool to stimulate the nervous system, but if used improperly it can have the opposite effect and dull, if not deaden, the nervous system.

Plyometric training consists of three very basic movements. Jumping movements characterised by two-foot landings is the most fundamental. Hopping is characterised by one foot landing. Hopping is more stressful due to the fact that bodyweight is supported on one leg on landing. The third, bounding, is characterised by alternate leg take-off. This is also quite demanding because all the bodyweight is supported on one leg in the landings. The complexity in plyometric training comes from combining these movements and their derivatives. In some sports it is the upper limb complex that is the focus of plyometric training; for example, jump press-ups, rebound medicine ball work, etc.

The prerequisites for effective use of plyometric training are coordination, balance, body control and awareness. Core control and core strength are also very important to maintain good dynamic posture during the movements. Leg strength relative to the level of the athlete's development is a must. It is not necessary to be able to squat a certain amount of weight, rather it is necessary to exhibit a certain degree of functional leg strength. If these prerequisites are at an acceptable level then the athlete is ready to start into a basic progression. Progression is essential to minimise injury and optimise training adaptation. Lead up activities done in a playful, game-like environment are a very important part of progression as well as good preparation. The key to progression is to teach landing first with foot position. The landing is on a full foot (mid foot contact), not on the ball of the foot or a completely flat foot. A mid foot landing will set the foot in a position to shock absorb and set up the utilisation of the elasticity of the muscles up the kinetic chain. This will teach how to absorb shock and set up the readiness for the any subsequent take-offs on multiple response activities. After landing, teach take-off which is triple extension of ankle, knee and hip, the summation of forces.

Plyometric training is classified based on the projection of the centre of gravity. The **in place response** is characterised by vertical displacement of centre of gravity. The **short response** is characterised by horizontal displacement of centre of gravity and ten contacts or less. The **long response** is characterised by horizontal displacement of centre of gravity with speed and more than ten contacts.

To get a better command of the process of putting the classifications into a coherent programme the *Plyometric Demand Matrix* (adapted from Radcliffe and Farentinos, page 42) was developed to govern progression (see table 14.2). The variables can be manipulated moving down the column or across. The suggested range of sets, repetitions and/or distance appears in each box.

	Low Impact	Medium Impact	High Impact	Shock
In-Place Response	3–4 sets 10–20 reps	3 sets 10–12 reps	2–3 sets 8–10 reps	2 sets 10 reps
Short Response	3 sets 10–12 reps 10–20 metres	3 sets 10 reps 10–20 metres	2–3 sets 8–10 reps 10–20 metres	2 sets 10 reps
Long Response	3 sets 10–20 reps 20–40 metres	2–3 sets 10–15 reps 20–40 metres	2–3 sets 10–12 reps 20–40 metres	NA

TABLE 14.2 A useful matrix in building progression into plyometric programmes by adjusting variables vertically or horizontally

For the athlete of advanced training age the numbers can be pushed up slightly as long as quality is not compromised. Keep in mind that this matrix is only a rough guideline and it must be adapted to fit the sport and the individual athlete.

Plyometric training considerations

Frequency – two to three times a seven-day microcycle depending on the phase of the year and the sport is acceptable. Low amplitude remedial in place movements can be done daily as part of a warm-up. Inter unit recovery is normally longer for plyometric work than traditional concentric or eccentric work.

Complexity – start with simple movements in place and then add combinations as the athlete achieves mastery. As far as sequence and compatibility with other components, plyometric training and strength training are very complementary. Plyometric training is also very compatible with speed development. Given this fundamental compatibility with other methods of high neural demand it is imperative to take into account the overall stress on the nervous system when combining methods.

Where in the programme –it must always be there! The number of contacts, the type of exercise and the complexity changes as the season progresses. Where in the workout is best? Generally, early in the workout before there is any fatigue. With the younger developing athlete put plyometric training before strength training and before sprinting. As the athlete advances in training age then the plyometric can be blended with the strength training during certain phases and even follow strength training. The sequence is very training age dependent.

Young developing athlete – there is no physiological reason why the young developing athlete cannot do plyometric training. The intensity should be low and the drills and exercises should be play-like. Games like hopscotch and jump rope are very appropriate as training and as lead-up activities. How is it best to assess intensity if it is so important? Wherever and whenever possible measure, time, video, watch and listen. It is important to apply sensible judgement when working with the growing athlete in terms of volume of impact and epiphyses (see page 33).

When problems do occur it is often because of inappropriate progression. Too much done, too soon or there was an inappropriate selection of exercises. Also poor technique in the actual execution of the exercises can create inappropriate stress. Strength deficiencies either in the lower extremities or the core, coupled with the previous two deficiencies can be a major factor in injury.

Circuit training

Circuit training is essentially interval strength training. A strength exercise is performed for reps or time and a certain rest interval is given and the athlete progresses to the next exercise. Circuit training was systematised in the UK in the 1950s. It is very effective, not just with sports and athletes where the strength endurance demand is high, but with speed and power athletes as a means of raising work capacity and changing body composition.

The goal of circuit training is to develop muscular endurance, which has the added benefit of improving work capacity. In team settings it is a very viable method because large numbers of athletes can train at one time. Circuit training also can be easily adapted to target specific areas of the body; i.e. leg, core or upper body, or address specific deficiencies. The goals of circuit training are: (1) Develop muscular endurance. (2) Increase work capacity. (3) Enable large numbers to train at one time. (4) Target specific areas or physical qualities.

In setting up a circuit-training programme, carefully consider the following:

- The circuit must be tailored to meet individual needs and rates of improvement.
- The exercises selected must be strenuous; small muscle group exercises are not appropriate.
- The exercises need to be simple, since skill will break down as the athlete fatigues.
- It is very important to standardise the exercise so that the athlete can measure progress regardless of the circuit criteria.
- It is important to recognise any bias in the circuit.

The actual circuit can be constructed in several different ways. Perhaps the most common circuit is a rep-based circuit where the athlete performs a set number of reps of a particular exercise and then moves onto the next exercise. This is the simplest form of circuit construction. It is also possible to construct a time-based circuit. The timed based circuit is set up so that the exercises are performed for a certain amount of time with a fixed rest interval. The load or exercise has to be carefully chosen so the athlete can work for the entire time prescribed. Progress is judged by the number or repetitions achieved. A combination of the two can also be used. For example, a good measure is to take total time for a rep based circuit to measure progress.

Circuit training should not be limited exclusively to the preparation period of training nor should its use be limited just to the sports that had obvious strength endurance demands. It is a training method that can significantly improve work capacity and impact significant body composition changes. The key is to understand sport demands and individual strengths and weaknesses and then design specific circuits that can be used throughout the training year as a tool to enhance work capacity and serve as a good routine breaker. There is no question that circuit training is a demanding form of training and because it is so demanding it must be used judiciously. The longest a block of circuit training should last is four weeks. For year round sports or where athletes are constantly on the move and having to maintain fitness levels in a variety of venues, a personal circuit is extremely valuable.

Strength and endurance training

Concurrent training for strength and endurance does not affect endurance gains, but it does significantly compromise strength gains and force development. Empirical evidence indicates that strength training will enhance endurance through improvement of structural strength. It will also retard muscle breakdown due to impact forces in running and contribute to speed development. The emphasis should be on neural development rather than hypertrophy.

Running as little as 4 kilometres a day has been shown to decrease vertical jump. Vertical jump is one of the best indicators of explosive power. If there is a need to combine the two components it is best to train the components separately on different days (Ward and Ward, 1997, p. 57).

Strength training for young and developing athletes

The common myths about strength training for the young developing are:

- Before puberty the young athlete cannot put on muscle mass or make significant strength gains because of the lack of androgenic hormones.
- It stunts growth because of stress on the growth plates.
- It will limit flexibility and hinder skill development.

Over the years these myths have grown without any basis in fact. Practical experiences over the years by coaches who work with young growing athletes completely refute each of these myths. In fact, in each case the opposite is true. The growing athlete who undertakes a comprehensive progressive resistance programme will incur fewer injuries than their counterparts who do not strength train.

Growing children and developing athletes are not miniature adults. Sometimes we are fooled by appearance. After puberty when the athlete's linear growth is greatest they look like adults, but they are still growing, therefore copying programmes from mature athletes can eventually lead to problems with injury and overuse. The principles governing strength training are the same for the growing athlete or the mature athlete.

The growing athlete is highly adaptable provided the stress is carefully applied in a progressive manner after a sound fitness base has been established. If a proper sensible criteria based progression is followed then strength training is a very appropriate activity for the growing and developing athlete.

The fact is that strength is a basic motor skill, which is an important precursor to other motor skills. To ignore strength development will only serve to limit the development of other key motor qualities such as speed, coordination and flexibility. Everything, regardless of the level of athlete, is related to broad fitness and activity base. Someone completely sedentary will be more likely to not make good progress and get hurt than someone who has been very active. It is generally acknowledged that youth today are not as active and fit as previous generations. They also tend to specialise in specific sports earlier; this has the effect of narrowing their range of motor skills as well as limiting their ultimate development in their chosen sport. The key is to do what is natural and playful first. If you watch children play in their natural environment they perform amazing feats of strength relative to their bodyweight. They push, pull, jump and throw with ease. If the object is too heavy they leave it alone. Nobody has to tell them it's too heavy! No one has to instruct on technique, they put their body into positions that are natural to achieve the desired outcome.

Strength training and weight training are not synonymous – weight training is part of strength training (resistance training). Strength training is an umbrella term that encompasses a spectrum of resistance modes from bodyweight gravitational loading on through to traditional weight training and Olympic weightlifting. All the modes are appropriate if utilised properly and are carefully taught as part of a progression over the course of the growing athlete's development. The key to all of this is to start where you can succeed with bodyweight gravitational loading and then to progressively add resistance as the growing athlete adapts to the stimulus of the current mode of strength training. A summary of suggested strength training loads is set out in table 14.1.

There are definite gender differences in regard to the need, response and adaptation to strength training. The growing female athlete is physically more mature than the male athlete at the same chronological age. A good rule of thumb is to consider the female two years advanced in physical development over her male counterpoint at the same age. The percentage of muscle mass is lower in women than in men 30–35 per cent for the female to 42–47 per cent for the male. Generally 11–13 for girls and 13–15 for boys are considered the optimum ages to begin formal training. This usually coincides with puberty where the production of anabolic hormones is considerably increased. The female must strength train earlier and keep the strength train threaded throughout the training year because of the differences in muscle mass and testosterone levels.

It is also important to consider motivation, emotional maturity, and cognitive development. These are essential qualities in taking instruction and following directions and the ability to follow a set prescribed programme.

Beware of one-sided training biased toward heavy lifting. This can have a negative effect as it takes the strength component out of context. The growing athlete can lift heavy after puberty.

Objective	Intensity of training load	Repetitions in each set	Sets in each unit	Training system	Recovery between sets	Time holding isometric	Evaluation procedures contraction	Probable event app. (possible event app.)
Development of maximum strength in events where single expression of maximum strength is required	Concentric 85% → 100% Eccentric •105% → 175%	1→5	A 5→8 N 2→4	Simple sets Super sets Stagger sets Pyramids-5 x 85%→ 1 x 100% Mixed sets /ecc.-conc.-isom.	4→5 mins	A 9→12 secs 80–100% N 6→9 secs 60–80%	Max. lift dynamometer	e.g. weight lifting shot discus hammer javelin (jumps) rugby front 5
Development of maximum strength in events where multiple expression of maximum strength is required	70%→85%	5→10	2→5	Simple sets Super sets Pyramids-8 x 75% ←→6 x 80% ←→5 x 85%	2→4 mins		Max. lift dynamometer	e.g. (circle throws) javelin high, triple, long sprints hurdles, rowing
Development of elastic strength where work is also done in other units for maximum strength	30%→50% or 55%→65% or 3%→5% body weight resistance exercises involving whole technique (e.g. gymnastics, jumping, etc.) or related plyometrics specific & special strength exercises	6→10 5→8 6→10 5→10	4→6 4→6 3→5 Performed as stage training 3→5	Simple sets Super sets Pyramid by intensity only. 10 x 30%: 10 x 40%: 10 x 50%: 10 x 55%: 10 x 60%: 10 x 65% Performed as stage training	3→5 mins		Standing long, triple, vert. jump, etc.	All explosive sports

A advanced athlete
N Novice athlete
*Advanced athlete only

Objective	Load	Repetitions	Sets	Organisation	Recovery	Notes	Test	Application
Development of elastic and maximum strength simultaneously	a 75% or b 3%–5% bodyweight resistance exercises involving whole technique or c alternating between 85% and elastic/plyometric equivalent	6 → 10	4 → 6	Simple sets / Super sets — Performed as stage training	3→5 mins / 3→5 mins		Standing long, triple, vert. jump etc.	All explosive sports e.g. hockey, rugby, soccer
Development of maximum strength base or strength endurance for all events	N 30%→40% / A 60%→65%	25%→50% Max. 15	4→6 / 3→5	Simple sets circuit / Simple sets stage	Optimal / 4→5 mins		Max. repetitions / Max. holding time, etc. Max. lift	General for all sports especially young or novice athlete
Development of strength endurance in those events with high demands for it	40%→60% / 50%→75% Max according to activity / loading the basic technique (e.g. hill running, swimming/ rowing dragging resistance, etc.)	3→5		Circuit training	30→45 secs	Not isom. but controlled lifts with 30%→50%, max. e.g. 6 secs flex. Performed as stage training	Max. repetitions / Max. repetitions per unit of time	All sports e.g. rowing, wrestling swimming cross-country skiing ice hockey steeplechase

TABLE 14.3 Overview of training units designed to address specific strength objectives

SOME SPECIFIC RECOMMENDATIONS TO CONSIDER WHEN IMPLEMENTING A COMPREHENSIVE STRENGTH-TRAINING PROGRAMME FOR THE YOUNG DEVELOPING ATHLETE

- Strength training should be part of a comprehensive fitness programme.
- The strength training programme should be built upon a firm foundation in movement skills.
- Young growing athletes are not miniature adults therefore we must adjust everything to the size, weight and maturation level of the youngster.
- Strength training programme should be bodyweight based, with the core strength and stability emphasised first.
- Overhead lifting or loading of the spine should be de-emphasised until sufficient core strength and stability is developed.
- The child must have the emotional maturity to accept instruction and follow a programme.
- Do not base the strength training programmes on chronological age; instead carefully consider biological age (maturation level).
- Always teach first then train. Do not assume that because it is taught that it is learned. Make sure that the skill or movement is mastered before you let the athlete begin to train with a particular exercise or method.
- Incorporate variety as much as possible to force adaptation and to maintain mental freshness.
- Machines are not necessarily safer, they must fit the athlete, and most do not.
- Qualified adults must supervise the programme.

Strength training for senior athletes

It is very important to carefully consider biological age, developmental age and prior activity level when implementing a programme for the senior athlete. The current, as well as recent activity level is a major determining factor in programme design. There are definite age related loss of strength and power factors due to: loss of cross sectional area; a loss of muscle fibres, primarily type II; expression of maximal is reduced, however potential still exists; and last but not least, a decreased ability of the nervous system to recruit. Postural 'anti-gravity' muscles and deceleration movements are even more important for the senior due to the effect of gravity on the ageing body. Force reduction is extremely important in order to effectively cheat gravity. A comprehensive strength training programme has been shown to have a significant effect on minimising the bone density loss that typically occurs with ageing.

Strength training for female athletes

Lingering stereotypes continue to hinder female athletes who want to strength train. The biggest myth is that strength training will develop muscles like a man. That fear is unfounded for the physiological reason that on average the female has smaller muscle fibres and lower testosterone than her male counterpart that does not allow her to get as big. The physiological facts are quite clear – there is a difference in muscle mass and a difference in muscle mass distribution. The female has less upper body mass than the male, in the lower body there is less difference, but still a difference. In absolute strength there is a fairly large difference between the sexes. In relative strength women are still not as strong as men in the upper body, but in the lower body the difference is significantly less. When the strength is expressed relative to lean body mass then the strength difference all but disappears. In regard to the menstrual cycle, strength training has no more effect than any other form of exercise. As far as training effect basically the same adaptation and responses will occur in terms of strength acquisition. The biggest limiting factor is in testosterone levels, at rest men have a ten times higher level which has implications on the ultimate ability of the female athlete to gain muscle mass.

For the female athlete the most important component of training for both performance enhancement and injury prevention is strength training. That is not to imply that the female athlete should *only* strength train, rather that strength training needs to be a factor that is always present in the female athletes' training programme regardless of the time of the training year or the stage in the career. It must be present in the context of the whole training programme and in concert with the themes and objectives of the overall programme.

The typical female athlete is usually deficient in this quality for myriad reasons. There is a tremendous ability to adapt to this stimulus with a positive spill-over to all other components of athletic fitness. There is also a very important positive psychological effect in terms of confidence and self-image improvement. With a well-designed strength training programme the female athlete can expect to achieve:

- gain in lean mass if that is the objective
- change in body composition – lose fat
- improved explosive power
- improved muscular endurance
- improved ability to handle bodyweight and control the body
- a reduction in injuries, especially lower extremity injuries.

SOME KEY POINTS

- The female matures earlier than the male athlete therefore it is important to begin strength training earlier. Start early, preferably before puberty. It has been an observation (not supported by research) that the female athlete who begins a sound well rounded strength training programme before puberty tends to be leaner after puberty.
- Strength train more often and continue throughout the competitive season because the drop off in strength is more dramatic when strength training is stopped.
- Separate the boys and girls during the middle school years. There is too much difference and it is discouraging to both.
- For those who have amenorrhea, a loss of bone density is a very real issue. Evidence is beginning to accrue that strength training can have a positive effect on bone density.

Machines versus free weights

Whether working with sophisticated exercise machines or free weights or other strength-related equipment, each has its advantages and disadvantages. Machines may be considered safer in one context but may cause forces to be abnormally transmitted on the other; or while offering an exercise which isolates a movement, machines can remove the value that free weights or other equipment bring in requiring stabilisers and synergists to exercise their function.

A balanced programme using what is available to athlete and coach is key, avoiding bias of any particular piece of equipment and maximising specific advantage which a given piece of equipment affords.

PERIODISATION OF STRENGTH TRAINING

Periodisation is simply planning (see chapters 19 and 20). Planning gives direction and purpose to the training – it is a systematic attempt to control the adaptive response to training in preparation for competition. Periodisation refers to the timing of the application of the training stimulus through systematic manipulation of the variables of volume, intensity and density. The goal is to have the strength/power at optimum levels at the time of the most important competitions or in an extended competitive season to stabilise strength/power at a level that can be utilised throughout the season. The key is how strength/power training is integrated into the total programme. Strength is only one component of athletic fitness.

To ensure an adaptive response periodisation necessitates an alternation of periods of accumulation and intensification. Accumulation periods are designed to create cellular changes and muscular hypertrophy with the work in this period characterised by medium loads and higher repetitions. Intensification periods are periods characterised by work that creates neural adaptation by recruiting high-threshold motor units though high loads and medium to low reps.

The type of strength training is dependent on the sport and the level of development of the athlete. The window of adaptation for a young developing athlete is quite large; generally they will adapt to a volume stimulus and not need any significant variability. As the athlete accrues training years the window of adaptation to strength becomes much smaller with the main stimulus intensity and more specific work with much more variation.

THESE ARE KEY ELEMENTS IN STRENGTH TRAINING PERIODISATION

- Incorporates a systematic approach that defines a strategy to distribute training loads in relation to competition goals.
- A defined structure for progression that incorporates a sequential building block approach and reflects the undulatory nature of the adaptive process.
- A set time frame for execution of the plan.
- Strength/power training must be integrated with all components of training.
- Systematic manipulation of the variables of volume, intensity and density.
- A method for monitoring training and evaluating competition results.

Periodisation of strength training: example

The following is an example of the periodisation of strength training for middle distance/distance runners:

Strength training phases – these phases must correlate with the running training. They must not detract from the quality of the running workouts so they should be sequenced after the running workout or as a second workout of the day. Intensity is the key throughout each phase; there is an emphasis on speed of movement with control. Reps are low on upper body because they are designed to build strength, not add bulk. There is a consistent thread of core (postural strength) in each training phase.

Foundational strength

Emphasis: total body and multiple joint movements with external resistance based on percentage of bodyweight and bodyweight.

Length of cycle: three to six weeks.

Frequency: four-day split routine.

Means: total body movements in a rep range of 4–6. Individual upper body exercises with resistance in a rep range of 6–10. With bodyweight the rep range is 6–10 for upper body and 20 reps for lower body. On lower body bodyweight exercises the speed is 1 rep per second – this is very important.

MONDAY AND THURSDAY – TOTAL BODY AND LOWER EXTREMITY

(key: KB = Kettle bell, DB = Dumbbell, BW = Bodyweight)

Single leg squat
3 x 6 each leg (standing)
Seated 2 x 6 each leg
KB swing 3 x 6 two arm
Jump shrug 4 x 6 (800 and 1500 only)
DB high pull 3 x 6
BW squat 3 x 20*

BW lunge 3 x 20* (10 each leg)
BW step-up 3 x 20* (10 each leg)
Front pull-down 3 x 6*
DB one arm rows 3 x 6 each arm*
Medicine ball total body throws
Over the back x 6, forward x 6, squat throw x 10

* Add one set per week until you reach five sets. Then stay at five sets for three or four weeks until you move to next phase of training.

TUESDAY AND FRIDAY – UPPER BODY

Assisted pull-up 4 x 4
TRX incline pull-up 4 x 6
Incline push-up 4 x 8
Bent arm pullover 3 x 8
Medicine ball wall throws
Overhead throw x 20

Soccer throw x 20
Chest pass x 20
Standing side to side x 10 each side (cross in front)
Standing cross in front x 10 each side
Around the back x 10 each side

Basic strength

Emphasis: Volume loading through push/pull/squat sequence work. Resistance is based on percentage of
   bodyweight.

Length of cycle: three to six weeks.

Frequency: four day split.

Means: DB complex + mini leg circuit, regular upper body.

MONDAY OR THURSDAY

DB Complex

DB High Pull x 6	5 Complexes
DB Alternate Press x 6	1:1 work:rest
DB Squat x 6	Pair off with partner
DB Row x 6	

Mini Leg Circuit

Squat x 3	
Lunge x 3 each Leg	Start with 3 circuits progress to 6,
Step-up x 3 each leg	No rest between exercises
Jump Squat x 3	

TUESDAY – UPPER BODY

Assisted pull-up 5 x 4	Overhead throw x 20
*Trx incline pull-up 5 x 6	Soccer throw x 20
Incline push-up 5 x 8	Chest pass x 20
Arm step-up 3 x 20	Standing side to side x 10 each side (cross in front)
Bent arm pullover 4 x 6	Standing cross in front x 10 each side
Medicine ball wall throws	Around the back x 10 each side
* PORTABLE BODYWEIGHT TRAINING TOOL	

WEDNESDAY AND FRIDAY

Medicine ball total body throws	Over the back x 6, forward x 6, squat throw x 10

Power endurance

Emphasis: high intensity work 30 seconds in duration with a 1:1 work to rest ratio in multiple sets using total body movements to involve as much muscle mass as possible.

Length of cycle: three weeks.

Frequency: as per the following, or restructure to GH workouts Monday, Wednesday, Friday; upper body Tuesday; total body throws Thursday.

Means: GH work.

MONDAY – GH WORKOUT

(Progress to five sets) 3 min rec between exercises
DB high pull 3 x 30 seconds – 30 sec rec between sets
Squat and press 3 x 30 seconds – 30 sec rec between sets
BW squat 1 x 30 seconds for maximum reps

TUESDAY – UPPER BODY

Assisted pull-up 5 x 4	Overhead throw x 20
Trx incline pull-up 5 x 6	Soccer throw x 20
Incline push-up 5 x 8	Chest pass x 20
Arm step-up 3 x 20	Standing side to side x 10 each side (cross in front)
Bent arm pullover 4 x 6	Standing cross in front x 10 each side
Medicine ball wall throws	Around the back x 10 each side

WEDNESDAY AND FRIDAY

Total body throws	Over the back x 6, forward x 6, squat throw x 10

THURSDAY – GH WORKOUT

(Progress to five sets) 3 min rec between exercises
DB high pull 3 x 30 seconds – 30 seconds rec between sets
Squat and press 3 x 30 seconds – 30 seconds rec between sets
BW squat 1 x 30 seconds for maximum reps

Strength endurance

Emphasis: work in the time range from 30 seconds to 60 seconds with recovery up to one to one, but more frequently one to one half to one to one third.

Length of cycle: three weeks.

Frequency: three days a week.

Means: circuit work, time and rep based.

MONDAY

45 sec work:15 sec rest
Alternate
Upper body exercise
Core exercise
Lower body exercise
800 go for 12 minutes total
800/1500 goes for 15 minutes total
Steeple & 5K go for 20 minutes total
10K go for 25 minutes total

TUESDAY OR THURSDAY

Medicine ball total body throws
Over the back x 6, forward x 6, squat throw x 10
Medicine ball wall throws
Overhead throw x 20
Soccer throw x 20
Chest pass x 20
Standing side to side x 10 each side (cross in front)
Standing cross in front x 10 each side
Around the back x 10 each side

WEDNESDAY OR FRIDAY

30 sec work:30 sec recovery
Same exercises as Monday to avoid confusion
800 go for 8 minutes – rest two minutes – 4 minutes
800/1500 goes for 12 minutes – rest two minutes – 6 minutes
Steeple, 5K & 10K go for 14 minutes – rest three minutes – 7 minutes

Recycle

Emphasis: each of the elements of the previous components is recycled through for short periods to stabilise or refresh as needed.

Length of cycle: three weeks.

Frequency: two to three days a week.

Means: each session will revisit the workout means from the previous cycles.

For example:

1 week foundation

1 week basic strength

1 week power endurance

1 week strength endurance

Mix it however you want to based on how they are progressing and what you think they need.

Hybrid

Emphasis: each component is touched on in a microcycle in order to stabilise strength components in peaking or tapering.

Length of cycle: three weeks.

Frequency: two to three times a week.

Means: combination(s) of each of the previous methods.

For example:

1 day foundation

1 day basic strength

1 day power endurance

This is totally by feel, women need to keep at least two days in, some men may have to drop strength training completely.

SUMMARY

Physical strength is the foundation on which all other physical competencies are developed. While it is important to understand types of strength it is of equal importance that such are seen in the context of natural movement patterns in general and of specific techniques. For example, increasing strength in major joint actions such as hip/knee extension or elbow and shoulder extensions and flexion clearly has a value. However, exercise selection must reflect the relationship of strength increases in these actions to enhancing intended efficient and effective movement. Hence the need to understand concepts of functional strength training when applying strength training principles.

Six key questions must be addressed together with comprehensive evaluation of the athlete's physical and psychological profile in determining the starting point for programme prescription, assessing potential and planning the journey to realise that potential. Specific considerations of programme design for growing female and senior athletes are outlined and specific issues around plyometrics and exercise machines are discussed. Examples of periodised strength training programmes affords coaches a useful reference framework.

REFLECTIVE QUESTIONS

1. Design a general strength circuit to include all major joint actions. Describe each exercise, its objective, apparatus and/or equipment and number of repetitions per exercise. The circuit should be performed three times. The total time to complete the three circuits is 30 minutes. You should consider and explain how you will decide repetition numbers for the mixed group of 16–18-year-olds and the basis of progression over twelve weeks – one circuit training unit per week.

2. If women respond to strength training essentially the same as men, why doesn't upper arm girth of female bodybuilders equal their male counterparts?

3. Design a specific strength programme for one of the following and discuss the bases of your exercise selection and prescription and for the equipment and/or apparatus used. The programme is for a six week pre-competition mesocycle (see chapter 21), two training units per week.
   a. A national level female medley swimmer (20 years).
   b. An international level male triple jumper (24 years).
   c. A club level male badminton player (17 years).
   d. An international level female rugby prop (28 years).

4. Review the exercise machines available at a fully equipped gym, listing the function of each and noting body position on the apparatus. Then prepare a discussion paper on the advantages and disadvantages of a strength programme designed to address the purpose for which the machine is designed using:
   a. Medicine balls, kettle bell and standard gym equipment (e.g. wall bars, beams, benches, climbing ropes, window ladders and vaulting boxes, etc.).
   b. Fully equipped weights room (i.e. Olympic Bard weights, squat rack, bench, dumbbells etc.).
   c. Both (a) and (b).

5. Create a wall chart for core strength exercises illustrating each exercise. Discuss why you have selected these exercises and, where relevant, justify the use of the apparatus/equipment you recommend. Are there possible age or gender differences given that those using your wall chart are 15–35 year olds? If so, what are they?

15 THEORY AND PRACTICE OF SPEED DEVELOPMENT

SPEED IN SPORT

Speed is the capacity of moving a limb or part of the body's lever system or the whole body with the greatest possible velocity. Maximum speed of a movement would occur without loading; thus, the discus thrower's arm will have greatest velocity in the throwing phase if no discus is held and velocity would be reduced as the weight of the discus increases relative to the thrower's absolute strength.

Speed is measured in metres per second, as, for example, in quantifying the value for speed of moving one part of the body's lever system relative to another; the forward speed of the body in sprinting or at point of take-off, in jumping; and the velocity of implements and balls at release or on being struck. The time taken to achieve a certain task may also be considered a measure of the athlete's speed. For example, speed might simply be the time taken to sprint 30m or it may be measured as the number of repetition runs in a shuttle run over 5m in 20 seconds. Equipment used to measure speed includes stop watches video-linked to relevant IT and software, photoelectric cells coupled to print-out devices, cinematographic techniques based on film speed, force plates, and so on.

Speed is a critical component of that complex requirement for achievement in competitive sport. It has four strands (figure 15.1). Strength in itself will not influence maximum speed of limb movement, but developing greater strength and applying it at speed will positively influence performance. There is a critical sequence in the progression of developing performance in this respect.

- Develop the general strength and mobility consistent with the technique(s) required.
- Learn sound technique(s).
- Develop related and specific strength.
- Learn to perform these at optimal speed.
- Develop general/related/specific strength to apply at optimal speed.

'Optimal' speed is as close to maximum as possible without compromising the technical model(s). In endurance sports, speed's role on the one hand expands the range of tactical variants. On the other, it is, as in the progression suggested above, within development of related and specific endurance.

Speed may be a determining factor directly, as in, for example, reacting to the starter's pistol, or indirectly, as, for example, in the development of kinetic energy in jumping. The difference between direct and indirect speed is that, with the former, 'optimal speed' is close to maximum, whereas with the latter, 'optimal speed' is a critical percentage of maximum which allows maximum expression of required strength. It is therefore important to bear in mind that speed increases may not necessarily lead to improved performance. The pattern of speed and acceleration of relative movements must be synchronised so that each part of the lever system can make an optimal force contribution. For example, there would be no point in making the discus arm so fast that it began to make its contribution before the legs and trunk, nor would it benefit the long

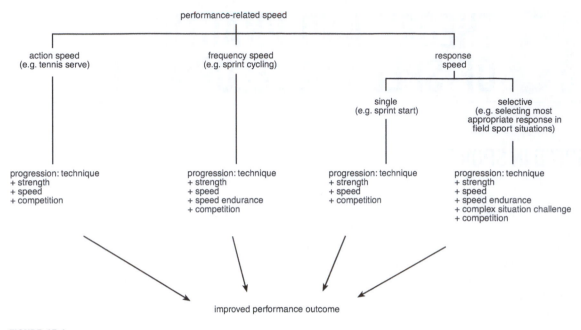

FIGURE 15.1 Four strands of speed

jumper to have so much horizontal speed at the board that there was insufficient time for the take-off leg to express the strength required for vertical lift. Speed development is, then, very much a matter of learning how to use it.

SPEED DEVELOPMENT
Speed in practice

There are seven areas in sports performance where training will enhance speed.

1. Response to a signal as, for example, in the sprinter's reaction to the gun, or the tennis player's reaction in volleying. In the case of sprinting, two aspects are noteworthy. First, reaction time (RT) is the time taken from the starter's gun to the commencement of force production. Another critical aspect to consider is the time taken from the starter's gun to clearing the blocks with the front foot, which is termed movement time (MT).

2. Capacity to accelerate: this is of particular importance to those athletes who must beat opponents across the ground or who must quickly reach a particular point on the court/pitch to execute a technique. Acceleration is especially critical where distances of a sprint are short.

3. Capacity to rapidly adjust balance following execution of one technique in order to prepare to execute another. This applies to every games situation.

4. Achievement of maximum speed (peak velocity): the athlete here is executing a given movement as fast as he can without compromising technique. Often speed is mistakenly thought of as an entity in itself, it is not. It is a sophistication of technique, where all demands of the technique are performed at the highest speed consistent with the general synchronised framework. Usain Bolt in producing the world record of 9.58s in Berlin (2009) reached a maximum speed of 12.27m/s. It is noteworthy that he reached 99 per cent of maximum velocity at 48m.

5. Capacity to maintain maximum speed once it is reached (speed maintenance). The ability to maintain speed is influenced by neural fatigue, coordination, and concentration. In 2009, Bolt maintained his speed of 12.2m/s for 20m (60–80m) in running his world record time of 9.58s.

6. Capacity to maintain anaerobic energy production: the rate at ATP is resynthesised via CrP breakdown and glycogenolysis will be limited by diminishing intramuscular CrP stores and acidosis resulting from high rates of lactic acid production. Appropriate training will minimise the influence of these factors on fatigue and allow the athlete to better maintain maximal or near maximal speed.

7. Making the correct decision quickly under pressure: in many sports, the difference between success and failure is determined by the speed at which a player or players solve a problem posed by the opposition; and a problem is then set for the opposition. The better the opposition or higher the level of competition, the less time a player has to make decisions.

These areas are embraced by the four strands of figure 15.1.

Strand	Areas
Action speed	(2) (4)
Frequency speed	(2) (3) (5)
Single response speed	(1) (2)
Selective response speed	(3) (5) (6)

Speed can be developed. The development of speed is dependent on several key factors, which are outlined below:

1. Innervation (figure 6.6, p. 109): a high frequency of alternation between stimulation and inhibition of neurones, and an accurate selection and regulation of motor units, makes it possible to achieve a high frequency of movement and/or speed of movement, married to an optimal expression or deployment of strength. This is the fundamental ability to move limbs at maximum velocity.

2. Elasticity (figure 6.8, p. 111): the capacity to capitalise on muscle tone via the elastic component of muscle has relevance to those sports demanding high starting acceleration (as in sprints and most field sports) or 'rapid strike' (as in sprinting and jumping). This involves a complex coordination of motor units, reflexes, elastic component and the ability to contract muscle at high speed. The characteristic is, however, identifiable and has been referred to in sports jargon as 'bounce'. Elasticity is connected to relative strength and elastic strength.

3. Biochemistry: ATP resynthesis during very high intensity exercise is achieved largely through the break-down of CrP and the anaerobic breakdown of muscle glycogen; as the duration of exercise increases, so too does the relative contribution of aerobic metabolism to meeting the rate of ATP resynthesis (Spriet et al., 1999; Van Loon et al., 2001). Muscle fibre type will also influence the speed of muscle contraction (MacIntosh et al., 2006).

4. Muscle relaxability: the ability of the muscle to relax and to allow stretch in speed exercises is fundamental to technique and to a high frequency of movement. Harre (1973) has said: 'If these qualities are insuffi-ciently developed, the required range of movement cannot be achieved in the course of the movement, particularly at the points of reversal of movement, as the synergists have to overcome too great a resist-ance.' So there are two thoughts to this: mobility/flexibility and coordination. Training that teaches the athlete to relax all muscles not directly involved with a given series of joint actions, even in fatigue, is then, of the utmost importance. Mobility work and focused application of psychoregulatory techniques for physical, mental and emotional relaxation are also clearly indicated here.

5. Focus and determination: the athlete must remain focused in the moment to produce maximum voluntary effort and subsequently achieve maximum speed. However, unlike the weightlifter who has a quantified target as the focus of his concentration, the sprinter has nothing more to go on than physical sensations, and the time recorded by an official. Human error may occur with the latter, so the coach must ensure that all possible information related to the performance is given to the athlete; if the information is accurate. Moreover, to provide a suitable stimulus/target to promote both higher levels of innervation, appropriate focus and simulated competition experience, speed work may be performed in groups, using handicaps, competitions, etc. to challenge the sprinters to run fast.

6. Environment: warm climate, altitude, footwear, running surface, low air resistance, clothing that enhances aero-dynamics, or anything which may oblige an athlete to learn how to move faster can assist speed development.

7. Aptitude, early development, and optimisation of development stages:

   - Elite speed athletes have a relatively high proportion of fast-twitch muscle fibres.
   - Optimal trainability of reactive/responsive and frequency speed abilities and optimal preconditions for motor learning are 8–11 (girls), 8–13 (boys) – with a 'peaking' at 9–10 (girls), 10–12 (boys).
   - During puberty (11–15 girls; 13–17 boys) there is improved trainability of the strength component of speed. Initial training of fast strength/elastic strength should be with low resistance. Maximum strength appropriate to speed performance is introduced later.
   - High-quality early technical schooling is essential in creating the right physical and timing framework(s) of coordination through which speed, then strength, then endurance may be applied. Nevertheless, it is important that over-schooling technical aspects might contribute to more mechanistic rather than fluent movements, which will contribute to the development of inappropriate motor patterns and subsequently slower performances.
   - Anticipation is the capacity to read situations from early perceptual cues in the environment – (psycho-logical precognition). It permits earlier choice of action options and so reduces response time whether for single or multiple action responses to the challenge of the situation. It profoundly influences action speed, single response speed and selection response speed.

Training for speed development

Speed development for track events has been extensively documented and will provide a useful base for the practice of speed development for other sports.

Intensity

The intensity of training loads for speed development commences around 90 per cent maximum. Here, the athlete is learning, at a relatively high intensity, those adjustments necessary to maintain the pace or rhythm of a technique while 'timing' is put under pressure. Gradually, the athlete moves towards 100 per cent. However, progression demands that the athlete attempts to exceed existing speed limits. Rehearsal of technique at intensities that break new ground is clearly not possible in great volume for reasons ranging from neuromuscular and metabolic fatigue to concentration. Thus, strategies such as pulling the athlete on an elastic rope or pulley system; reducing the weight of implements; reducing the time scales for making choices of action can be effective in having the athlete sprint at intensities greater than 100 per cent. Contrast training (Matveyev, 1981) can be an effective method for challenging the speed barrier. In contrast training, athletes complete a combination of some added resistance (e.g. headwind; sled; hills), some assisted (e.g. pulley system; running with the wind/downhill), and then under 'normal' conditions.

Depending on goals, improving speed depends on long-term development – a continuing cycle that may run over several months or even years (see chapter 21). The sequence of development is:

- develop a level of general conditioning, which permits learning a sound basic technique;
- learn a sound basic technique;
- develop a level of related and specific conditioning, which permits progressive sophistication of technique;
- develop technique at speed.

Technical components should be learned and stabilised at slightly slower speeds (i.e. 90–95% maximum). Nevertheless, from the outset the athlete should be encouraged to consolidate technique as he progresses from 90 towards 100 per cent and beyond. This is necessary because the transfer of technique learned at a slower speed to the demands of maximum speed is usually very complex. It is suggested that over the course of the season that the sprinter builds his race from start to finish. For example, early in the season he might perfect his technique over the first 30m (building from 90–100%) and then gradually extending that to 50–60m; and then eventually over the 100m distance. Another approach is to run a distance of, say, 75m, concentrating on the perfection of running action for 30–40m and then raise the speed of running for 20m and then focus on high stride frequency and 'spinning the wheels'. A hurdler strides over three hurdles with 5–7 strides between, then sprints over three hurdles with the normal three stride pattern. A tennis player brings the speed of service down to that which allows him to place the ball accurately in the service court, and to 'feel' the synchronisation of each element in the technique. The idea is to relate to the timing of the technique as a basis for development; then to progress pace but within the constraints of sound technique. Finally, the athlete masters that level of speed that permits him to select a given pace within his range, and which is sufficient to overcome the challenge of his opposition.

There should be no fatigue factors in speed training because it is essential for the nervous system to be in a state of optimal excitement. Consequently speed training will follow immediately upon relevant warm-up. Endurance or strengthening work may follow, but never precede, speed training. In addition, recovery between exercise bouts must be sufficient for the athlete to be able to perform the subsequent sprints relatively free of fatigue.

Training extent

There is an inverse relationship between the intensity and duration of exercise. If the athlete is working at maximum intensity, duration (or volume) of the exercise will be relatively low and the number of repetitions may be few. Nonetheless, it may be necessary for the athlete to rehearse a technique frequently at high intensity, if new levels of speed are to be stabilised. The following points may serve as a useful guideline to making decisions on extent.

1. Sprinting with appropriate technique can be repeated in high volume and high intensity only if presented in small 'learning packages'. This ensures the highest speed of execution and adequate recovery between bouts that, in turn, allows the athlete time to consolidate neuromuscular memory patterns. So, a large number of sets with small numbers of repetitions of very high intensity is possible provided recovery periods between exercise bouts allow for near complete restoration of CrP and a return of pH in the exercising muscles to normal resting values. Total volume of high intensity speed work should be around 300m.

2. In sprint training, the minimum distance to develop acceleration is that which allows the athlete to achieve near maximum speed. For most athletes this is around 30–40m. However, in other sports there are constraints imposed by the confines of the playing area. In some sports, then, the athlete must learn to achieve maximum acceleration over a very short distance (5–10m) and 'arrive' at the conclusion of such a burst of speed, prepared to select and execute a high precision technique. Soccer, tennis, and basketball are examples of such sports.

3. Where maximum speed is being practised, a limiting factor to effective rehearsal can be the exhausting process of accelerating to maximum speed. For example, in long jump and in games where passing must be practised at the highest speed, the athletes must lift their pace from being stationary to the pace required. This is demanding on the neural system. To overcome the problem, some athletes practise from longer rolling starts or with the assistance of downhill starts. This means that although the athlete will look to distances of 10–30m to practice maximum speed itself, it may be necessary to have 20–40m roll-in to reach that speed.

4. Optimal values can only be determined by individual testing on how long maximum speed can be held. The initial challenge is, of course, to achieve maximum speed. It has already been pointed out that Bolt could only maintain his maximum speed for 20m. However, for world class sprinters, male and female, this is normal. Coordination and concentration appear to be the keys to extending this distance, so it may be possible that athletes can learn to maintain maximum speed from 60m to the 100m finish.

5. In sprinting, most athletes require 5–6 seconds to achieve maximum speed. This suggests that distances of 40–60m (dependent upon age) are required to develop the linking of initial acceleration and the 'pick up' to maximum speed.

Training recovery

Recovery periods between maximum exercise bouts must be adequate to allow near complete resynthesis of CrP stores and for muscle pH to return to near normal, but short enough to maintain excitement of the nervous system and maintain optimal body temperature. Given a reasonably warm climate, the interval between each run should be 4–6 minutes, which creates problems for athletes living in countries with long cold winters.

In the interest of gaining optimum advantage from each run, it might be advisable to allow this interval and to 'warm-up' before each run. Sets should again be used with, say, 3–4 runs per set and 2–3 sets per unit.

For 100 per cent recovery of the neuromuscular system from a maximum speed or elastic/fast strength or speed endurance unit, approximately 48 hours is required. A further 24–36 hours is required for the peak of over-compensation (Grosser, 1991).

Units (training sessions)

The total number of runs per unit, as indicated above, should be between 6 and 12, although this will depend on the athlete. The number of training units in each weekly microcycle (microcycles, mesocycles, macro-cycles and units are explained in chapter 21) will vary throughout the year, but at least one unit of speed training per microcycle should be included in mesocycle 1 of the annual cycle (see p. 314) with 2–3 in meso-cycle 2, and 2–4 in mesocycle 3, irrespective of the sport. With endurance sports, speed work will range in intensity from maximum to racing pace and unit distribution will vary according to racing distance, phase of the year and the athlete concerned.

Against this background of sprint speed development, six basic principles (Stein, 1998) may be considered as the foundation of speed training method:

1. **Quality first** – all speed training is at the near maximum and super maximum level. This places high demands on the neuromuscular system. That means high intensity exercise bouts need to be combined with low overall training volume and involve sufficient recovery periods between both bouts and also separate training sessions.

2. **Technical precision without compromise** – whether as a whole technique or as a drill, the technical execution must be precise – rehearsed practise makes permanent.

3. **Specificity** – the speed component of performance is the focus of specific exercise rather than related or general. 'These special exercises should simulate the spatial, temporal, dynamic and energetic character-istics of competition as closely as possible.' (Stein, 1998). The importance of specificity (e.g., simulated competitions) is central to effective speed development. This does not negate the value of drills, which isolate speed of particular joint actions (e.g. sprint drills programmes of Seagrave, Mach, and others). Speed drills can facilitate learning and execution of the full technical model; however, drills should be performed at speed and segued into a sprint or full form of the desired movement to facilitate learning.

4. **Speed development depends on several factors** – the seven factors set out on pages 256–7 must be under-stood and built into a speed development programme.

5. **Speed training must include constant feedback** – feedback is central to the learning process. Both objective (e.g. video analysis; stride length x stride frequency relationship) and subjective feedback (e.g. perception of maximum speed; kinaesthesis or 'touch' on the ground) are critical to the learning process in the development of speed.

6. **Speed development depends on high motivation with minimal external and internal pressures** – it is essential that the athlete be actively engaged in affording full mental effort to executing maximum speed to benefit from speed training; that is, a relaxed and focused mind and fluent movement patterns will foster

the production of maximum speed. This attentional focus in the moment necessitates an adaptive motivational climate, which is created by the coach to support the learner and learning minimising controlling influences on the joy (intrinsic motivation) of running fast (Mallett, 2005).

These principles help design speed development in any sport. The following are specific examples:

For acceleration development

- Different starting positions sprint from 10–15m (especially in team sports) to 50/60m; this may also involve responding to cues in the environment and then chasing/competing for the ball.
- Facilitated movement – sprinting downhill, pulled by elastic/pulley system.
- Resisted movement* – uphill sprint, resistance towing (maximum 5–8% bodyweight; excessive loads can compromise technique).
- Competitions – handicap starts; chasing others; short shuttle relays.
- Varied speed runs – sprint drive – 10–20m; hold form 20m; lift pace 20–30m.
- Extreme short sprints – 5m; 10m; 15m; 20m.

(* When resistance is used it should not exceed 5 per cent of the normal situation in these or other technical/strength speed practices. If it does, the technical model is compromised and compensatory movements are introduced.)

For developing capacity to maintain maximum speed

- 'Flying' sprints – gradual acceleration to 30m and then hold speed for 10–30m.
- 'Build-up' sprints – 25–60m then focus on turning over (maintaining high stride frequency) or using cues like 'cycling downhill and spinning the wheels'.
- Coordination light stride runs (focus on fast and shorter arm swings to promote stride frequency).
- Isolation and dynamic/elastic drills – hopping, high knee running, 'prancing horse' (skip) runs, heel flicks, skip drills fast ankle flexes on spot that once developed transition into the 'real deal'.
- Sprinting downhill on 2–5° gradient.
- Facilitated (pulled) sprints – elastic rope, pulleys, super speed motorised treadmill.

For frequency speed

- Maximum speed frequency repetitions should be worked for 8–10 sec (elite performer); 6 sec (youth) in these practices.
- Active ankle work – isolation and elastic drills.
- Skipping rope workouts maximum speed.
- Low obstacle or ground marking precision/speed movement – sprints on flat, uphill, downhill.
- Alternate side speed hopping across a line.
- Alternate forward/backward hops across a line.
- Sprints/fast foot movements across hoops/tyres on ground; rope/stick ladder on ground; speed grid – 3m × 6m (18 × 1m × 1m squares) – stepping/hopping challenges.
- Speed change sprints.

- Direction change sprints through a cone grid (3m separating cones in any direction).
- Contrast method (Matveyev, 1981) – resisted activity immediately followed by normal or facilitated activity.

Young athlete speed development

When developing speed in young athletes, the learning situation should be modified to permit maximum speeds by using:

- lighter equipment
- smaller equipment
- bodyweight supports
- reduced dimension areas
- isolated action speed then building towards multiple action and selective response. Response speed may be developed by challenging response speed to optic, acoustic or tactile signals.

Throwing

Speed in throwing can be developed by using lighter implements. Insufficient research data is available to provide detailed information, but the following points may serve as guidelines.

1. If the implement is too light, there is the risk of injury and disruption of the normal motor patterns of technique. Using implements approximately 5 per cent heavier for a set of repetitions followed by 5–10 per cent lighter, and then the normal weight on a set-for-set basis, improves speed. This mix can be extended to include specific strength work with implements heavier than the normal implement.

2. Rebounding work or plyometrics should be considered as speed-related training. Work in this area may effect a faster transition from yielding to the power of approach, shift or turn, to overcoming the load of impetus when moving levers (legs, hips) through the throw. This is particularly so for javelin, where increased speed of approach will place a considerably greater load on both legs. It is as if the athlete must concentrate on 'bouncing' out of the entry into the throw, rather than accepting the momentum of approach or shift. The danger is that to 'accept' is often to 'cushion' and this decreases speed and the elastic use of kinetic energy.

3. Speed should only be pursued within the limits dictated by the athlete's technical ability. The fundamentals of technique must not be abandoned in the pursuit of speed.

Jumping

The development of speed in jumping should be considered in two parts: development of approach speed (e.g. sprinting), and the development of the ability to use kinetic energy of increased approach speed. The previous discussion of sprinting speed should be applied to the development of approach speed, bearing in mind that the approach run must be consistent, even with advances in speed. The problem of using this increased speed is best solved by learning the new motor pattern of a faster passage over the take-off foot, and then progressing to the application of strength at this increased speed. The high-energy cost of acceleration means that flat-out approach runs from scratch are inadvisable. The areas of practice that should be explored are:

- downhill approach to take-off
- fast 'touch-off' take-offs
- rolling start approaches
- pole plant in sand following the above (landing area placed over long jump pit/pole vault)
- faster high jump approach onto extended landing area
- increasing the speed of the non-jumping limb movements relative to the jumping limb.

Ultimately, the ability to use the kinetic energy of the approach is strength related and consideration must be given to elastic strength work, rebound work, and depth jumping. Relative strength rather than absolute strength is critical.

In some sports, speed development offers a different type of challenge. Two examples are given below: swimming and tennis.

Swimming

Specific endurance is the single most important conditioning requirement in competitive swimming. The 50m sprint event brought to the sport speed demands within the traditional technique-strength-endurance framework previously only associated with water polo. When 50m sprints were introduced, maintaining speed and maximum speed required focus and improvement.

The process sequence for speed development training is:

- A foundation of swimming-specific basic strength and aerobic endurance.
- Increased related strength (therefore hypertrophy) via the weights room and in the water.
- Increased specific strength by swimming against resistance (therefore increased fibre recruitment).
- Facilitated (via pulley, etc.) super-maximum speed training to oblige increased stroke/impulse frequency.
- To build-in speed endurance.

Individual repetitions within sets in a speed-training unit last 6–8 seconds max.

Intervals are between 3–5 minutes.

Total repetitions within a training unit are 4 minimum–20 maximum.

In other sports it represents a very complex challenge.

Tennis

Tennis is one of the most demanding and complex sports in terms of top competitive performance. A player's abilities are a mixture, requiring high levels of specific competence at technical, tactical, strategic, psychological levels and in strength, endurance and speed.

The game has significantly changed in the past couple of decades and the physical demands on players, particularly at the elite level, are considerable.

Materials were optimised in areas such as stiffer rackets, changing court surfaces and ball technology. On top of this there has developed a more aggressive playing attitude and changing anthropometry and physical condition in both men's and women's tennis. As a result, speed has become a key component in a player's performance armoury. A player is dependent on speed for:

- returning the ball on court one more time than the opponent
- sprinting to get to the ball
- reading the game better than the opponent
- psychological construction of a tactical plan and for changing it
- preparing for and executing a stroke then moving to reduce the opponent's choice of response
- the pace of the player's game and response to the opponent's pace
- speed given to the ball; taking the ball earlier; response in volleys, etc.

Energy production/demands is also an issue, of course, as shortcomings in meeting energy demand shifts the game from one of speed/strength to one of strength/endurance. The average duration of rallies is 10 seconds and time between 20 seconds. Maximum sprinting distance is 14m – but the average is around 4m. There are also two minute pauses after every other game. So the energy requirements are in the main closer to those of a sprinter than an endurance athlete. That said there must be a sound aerobic base to reduce the possibility of cumulative fatigue. So what sort of speed work does a tennis player require?

- short sprints to optical/acoustic signal – 2m–15m
- varied distance short sprints 5–20m in 10–90 seconds sets of sprint/skip-walk-jog
- court sprints over marked routes
- shadow/mirror sprints
- volleys under pressure in 5–15 seconds sets, with two feeders; with a 360 degree turn between, or sitting/ squatting/kneeling between; with back to feeder and responding to sound; standing or covering 2.5m right and left, etc.

Sprinting exercises
- Sprinting drills.
- Flying sprints 10–30m.
- Standing start sprints; sprinting from 'dancing' on the spot 2–10m.
- Facedown lying sprints 2–10m.
- Fast feet drills for 6–8 seconds in one position, with turn, etc.
- Plyometric/elastic strength routines – hopping, bounding, two-feet jump.
- Multidirectional 'sprints' – side, forward, back, diagonal, etc.
- Fan sprints.
- Potato races; shuttle sprints.
- Performing these practices with racket to play strokes either shadowing or actual.

Tennis-specific speed
- Rapid serves, forehands, returns under time pressure (10–20 seconds).
- 12 repetitions of 3–4 winning shots hit either forehand or backhand from half court.
- Tennis strokes with squash/badminton racket and soft balls.
- Fast shots in specific situations – fast lobs, smashes, returns on the run.
- Working through 3–4 identical tactical sequences under time pressure.

THE SPEED BARRIER

Saziorski (1971) suggests that a 'speed barrier' can arise if the young athlete trains exclusively on sprint exercises, or if the advanced athlete neglects the use of special exercises for the development of elastic strength. Osolin (1952) tends to agree by stating that due to establishing a 'kinetic (motor) stereotype' by working at maximum intensity (e.g. training with the same group at all times) the development of speed may be made more difficult, or even prevented. However, he offers a note of optimism by suggesting that practices such as 'forced speed' (e.g. catapulting the athlete with the use of an elastic rope), or 'assisted speed' (e.g. altitude sprinting, downhill runs, or wind-assisted runs), or lighter implements, or increased competition demands, etc., will break an athlete's existing speed barrier; if, the technical model is not compromised.

Upton and Radford (1975) appear to support this notion of a speed barrier and explain: 'The benefits of teaching methods that stress fast limb movements and the sensation of speed (e.g. by towing) may well result from improvement of neuronal programmes, increased motoneuron excitability and more synchronous firing of motoneurons.'

This observation highlights an often neglected cause for speed barriers – the failure to involve efficient 'neuronal programs ... and more synchronous firing of motoneurons'. The introduction of sprint drills to the conditioning programme may be an attempt to establish motor unit programming. Ballreich (1976) claims that '... sprinting for top level sprinters can probably best be improved by developing its technical (coordination) rather than its conditioning (power) component'.

Endurance and speed training

Speed and endurance exist on a continuum and depending on the competition demands, an athlete's training may need to develop a capacity to repeat high intensity exercise while maintaining speed. Adaptations to endurance training include improved delivery and use of oxygen at the exercising muscle; given that resynthesis of CrP is dependent on oxygen and that removal of lactic acid from muscle is also dependent on aerobic metabolism, endurance training will improve the muscle's capacity to recover from high intensity (sprint) exercise. Thus, endurance exercise will allow a sprint athlete to recover faster between bouts and theoretically allow that athlete to engage in higher quality sprint training sessions. Training that combines speed work within an endurance session can involve repeated bouts of exercise interspersed with brief recovery bouts (that intentionally will be too short for complete resynthesis of CrP and restoration of normal pH values in the muscles). This type of training will not only lead to improvements in endurance capacity, but it will also result in an improved capacity for the muscles to accommodate the inevitable acidosis that will occur with sprint exercise. Thus, there are clear benefits to the athlete in the capacity to undertake high intensity exercise and also the capacity to perform endurance exercise. This type of training will clearly benefit those athletes who compete in sports that involve multiple sprints.

Speed endurance will be addressed in the next chapter, however units that will develop this characteristic are shown below.

1. Repetition runs at sub-maximum to near maximum intensity. Long recovery periods are necessary between runs of near maximum intensity to ensure that quality is maintained, while shorter intervals are required where runs are of sub-maximum intensity. Sets of runs with 2–4 minutes between runs are recommended, but these will of necessity be short sets (e.g. 2–4 runs) to maintain quality. Between sets,

longer intervals of 10–15 minutes should be introduced and it is recommended that at least half of this interval is active.

2. Stress loading at maximum or near maximum intensity (for the distance used) over distances between ⅔ × and 2 × the racing distance.

3. Stress loading at maximum racing speed over stretches of up to 10–20% longer than the racing distance.

4. Varied speed runs where the tempo or intensity varies in the course of the run, e.g. 150m of 50m acceleration, 50m hold, 50m acceleration.

5. High repetition, short distance sprints (30–60m) where maintaining maximum striding rate is emphasised, e.g. 6 × 6 × 40m – incomplete recovery in sets.

6. Competitions.

A microcycle of 2–3 units per week should be used in mesocycle 2, but 1–2 units per microcycle will be adequate as the competition density assumes an endurance training role of its own.

Speed endurance practices for sports other than pure sprinting are poorly documented, but the endurance factor must be borne in mind. Five sets of top class tennis frequently exceed five hours (e.g. Isner v Mahut, at Wimbledon 2010, took 11 hours 5 minutes); vault and high jump competitions can last over six hours, qualifying throws/jumps may be separated by 60 minutes, athletes declining to jump may cause an athlete to have several jumps/vaults in rapid succession, a qualifying contest and final in one day can necessitate nine throws/jumps at maximum intensity; field games last from 60 to 90 minutes; boxing (professional) may last 75 minutes; sailing lasts hours, etc. In Formula 1 races, the heart rate of drivers is, for approximately 90 minutes, in the range of 175–185 beats per minute. These factors may mean speed endurance and strength endurance work for all sports where there is a demand for speed (particularly repeated speed) in the presence of fatigue. For example in throwing:

- rapid succession throws with normal implements being fed to the athlete (full throws, isolated action and standing throws)
- rapid succession throws with medicine balls or lighter implements, as above
- single throws separated by 15–60 minutes, etc.
- track workouts followed by throws
- maximum repetition simulation throws per 30 seconds, etc.

Or in jumping:

- rapid succession short approach jumps
- rapid succession 'stepdown' jumps (e.g. 21 stride, 17 stride, 13 stride, 9 stride) with walkback recovery
- speed bounding/hopping, etc., over 30m
- jumping circuits over 400m (50m bound, etc.)
- single jumps/vaults separated by 15–60 minutes, etc.
- fast agility work on ropes, bars, etc., for simulated work on the pole.

Or in games:

- rapid succession strokes in tennis/squash
- continuous pressure passing/lay-up practice in basketball
- unopposed non-stop rugby/soccer/hockey
- high speed games without breaks at altitude
- conditioning work followed by continuous speed work under pressure.

Attitude and speed training

In the intensely interactive world of team games, combat sports, racket games, etc., in order for speed of individual or team performance to be delivered instinctively under the pressure of competition, it must be repeatedly rehearsed in training. Successful performance is not only due to speed of movement across the ground and speed of choosing correct action options, but also speed of thought and interpretation of situations. A player giving or passing the ball to a colleague must be thinking about, and moving immediately to, a position to support the person receiving the ball. This means having this attitude in even simple practice situations. Without doubt it contributes immensely to the rhythm and speed at which a given team will play in competition.

Risk of injury

Speed work must be preceded by a full warm-up. Some 35–50 per cent of warm-up mobility work must be dynamic mobility exercise. Maximum speed training will be developed on a basis of sound technique and relevant strength. In other words, speed training is introduced only when the athlete has been prepared for it. In cool/cold weather athletes should wear tights and warm but non-restrictive clothing. The advice of a physiotherapist should be sought to agree use of embrocations/creams. At the earliest signs of cramp or pain, activity should stop.

SUMMARY

Speed of whole body movement, or of individual joint actions, is a decisive factor of successful performance in many sports. While speed is frequently the product of a coordinated sequence of strength expression of joint actions, the development of speed is not synonymous with the development of strength. In speed-dependent sports, it is important that speed of technical performance is introduced early. However, this must not compromise the basic technical model. Speed is considered under the heading of 'conditioning training' in many programmes, due to the possible combination of speed with strength, endurance and/or mobility. However, it may equally be considered as a sophisticated extension of technical training. Practices for development of speed are specific to the technical demands of a sport. Such demands vary according to the involvement of strength, endurance and mobility, the synchronised use of varied speed of joint action, and the requirement for optimum or maximum speed.

REFLECTIVE QUESTIONS

1. Discuss the contribution of each of the following to sprinting speed.
   a. Technique
   b. Strength
   c. Speed (reaction and leg speed)
   d. Endurance
   e. Mobility
   f. Psychology

2. 'Speed in interactive sport from individual combat to team games is as much about decision making as movement.' Discuss this statement and outline how you will develop both aspects of speed in one of the following:
   a. An epee specialist in fencing
   b. A midfield player in soccer
   c. A doubles player in tennis
   d. A keirin cyclist

3. Because accelerating to maximum speed is an exhausting process, athletes may only have limited opportunity to learn techniques at high speed in a given training unit. Review how this may be resolved to increase repetitions in a training unit in different sports and list your findings. Using the bases on which these solutions have been designed, discuss ideas for such technical training in three sports of your choice.

4. Under pressure in the final 10–20m of a track sprint, an athlete endeavours to increase his stride length by pushing harder on each stride, yet his opponent appears to accelerate past him. Discuss why this is an error on the athlete's part in sprinting, yet may have been the right thing to do in the final 10–20m of an endurance race. What coaching advice would you give the athlete? Sggest practices to help him.

5. Discuss the merits and demerits of reaction/response games as a basis for speed development.

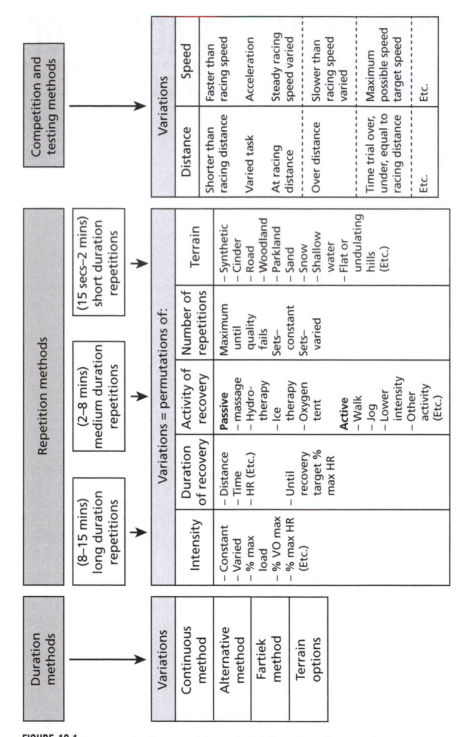

FIGURE 16.1 Summary of endurance training methods (adapted from Harre, 1973)

sand). Like the alternating pace method, anaerobic periods provide a strong stimulus for the improvement of VO_2 max. In addition, the demands of terrain improve strength endurance and proprioceptive balance.

Repetition

These methods offer a wide variety of possible training effects, due to the manipulation of a number of variables:

1. Duration of the training run (in distance or time: classified as short, medium or long).
2. Duration of the recovery period (distance or time).
3. Intensity of the training run (m, seconds, % VO_2 maximum, speed, etc.).
4. Number of repetitions and sets.
5. Activity of recovery (walking, jogging, passive).
6. Terrain for training (uphill, track, sand, surf, etc.).

Training needs to be specific to the type of endurance required for a given sport, but the effect of adjusting one or more of these variables can produce significant improvements in performance. The following are examples of training practices in which a number of variables can be changed.

Interval training

This type of training is extremely effective for rapidly improving aerobic endurance. Using the variables described above, interval training might look like the following:

1. 200m target pace running.
2. 200m active jog recovery.
3. Intensity sufficient to raise HR to approximately 180 beats/minute.
4. Progressive increase in repetitions.
5. Jogging for 90 seconds – returning HR to approximately 120 beats/minute.
6. Track.

This example session is known in sports jargon as slow–fast 200s, and results in a more rapid improvement in aerobic capacity compared to longer duration, continuous training (long steady distance). This type of training is physically demanding and engages all muscle fibre types; recovery between bouts is carefully managed to create a planned level of fatigue. However, it is this fatigue (and the repeated exercise that occurs under fatigue conditions) that provides the stimulus for adaptation both to the cardiovascular system and also at the muscle. Exercise for short periods at or above VO_2 max can evoke greater changes in aerobic capacity compared to those changes that occur with continuous submaximal exercise.

Speed endurance training

This develops the athlete's ability to produce high quality performance despite reduced levels of CrP and acidosis in the muscle. There are an infinite variety of units for this objective and their value may only be truly assessed by studying their place in a training plan. For example, in the month of August, a girl running $4 \times 200m$ in 27 seconds with 30 seconds recovery may have progressed in intensity and density, but regressed in extent from a unit performed in January of $10 \times 200m$ in 30 seconds with 75 seconds recovery. Of all types of track training, the control of these units is the most difficult, and coaches tend to use past experience as the main key for adjustment. Broadly speaking, the following general rules apply:

1. Increase the total extent (number) of repetitions (e.g. 4 × 200m to 12 × 200m).

2. Using a given recovery time, standardise an intensity of run over the training distance (each run aims at a given time, e.g. 12 × 200m in 34 seconds with 75 seconds recovery).

3. Gradually increase intensity (make runs faster, e.g. 12 × 200m in 34 seconds to 30 seconds with 75 seconds recovery).

4. Reduce the total extent (number) of repetitions (e.g. 12 × 200m in 30 seconds with 75 seconds recovery to 2 × 4 × 200m in 27 seconds with 75 seconds recovery and 15 – 20 minutes between sets).

5. Gradually increase density (shorten the recovery, e.g. 2 × 4 × 200m in 27 seconds with 75 seconds to 30 seconds recovery).

This type of work seeks to maintain quality and striding rate, and work sets are often used. If the times for repetitions fall off in the course of the unit, the training is moving towards strength endurance rather than speed endurance. All progression must guarantee the maintenance of quality. It should be noted that within a unit, varying pace may be used in separate sets – hence units such as 'step- downs'. For example:

- 3 × 300m in 48 seconds with 100m jog recovery in 60 seconds (jog 100m in 60 seconds between sets)
- 3 × 300m in 45 seconds with 100m jog recovery in 60 seconds (jog 100m in 60 seconds between sets)
- 3 × 300m in 42 seconds with 100m jog recovery in 60 seconds

Or again, varying distances may be incorporated with varying pace within a unit. For example, the following comprises one set of a three set unit, with 100m jog between sets and repetitions:

- 600m in 108 seconds
- 400m in 68 seconds
- 300m in 48 seconds
- 200m in 30 seconds
- 100m in 14 seconds

These two unit variations are a means of educating the athlete in pace judgement and in the physiological demands of pace change. Speed endurance training, in making complex demands upon the athlete in terms of energy provision, coordination, and strength, creates a stimulus for the complex adaptation required of middle distance athletes. The repeated high intensity nature of interval training engages all the energy systems and all muscle fibre types in those muscle groups being used. In addition, adaptations within the muscle involve increases in both aerobic and glycolytic enzyme activities and also improvements in muscle buffering capacity (i.e., the capacity of the muscle to manage decreases in pH). Changes in the capacity of the cardiovascular system to deliver oxygen to the exercising muscles also result.

Strength endurance training

This is training to develop the athlete's ability to apply force when acidosis in the muscles is resulting in fatigue and weakness. Quality demands are reduced and replaced simply by the task of completing the training unit. Recovery periods are normally very strict and, although the intensity of the run is seldom monitored, the athlete must run as hard as possible. Thus we have units such as:

Circuit training

- $2 \times 4 \times 100m$ 'back to back' (30 seconds recovery)
- $2 \times 5 \times 80m$ 'turnabout' (shuttle running)
- $6 \times 150m$ hill run (jog recovery 90 seconds)
- $5 \times 80m$ sand dune climb (walk down recovery)
- $6 \times 200m$ in surf (passive three minute recovery)
- $4 \times 200m$ skip B (high knee and clawing action; passive three-minute recovery) resisted performance of a given activity in the climate of endurance factors, i.e.
- $6 \times 50m$ swimming and towing a drag, $8 \times 500m$ rowing and towing a drag.

Strength endurance sessions improve the athlete's ability to keep going when lactate is high and, although annual training plans vary, such units may be best inserted between mesocycles 1 and 2, and/or late in mesocycle 2 (see chapter 15). This type of training is extremely demanding and recovery from these sessions needs to be carefully monitored. Athletes need to avoid attempting too many strength endurance sessions within the same microcycle, as inadequate recovery between each will increase the risks of overreaching, compromised function and also injury.

COMPETITION AND TESTING

Competition and testing provide the necessary feedback and stimulus for an athlete to further improve endurance capacity. Goals and tasks to be set may include:

- Time trials at distances equal to, less than, or in excess of the racing distance.
- Specific task runs where the athlete must reach a certain point in a given time, then finish at a maximum intensity (e.g. 600m where the athlete must reach 400m in 60 seconds, then sprint to finish).
- Standard training units where the athlete attempts to perform a given unit prior to being tested.
- Competitions themselves, e.g. indoor, cross-country, etc. It is also possible to give an athlete a specific task within a competition – say in one mile, to reach the bell in 3 minutes 3 seconds – then break four minutes for the final mile time.
- Maintenance of high rate of execution and accuracy of a given technique.

The methods used by athletes to improve their endurance capacity will be influenced by a number of factors. These include:

- the competition demands of the sport;
- the individual athlete's training status;
- the stage of development of the athlete (age, gender, anatomy, physiology, etc.);

- the long and short-term objectives of training;
- the limitations of the training environment;
- the demands of the non-athletic environment;
- the athlete's own personality.

The competition demands of the sport

The duration and intensity of exercise influence the relative contributions of aerobic and anaerobic metabolism in meeting the demands of various events, as shown in table 16.1. While training should be for the most part specific to the particular demands of an event, especially close to competition, it is important that athletes train over a wide range of distances in order to maximise adaptations to all physiological systems that will be involved in the event. A carefully planned periodised training programme will allow for different areas to be developed in a pre-competition phase.

Distance in m	Aerobic	Anaerobic
200	5%	95%
400	17%	83%
800	34%	66%
1500	50%	50%
5000	80%	20%
10,000	90%	10%
Marathon	98%	2%

TABLE 16.1 Aerobic v anaerobic contribution to energy requirement according to distance run.

Short-term endurance: the endurance required for covering efforts of 45 seconds to two minutes duration. Obviously, there is a high involvement of the anaerobic energy systems in such efforts. Speed endurance and strength endurance are critical to short-term endurance.

Medium-term endurance: the endurance required for efforts of two minutes to eight minutes duration. Again, while the anaerobic energy systems are heavily involved, there is also a significant contribution of the aerobic energy system to meeting the exercise demands – a steady state will be maintained for most of the time. Strength endurance and speed endurance determine medium-term endurance efficiency since a relatively high resistance, represented by the amount of force which the athlete must apply, must be expressed at a relatively high frequency over the whole period. Although present world times fall outside this range, steeplechase may be considered as having very high medium-term endurance demands.

Long-term endurance: the endurance required for efforts in excess of eight minutes duration and during which time there is no essential decrease in speed. The aerobic system is largely responsible for maintaining energy production in the muscles. This type of endurance should be considered as virtually synonymous with aerobic endurance/heart endurance.

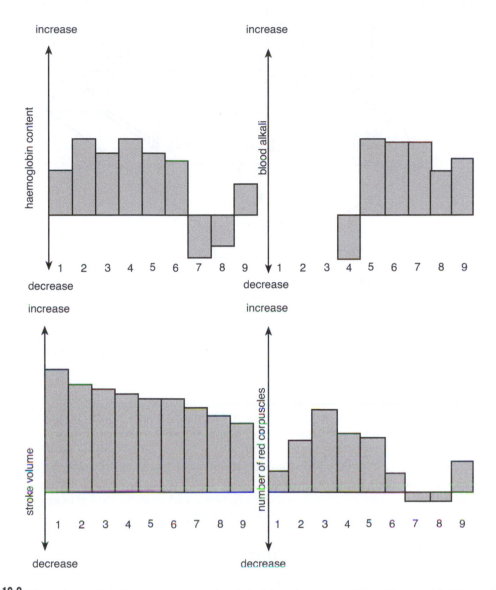

FIGURE 16.2 Effects of certain training programmes on selected physiological parameters (adapted from work by Viru, et al., 1972). (1) Sets of 4–5 runs with 1.5–2 min recovery; 7–10 min between sets. e.g. 3 × 4 × 150m (75%). (2) Complex training involving various sessions. (3) Long steady distance. (4) Fartlek. (5) 2–5 flat out runs – full recovery. (6) Interval sprints (40–50m sprint/jog). (7) Hill runs up 15° gradient. (8) Intensive interval runs 100–200m at 80–90% with 1–3 min recovery until quality drops. (9) Extensive interval runs – such as slow/fast 200m.

Speed endurance: the endurance required to resist fatigue due to loading at sub- maximum and maximum intensity (approx. 85–100% maximum intensity). Exercise is being performed above the anaerobic threshold and this results in acidosis within the muscle; interval training will improve the muscle's capacity to manage the acid load and this will delay the rate of fatigue experienced by the athlete exercising at this intensity.

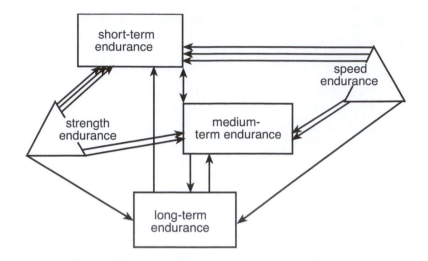

FIGURE 16.3 Inter-relationship of various areas of endurance

Strength endurance: the endurance required to resist fatigue when pH in the muscle is falling; determination to maintain exercise in this fatigued state can be trained also. The schematic relationship of these different endurance capacities is represented in figure 16.3.

Yet another school of thought holds that all endurance events are founded upon an extensive base of aerobic efficiency – so much so that approximately 67 per cent of the training year is devoted to duration methods and their derivatives, and approximately 20 per cent of the training year to the specific demands of a given endurance sport, as well as 13 per cent to competition. Aligning the training programme with the known demands of the event is essential and with significant advances being continually made in understanding how different training methods influence adaptations across a variety of physiological systems, approaches will continue to change. In addition, whatever training practices are adopted, the risks of injury and compromised function need to be minimised in the overall periodised plan.

The individual athlete's training status

Anthropometric measures, concentrations of various blood markers, anaerobic threshold and VO_2 max data can provide useful information to the coach as to the effectiveness of a training programme. These laboratory data will be of most value when considered with personal best performances at commencement of training, how long the athlete can run at a predetermined speed (e.g. 20 seconds/100m), and standard training programme (e.g. the athlete runs 5 × 500m at a speed of 90 seconds/500m with a fixed recovery period). Before and after each repetition, and the total training programme, heart rate and lactate measures are taken.

Clearly, sheer volume of a repeated action, such as running or other activities where there is persistent impact on components of the musculo-skeletal system, has high potential for over-use or stress related injury. Hence introduction of non, or very low, impact alternative workouts either to reduce the risk or to ensure minimal loss of general endurance capacity. Cycling, rowing, cross-country skiing, aqua jogging and swimming are among the more frequently used alternatives, applying adaptations of duration and repetition methods listed in figure 16.1.

The stage of development of the athlete

Pre-pubertal athletes can engage in endurance, sprint and even degrees of resistance training. However, children should avoid early specialisation in particular events; a wide variety of enjoyable activities will allow for a broad development of physical qualities. Avoiding early specialisation will not only reduce pressure on the child but there will also be a reduced risk of over-use injuries.

Long-/short-term objectives of training

The athlete will have some ultimate goal in mind as a supreme raison d'être for training. This may be an Olympic final, a world record, etc. However, he will also have landmarks that must be reached en route. This may be a particular level of performance, a victory at a national championship, etc. Programmes will therefore be constructed to meet the various goals, each leading towards the ultimate goal, rather than ending in themselves.

Limitations of the training environment

The proximity of hills, beaches, plough, surf, ideal stadia, basic stadia, gymnasia, sports halls, etc., must all be taken into account, together with their training value potential. Not every athlete has access to the ideal complex of training facilities so a programme may have to be created imaginatively in a situation that is not ideal.

Demands of the non-athletic environment

The problems of other commitments, e.g. to family, business, education, social scene, cultural pursuits, and so on, must be solved with the assistance of athlete, coach, and a carefully constructed plan.

The athlete's own personality

According to Harre (1973) (see also chapter 10), duration methods encourage development of buoyancy and elasticity of mind. Buoyant behaviour 'includes all those volitional controlling qualities of personality that help to overcome inward and external difficulties and problems, by a consistency in readiness to make an effort of will'. On the other hand, he suggested that interval training develops that form of control, which he refers to as 'impetus of will'. By this he means a fluctuating, varying nature. He goes on to point out that only in consideration of specific demands can buoyancy and impetus of will have a positive or negative value, and that they can be present as integrated behaviour patterns in an athlete.

Working from strength v compensatory work

There are two poles of opinion when attending to the specific needs of an endurance athlete. The first looks to building a programme based on the athlete's strength, and by so doing gradually make ground on his weakness. The other looks to focusing on the weakness, and building a compensatory programme. This method is founded on the belief that the athlete's strengths need little work to maintain a high level, and the weaknesses can therefore be afforded more time – and brought up to the same level as the strengths. To give an example, if an athlete can run 200m in 23.00 sec, and 800m in two minutes, it is clear that endurance should be worked on. The 'working from strength' coach will build his programme around repetition work over 100m, 200m, and 300m, gradually introducing longer repetitions and long runs. The 'compensatory'

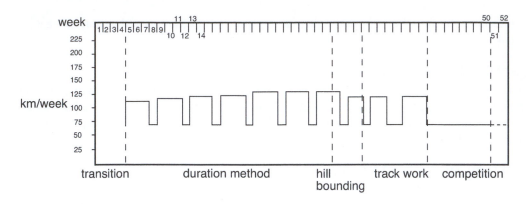

FIGURE 16.4 Interpretation of Lydiard method of planning endurance training (from Sinkkonen, 1975)

coach will look to longer endurance work and longer repetitions from the outset. Working from strength fits better into Harre's idea of building programmes according to the athlete's personality. Moreover, at a most fundamental level, it ensures that the athlete enjoys a positive motivational profile through a period of hard work.

Examples of endurance training plans

But what of the plan itself? It would appear that whatever it might be, it must fall into one of two categories: the Lydiard method or the complex method. The former has now appeared in many forms and varieties, for example that used by Kari Sinkkonen with the Finnish distance athletes in 1975 (figure 16.4), or any of the African systems. The latter has new varieties every day!

Every athlete and coach evolves a different interpretation of the complex method, but for the sake of illustration, figure 16.5 includes a variation on the model (referred to as 'the Oregon method') used by Bill Bowerman of the University of Oregon.

Altitude training in practice

Living and training at altitudes of between 1500m and 3000m for 2–3 weeks at a time is an approach taken by competitive endurance athletes to potentially improve their sea-level performance. Hypoxia at moderate altitude elicits an increase in the production of erythropoietin (EPO), a hormone which is responsible for regulating the production of red blood cells. Even if there is a small increase in the number of red blood cells, this will improve the oxygen carrying capacity of the blood, raise VO_2 max and improve endurance performance. Research has consistently found that there is considerable variation in how individuals respond to hypoxia; some have a strong EPO response while others show very little change. Perhaps the most significant issue with altitude training is that the intensity at which individuals can exercise in hypoxic environments is reduced and this will lead to a lower training stimulus. To overcome this, exercise scientists have developed altitude tents and 'houses' in which a hypoxic environment is created at sea level. Athletes essentially sleep and relax in these tents or houses (to potentially gain increases in EPO and red blood cell mass) but train normally at sea-level – so as to maintain an adequate exercise stimulus. This particular approach is known as 'living high, training low' or HiLo.

If athletes do ascend to moderate altitude for an extended period of training, the following may be helpful.

Pace for the month   62 sec / 400 m   Next month 61 sec / 400 m

	Week 1	Week 2	Week 3	Week 4
Sunday	20 miles continuous			
Monday	8 x 400m: 62: jog 400 m	10 x 400 m: 62: jog 200 m	8 x 400 m: 62: jog 100 m	10 x 400 m: 62: jog 100 m
Tuesday	10 miles alternating 800 m jog between sets	as before	as before	as before
Wednesday	2 x 5 x 300 m: 46.5: jog 300 m	3 x 4 x 300 m: 46.5: jog 200 m	4 x 3 x 300 m: 46.5: jog 100 m	5 x 3 x 300 m: 46.5: jog 100 m
Thursday	Fartlek – 60 mins			
Friday	10 miles continuous			
Saturday	Competition-training / cross country / time trials / indoors / etc.			

FIGURE 16.5 Interpretation of complex method of planning endurance training.

1. Altitude exacerbates infections and dental problems, so a complete health check is required before athletes can participate in an altitude camp.

2. Athletes should have a trial period at altitude outside the competition season before using it as final preparation for a major championship. This affords the opportunity to learn what suits a given athlete.

3. The ideal period for altitude training is 2–3 weeks.

4. Athletes should first be tested at sea level to establish different speeds for endurance training at altitude. Once this information is recorded (in metres/sec), subtract 0.20–0.30 metres/sec and these are the speeds for use at altitude. For example: 4.70 metres/sec – sea level = 4.40–4.50 metres/sec – altitude.

5. In the first three days at altitude, athletes should keep things at the intermittent walk/jog level to allow gentle adaptation. This is essential for first time trainers at altitude, but even established altitude trainers should have two days like this. The pattern should be:
   Days 1–3/4   acclimatisation, e.g. instead of 2 × 60m runs – 4 × 30m runs.
   Days 3/4–18   hard training – normal programme but gentler progression; longer recoveries, etc. (bearing in mind note 5).
   Days 19–21   assimilation and recovery – lower intensity and extent.

6. Athletes dehydrate more readily at altitude so extra fluids must be available for consumption. Athletes also require higher intakes of carbohydrate because glycogen use at altitude is greater than it is at sea level.

7. After the end of altitude training athletes may feel unwell and, although tired, will have difficulty sleeping. For these first 2–3 days back at sea level, training loads should be lower. After this period the athlete will feel much better and performance capacity increases.

8. Athletes may experience quite significant improvements in performance around 3–4 days after returning to sea level but then performance is likely to deteriorate for a week or so. However, there will be a return to improved performances from the 10th, 11th, or 12th day which can continue for about four weeks.

Around 85–90 per cent of all experienced altitude trainers produce their best results after 3–4 days and after 18–24 days.

9. Ultraviolet radiation is more intense at altitude. Suncreams/blocks and sunglasses should be worn.

10. Warm clothing should be taken for evenings and for immediate post-training.

11. An extra 1–2 hours sleep should feature in the training period at altitude.

12. The most used altitude facilities are listed below in table 16.2.

	Venue	Country	Altitude (m)
1	Belmeken	Bulgaria	2000
2	Tsahkadzor	Armenia	1970
3	Font Romeau	France	1895
4	St. Moritz	Switzerland	1820
5	Sestriere	Italy	2035
6	Piatra Arsa	Romania	1950
7	Issyk Kul	Kyrgyzstan	1600
8	Zetersfeld (Lienz)	Austria	1950
9	Addis Ababa	Ethiopia	2400
10	Nairobi	Kenya	1840
11	Ifrane	Morocco	1820
12	Kunming	China	1895
13	Mexico City	Mexico	2200
14	Toluca	Mexico	2700
15	Colorado Springs	USA	2194
16	Keystone	USA	2835
17	Flagstaff	USA	2300
18	Bogota	Colombia	2500
19	Boulder	USA	2000
20	La Paz	Bolivia	3100
21	Quito	Ecuador	2218
22	Davos	Switzerland	1560
23	Pontresina	Switzerland	1900
24	Crans-Montana	Switzerland	1500
25	Kaprun	Austria	1800
26	Silvretta	Austria	1800
27	Medeo	Kazakhstan	1691
28	Kesenoyam	Russia	2000
29	Pzhevalsk	Kyrgyzstan	1800
30	Tamga	Kyrgyzstan	1700

TABLE 16.2 Altitude training venues

SUMMARY

The preparation of endurance training plans and their progressive units (from the wide range of training practices) is a most interesting and rewarding exercise for the coach. Our well-documented knowledge of related physiology offers an excellent framework within which to apply training units consistent with the laws of specificity, overload and reversibility. Thus, with insight, the coach may accurately evaluate the endurance demands of sports (ranging from the marathon to ice hockey) and create a training programme geared to adapting the athlete's physiology to meet these demands.

The female athlete must have aerobic training emphasised in her training plan. Nevertheless, the coach should be aware that it is not sufficient to compensate for weaknesses and that he should build upon strengths when planning training.

REFLECTIVE QUESTIONS

1. Your athlete insists that a simple mode of cross-training exercise improves aerobic fitness for all physical activities requiring a high level of aerobic fitness. Give your opinion regarding the effectiveness of single mode cross-training exercise.

2. For their assault on Mount Everest, elite mountaineers take three months to establish base camp at 4216m, 4953m, 5410m, 6086m and 6604m before their final ascent. Explain the physiological rationale for a stage ascent approach to mountaineering.

3. In the 1970s, female 800m and 1500m athletes in former Czechoslovakia were not performing well at international level. Their times over distances up to 400m were good so it was decided that endurance work such as cross country and long steady runs should have programming priority. This produced negligible improvements. So instead, the athletes' programmes were changed to be based on interval and repetition workouts using 100m, 200m, 300m and 400m. The improvement was dramatic. Why? Discuss possible explanations for the difference.

4. For major competitions in hot Mediterranean summer venues, Kenyans and other high performance African athletes have frequently finished their preparation prior to travelling to the competition venue in Scandinavia. Discuss possible explanations for this.

5. Your national level female triathlete has a stress fracture of the lower fibula. In order to maintain endurance fitness, identify those activities that the athlete may pursue without irritating the injury and design a training programme for eight weeks for two of these activities (not including swimming or cycling!). You should clearly indicate the specific training effect you intend (e.g. aerobic capacity; lactic anaerobic capacity) and particular physiological measures (e.g. increase in RBC count; improved OBLA score) and how such would be assessed. Finally, also discuss which, if any, would have most relevant technical advantage for the athlete.

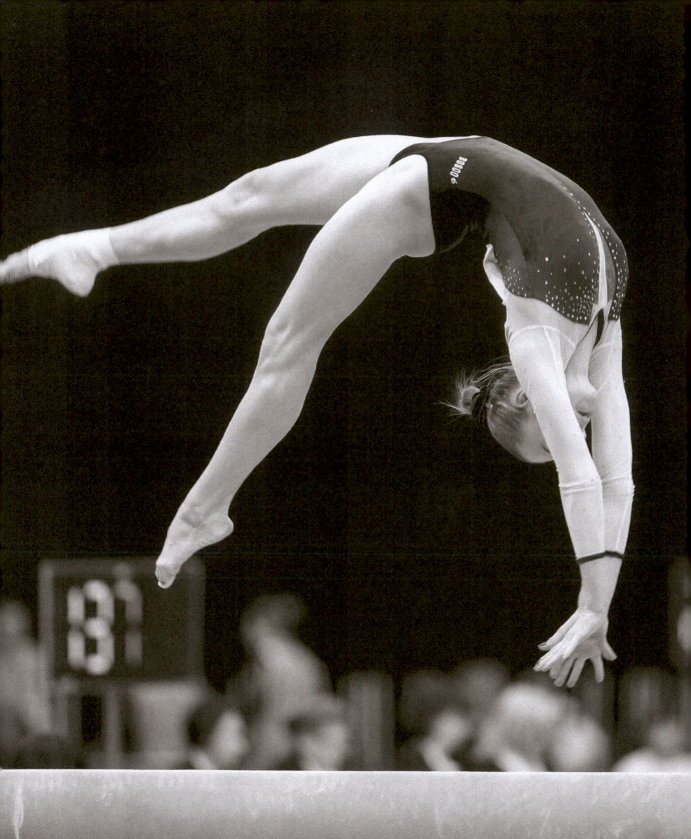

17 THEORY AND PRACTICE OF MOBILITY DEVELOPMENT

MOBILITY CLASSIFICATION

Mobility is the capacity to perform joint actions through a wide range of movement. In sport, it should be considered in the light of an optimum application of strength throughout a range of movement appropriate to the demands of a given technique. Mobility is measured in degrees, radians or centimetres. Passive values are greater than active values and the reduction of the active-passive difference is often used as a criterion of achievement. There are three distinct varieties of mobility: active, passive and kinetic.

Active mobility: the capacity to effect movement by contraction of those muscles which naturally cause the movement. In figure 17.1, the athlete is flexing the femur on the pelvis by contraction of the hip flexors. In this instance, the neuromuscular pattern provides stimulation of the hip flexors (protagonists) to contract, and inhibition of the hip extensors (antagonists). The relaxed hip extensors are consequently 'stretched'. This represents the classical reciprocal inhibition.

Passive mobility: that movement which is effected by expression of external force on the joint action (e.g. apparatus, the weight of the body, a partner). In figure 17.2, the femur is being flexed on the pelvis by the combined effects of bodyweight and resistance of the wall bars. In this instance, the neuromuscular pattern stimulates neither the hip flexors nor hip extensors to contract. There is a variant of passive mobility which merits special mention here. This involves inhibition of reflex contraction in the antagonist muscles. This is referred to more in terms of training method than a sub-classification of mobility, as 'proprioceptive neuro-muscular facilitation' (PNF method).

Kinetic mobility: that movement which is effected due to momentum of one or other or both of the levers involved. In figure 17.3, the femur has been flexed on the pelvis by the momentum of its swing. In this instance, the neuromuscular pattern provides stimulation of the hip flexors (protagonists) to contract forcefully, and inhibition of the hip extensors (antagonists). However, as the movement reaches the limit of extensibility of the hip extensors, the muscle spindle reflex mechanism may initiate a reflex contraction of the 'overstretched' hip extensors. Consequently, this type of mobility presents the possibility of muscle damage, not only when it is applied as a means of developing mobility in general, but also when it is applied as an essential feature of technique. Kinetic mobility is also known as 'ballistic mobility' and 'bouncing mobility' and has also been covered by the umbrella title of 'dynamic mobility' (discussed below).

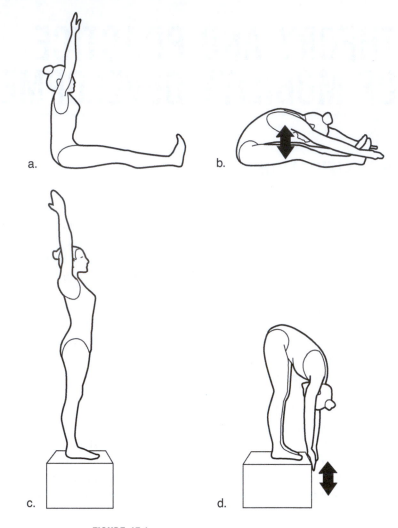

FIGURE 17.1 Examples of active mobility exercise

Factors influencing mobility

1. The elasticity of muscle and tendon of those muscles being stretched (but note that increased strength of a muscle does not reduce its extension capacity).

2. The elasticity of ligaments supporting the joint involved. This presents one of many coaching dilemmas. The ligaments provide joint stability but the characteristic to be developed is joint mobility. Ligaments do not display any apparent elasticity but, given extensive exposure to stretch, may be extended to a new length. This, while providing increased mobility, reduces the stability of the joint. Consequently, great care must be taken to ensure that those muscles which cross the joint are strong enough to provide some compensatory stability to protect it from injury.

3. The structural barriers of any muscle hypertrophy, or any skin and tissue folds which prevent freedom of joint range (e.g. 'spare tyres' – in hip flexion).

4. Structural barriers of joint construction and bone.

5. The strength of the protagonist in active and kinetic mobility.

6. The capacity of the neuromuscular system to inhibit the antagonists (those muscles being stretched).

7. The degree of technical mastery of the movement concerned, especially if the movement is one of several which comprise a sports technique.

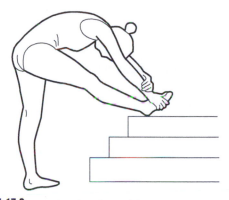

FIGURE 17.2 Examples of passive mobility exercise

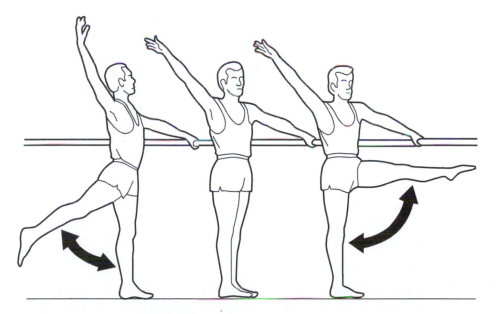

FIGURE 17.3 Examples of kinetic mobility exercise

8. The athlete's internal and external environment (table 17.1).

Conditions	Time	Result in mm
After night's sleep	8.00	−15
" " "	12.00	+35
10 min with body exposed at 10°C	12.00	−36
10 min in warm bath at 40°C	12.00	+78
After 20 min loosening up	12.00	+89
After tiring training	12.00	−35

TABLE 17.1 Alterations in mobility under different conditions from Osolin (1952).

9. The effect of recent injury in the muscles or joints concerned, or of fibrous adhesion of an old injury which has caused the athlete to be restricted in a given movement for a considerable period.

10. The restrictions of inappropriate clothing.

11. The athlete's age and stage of development. After the age of approximately eight years, mobility will gradually reduce. Mobility training is therefore essential to the athlete.

12. Structural adaptation to occupational postures (e.g. stooping over a machine, studying in a cramped position) or muscle habits may reduce free movement in certain joints.

Role of mobility

Mobility is fundamental to the efficient performance of any action, both in nature and degree. Poor mobility development will present the athlete with several problems.

1. The learning of sports techniques is difficult and in some cases impossible. This prevents the athlete from successful participation in certain sports. Moreover, the coach may believe an athlete's inability to perform a given technique is due to poor motor learning, lack of strength, etc., when in fact the problem may be quite simply that the athlete has insufficient mobility to assume a requested position.

2. There exists the very real problem of injury due to muscle, tendon or ligament strain. For instance, when the athlete attempts to exceed his mobility range, there can be strain of other muscles and tendons which are employed to compensate for poor mobility in a given range, or strain of ligaments which become excessively loaded when a restricted range of movement demands extraneous compensatory and balance adjustments.

3. The development of other characteristics (e.g. strength and speed), or their effective application in technique, may be retarded. Ultimately, in terms of results and execution, this will lead to poor technical performance.

4. The range of movement through which force may be applied (e.g. throws, golf swing, tennis strokes, stride length, etc.) is reduced and consequently the total performance is impaired.

5. If the quality of a given movement is reduced due to lack of mobility, that movement cannot contribute fully as a component of more complex or similar movements. Thus the total movement potential of the athlete is reduced.

6. A lack of mobility in any joint action imposes an extra workload and tension on those muscles compensating for this deficiency. The result is more rapid tiring and a reduction of performance capacity.

7. Before performing in speed, elastic/fast/strength training or competition, kinetic mobility should predominate in warm-up. This supports the energy resource and neuromuscular dynamics of the activity to follow. Sustained slow stretching, whether as active or passive mobility, inhibits both resource and dynamics.

The net result of all of the above is that a lack of appropriate mobility reduces the athlete's 'sphere of influence' in game situations, and his adaptability and technical efficiency of sports performance. Moreover, it increases the athlete's risk of sudden injury and unnecessary cumulative strain of muscle, tendon and ligament. A lack of mobility, then, has far reaching effects. The athlete must develop and maintain a level of general mobility to gain maximum advantage from training, freedom from the risk of injury and attainment of a certain level of specific mobility, in order to meet the demands of technique.

MOBILITY TRAINING

Training to develop mobility must also obey the laws of specificity, overload and reversibility.

Specificity: training must focus on a particular joint action and the active, passive or kinetic nature of the mobility required in that joint action. 'Specific' here refers to athlete, joint action and technical demand.

Overload: the range of movement will not be maintained unless the existing limit is reached regularly, nor will it be improved unless that limit is exceeded. For instance:

- Active mobility exercise is acceptable for maintaining a range of movement, provided strength of the protagonists is not lost. It has only limited value for developing mobility and implies increased strength of the protagonists and work in the end position, i.e. at the existing limit of the range of movement.
- Passive mobility exercise, given appropriate external force, will maintain or increase the range of movement.
- Kinetic mobility exercise makes its greatest contribution by relating mobility which is achieved through active or passive exercise, to the dynamics of a sports technique. However, as a carefully supervised type of exercise, it may also improve mobility.

Reversibility: mobility status is lost more slowly on cessation of regular specific training than other characteristics. Nevertheless, it is gradually lost so the athlete should include mobility training either as an introduction to a unit, or as a unit in its own right.

Mobility unit construction

There are virtually thousands of mobility exercises to choose from but, for the guidance of coaches, a summary of points relative to mobility unit construction is included here. Obviously, the coach must understand the specific joint actions to be mastered by the athlete and, as always before selecting training units, the laws of specificity, overload, and reversibility must be obeyed. The following order of events should also be observed.

1. Raise body temperature by jogging, striding, and gentle warm-up activity in natural fibre sweat suit (if air temperature is 22°C or higher) or in a natural fibre sweat suit plus wet suit (if the temperature is 21°C or lower). The purpose of this warm-up is to settle the body temperature at 37.5–38.5°C.

2. Active and slow, sustained exercises for each joint action.

3. Passive exercises with partner, apparatus, bodyweight, etc.

4. Kinetic exercises and combined elastic strength/mobility exercises (experienced athletes only).

5. Specific exercises related to the whole technique(s), and whole techniques up to competition or training performance speed.

When the activity to follow is not speed or elastic strength dependent, the priority of each item is approximately: (1) 25%, (2) 20%, (3) 20%, (4) 10%, (5) 25%.

If the following activity is speed or elastic strength dependent, the priority is: (1) 25%, (2) 10%, (3) 15%, (4) 25%, (5) 25%.

Mobility work should always precede other training and never be practised in a state of fatigue (following strength or endurance training, etc.) unless gentle active mobility is used. Like all training, mobility must be carefully supervised while the athlete learns training discipline (e.g. no experimentation, no interference with other athletes, no lazy 'compromised' movements, etc.).

Especially with the young athlete, all joint actions must be afforded mobility training as the basis upon which specific mobility training will develop. With the advanced athlete, general mobility training holds high priority in mesocycle 1 of the annual cycle and should be included (possibly in warm-up for other training units) throughout the year. Highly specific mobility is for advanced athletes only.

However, all levels of athlete require a complementary development of strength, but in separate training units. The advanced athlete may combine mobility and strength work in kinetic mobility exercises, but this work should be supervised and never taken to the point of fatigue.

Sets of exercises should comprise 10–15 repetitions, since only after several repetitions is there any visible increase in range of movement. The recovery period between sets must not be long enough to permit temperature reduction. It may also be active (walking, jogging, general stretching) or passive (relaxing in warmth). When active or passive mobility exercise is used in training units, the end position of stretch should be maintained for 6–10 sec in each repetition. Several authorities recommend daily or twice-daily units of mobility training. Personal experience suggests that general and/or specific mobility work as part of warm-up for daily training units, supplemented by separate units within the microcycle where mobility is trained exclusively, is sufficient for athletes in the majority of sports. Exceptions are sports such as gymnastics, where daily mobility units are essential.

PNF method would be used at stage four in the training unit. It must be used with care, and partners should be mature, responsible persons, trained in the application of the method. The athlete's partner slowly forces the relevant limb to the existing comfort limit of a range of movement. When the athlete feels discomfort, the movement stops and the partner then offers a resistance so that the athlete can perform an isometric contraction against the original direction of movement. This is held for 6–10 seconds. Athlete and partner rest for 30 seconds then repeat the exercise 3–6 times. An extension of this method, referred to as 3 PIC, requires the athlete to contract the protagonist muscles for 3–6 seconds immediately following the isometric contraction. The partner then recommences the cycle of forced stretch, isometric contraction against the direction of stretch, and active contraction with the direction of stretch. The cycle is repeated 3–4 times before resting for 30 seconds and going through the exercise again. The total number of repetitions of the exercise is 3–6.

Mobility derivatives

Fleishman (1964) distinguishes between 'extent flexibility', which is defined here as mobility, and 'dynamic flexibility', which is an ability to perform repeated contraction and stretching of muscle. This derivative of mobility appears to embrace innervation, as previously discussed and kinetic mobility. Thus, dynamic flexibility may be more accurately thought of as a specific 'functional' or 'applied' mobility. This moves close to the areas of 'agility' and 'quickness' which links technique, speed and mobility. These complex characteristics are derivatives of the basic fitness characteristics. Listing and explaining all of them is impossible due to lack of standard definitions.

SUMMARY

Basic to a development of the technical model, or models demanded of a sport, is a wide range of movement in all joint actions. A limited range of joint action compromises movement potential for the interpretation of technique, and the range through which force is applied is a critical factor in determining the nature and degree of force expression. The structure of joints, elasticity of soft tissues, and neuromuscular coordination are significant. The most important factors determining active, passive or kinetic mobility are specific exercise, joint structure, elasticity of soft tissue surrounding joints, neuromuscular coordination and temperature.

REFLECTIVE QUESTIONS

1. To add variety to your training programme without losing tight focus on exercise specifics, create three mobility programmes which cover all main joint actions. So the first exercise in each programme will provide stretch through the same joint action; the second in each programme through the next joint action; etc. To simplify things, start with the neck and work down the body to ankles/feet. Limit yourself to 20–24 exercises, so 60–72 in total.

2. Discuss the advantages and disadvantages of combining mobility work with relaxation techniques such as autogenic training or hatha yoga.

3. Traditionalists would argue that 'sustained slow stretching' should always feature strongly in all warm-ups to protect against the potential injury risk of dynamic kinetic exercise. Design a warm-up routine for female sprint hurdlers which would protect without losing the value of dynamic kinetic content.

4. Present arguments for and against the statement: 'Lack of mobility is the prelude to loss of strength, as there is disinclination to exercise throughout the desired range of movement, which may eventually lead to disinclination to exercise that joint action.'

5. In sports such as gymnastics, extensive mobility work is done with young children up to the age of eight years. Clearly this creates greater movement potential in pursuit of technical excellence. Discuss the merits and demerits of such early age development focus.

18 EVALUATION IN SPORT

'Possibly the only sustainable competitive advantage we have is the ability to learn faster than the opposition.'

Arie de Geus

Being prepared to persistently learn faster is on the one hand a matter of attitude and conscious decision; and on the other, of having in place a process to do so. That process is an evaluation programme which variously affords opportunity to preview, review, monitor, control, align, re-align and debrief. It belongs to a responsible strategy in pursuit of agreed objectives.

There are several variations to designing such a strategy. The acronym OPERA summarises a sound basic five step approach for coaches:

Objective: Measurable agreed intended outcome goals; or performance/progress goals; or process/technique/quality goals.

Plan: Detailed plan to bridge the gap in status between the desired outcome and where they are now.

Execution: Deliver the plan.

Review: Measure and monitor as frequently as is consistent with keeping the process on track.

Adjustment: Make necessary changes to re-align with the objective.

It is the evaluation programme which ensures a constructive dynamic in the strategy.

EVALUATION PURPOSES

Mass longitudinal screening techniques, sometimes referred to as performance bioprofiles, assess the athlete's status in all appropriate quantifiable parameters and environmental factors relevant to development stage and performance in a sport. Such information, married to the athlete's training programme and competition performance over several years, will benefit the athlete and future generations of athletes when there is constructive communication and exchange of information between coaches and performance science research professionals. The six steps in this are:

1. Selection of characteristics/capacities to be measured.
2. Collection of all relevant data.

3. Measurement and analysis.
4. Translation to action options.
5. Selection of the best option.
6. Delivery of the option in practice.

Advances in information technology have dramatically enhanced intelligence through each step. So what are the purposes of evaluation in practice?

1. **To assess the athlete's aptitude/talent for a given sport:** This purpose is often referred to as 'talent spotting'. For the most part it remains a combination of subjective opinion by those experienced in identifying talent such as 'scouts' in professional sport; and a growing volume of objective performance-related science. Indices of aptitude/talent may be derived from collective evaluation of the following:

   - The status of the athlete's performance of the given technique/sport, with respect to existing norms according to age, gender, etc.
   - The athlete's status in those capacities characteristic of the given sport (physiological, physical, anthropometric, etc.).
   - The speed at which the athlete improves performance during the period of instruction.
   - The early ability to reproduce consistently good performance (stability).

   Clearly, the most important condition for diagnosing aptitude/talent is regular participation in the sport concerned.

2. **To plan the athlete's developmental programme:** only by exposing the athlete to a comprehensive battery of tests and comparing the athlete's status with norms according to chronological age, developmental age, gender, etc. and training against intended outcomes can the coach begin to plan an athlete's development programme. This, of course, will also be seen in the context of environmental factors such as:

   - support, e.g. physiotherapy, performance science, financial
   - occupation, e.g. student, mother, labourer
   - social, e.g. family, institution, religion
   - training, e.g. facilities, equipment, venues
   - nutrition, e.g. calorie intake, balance, nutritional supplements
   - lifestyle, e.g. sleep quality, recreation, lifestyle management.

3. **To assess the effect of training systems on performance:** here, the athlete's status in those parameters which are to be developed by the training system, from general competency platform to specific performance structure, is compared with performance norms in the sport. The results are also compared with previous results in the same testing situation. The contribution to the performance of the athlete's status in each parameter measured is thereby assessed. In addition to assessing the system, coaches must also apply reflective learning to assess their professional effectiveness in contributing to the outcome of the training/system evaluation.

4. **To assess the efficacy of training systems in developing specific parameters:** as the athlete works to develop strength, speed, etc., via various specific training units, the athlete's status in these parameters must be constantly monitored. Evaluation of results will allow any necessary adjustment of loading within each training unit.

5. **To establish homogeneous groupings for training:** it is reasonable to group athletes according to physical capacities such as speed, strength, endurance, or by technical ability or general/specific competency battery profile etc. Evaluation will enable the coach to form those groups to the best advantage of their members.

6. **To assess knowledge of a given sport, sports' values and sport's role in society:** the athlete must not only understand techniques, tactics, training principles and rules, but also the high values that shape behaviours in sport and why sport is a valuable part of life in the local and global community. Although it is not commonplace to test the athlete's command of this knowledge, it is important and may be seen as part of the training process.

7. **To establish the characteristics demanded of a given sport:** a detailed study of biomechanics, physiology, psychology, etc., provides some insight into the demands of a given sport. However, by evaluating the status of successful athletes in physical, physiological, and other parameters, a more substantial link between athlete and sport can be established. Because there can be a very clear overlap between some sports, exercising this purpose of evaluation may find athletes comfortably and successfully switching sports (e.g. rowing to cycling; track sprinting to pushers in bobsleigh).

8. **To enrich the motivational climate** throughout the athlete development pathway.

Performance parameters in evaluation programmes

Possible parameters which may be tested or assessed in evaluation programmes are clearly specific to athlete and sport. They must also be appropriate to the training systems used. They include:

General

- Endurance – aerobic and anaerobic
- General movement – motor coordination, agility, balance
- Anthropometrics and body composition
- General fitness battery
- Mobility
- Strength – general, maximum, elastic, endurance, core, power
- Speed and reaction time
- Psychology
- Nutrition and hydration

Sport specific

- Endurance
- Strength
- Mobility
- Technique(s)
- Aptitude/talent
- Tactical
- Psychology

Tests are not ends in themselves, but a means of evaluating an athlete's status. In short, testing procedures assist the coach in understanding the athlete's training status and development, and in making training programmes more efficient.

Phase	Descriptor	Application	Current technology examples
WHAT DOES IT TAKE TO WIN?			
One	**Competition analysis**. A description of the winning characteristics behind successful performances	Typically includes split times in racing sports; event frequencies in team sports; deterministic models in high technology sports using 1st principles physics relationships.	GPS measurement systems, e.g. GP Sports, Catapult, Statsports.Software based analysis tools, e.g. SportsCode, Quintic, Dartfish
Two	**Technique analysis**. Measurement and assessment of the underlying mechanics that can explain the competition analysis.	Typically includes race analysis that explains the outcome times such as step length, step frequency, contact times and forces in racing sports. Also includes more detailed mechanics to describe joint motions and forces underpinning skill execution.	Optojump for running analysis. Kistlet Force plates. Coach's eye. Markerless kinematics such as Organic Motion.SRM cranks for cycling. Hawkeye projectile tracking.
Three	**Physical and physiological analysis**. Measurement and assessment of the underlying physiology that supports the mechanics of competition analysis and race analysis.	Typically includes an assessment of maximal physiological capacities and their efficiency under various exercise stresses.	VO_2 max and other max capability assessments. Speed-HR-lactate assessments through step test assessments from sub max to max stress.
WHAT IS YOUR JOURNEY TO SUCCESS?			
Four	**Training analysis.** A description of the actual versus planned training that explains the process leading to competition performance.	Typically includes measurement of the periodisation process, volumes, intensities, types and the cumulative load being applied as a measure of stress.	Excel spreadsheets. Custom training software, e.g. Strava, Mapmyrun / ride, Sportlyzer, Restwise.
Five	**Acute training monitoring**. A series of descriptive responses from each training session that can be used to monitor acute responses to a training session.	Typically includes heart rate assessments, lactate assessments, core temperature, session RPES etc. to understand responses to individual training sessions.	Polar heart rate monitors. Lactate pro monitors. Power measurements from SRM cranks. Vitalsense vital signs monitors.

TABLE 18.1 A performance framework for applying technology to athlete and coach development. The steps and processes used to describe, understand and breakdown performances and the role technology has in the process to deliver an efficient and effective decision making process in field-based environments.

Phase	Descriptor	Application	Current technology examples
Six	**Chronic training monitoring**. A series of biomarkers from blood, saliva, urine that are used to monitor cumulative changes pre and post training blocks or around consistent training stresses on a weekly basis to monitor stress-adaptation.	Typically includes various biomarkers from endocrine, immune and metabolic systems	Salivary cortisol, IgA and free testosterone using near real time multiplex biochemistry methods, e.g. Randox.

WHAT ARE THE RISKS TO THE JOURNEY?

Phase	Descriptor	Application	Current technology examples
Seven	**Injury and illness surveillance.** A descriptive process that collates critical risk factors at the time of an acute injury using international consensus methods.	Typically includes collection of data such as injury type, location, severity, functional events at time of injury.	Can range from excel based recording systems to software based recording systems e.g. Smartabase, Edge 10, Kinetic Athlete, KItman labs.
Eight	**Functional risk assessments.** A series of assessments to describe the 'health' and condition of muscle, joints and soft tissue during static and dynamic sports specific movements.	Typically includes an assessment of joint motion, joint forces at different joint speeds, body symmetries, functional movement control etc.	Includes such methods as isokinetic dynamometers, goniometers, force plates, kinematic assessments, gait analysis etc.

HOW DO WE LEARN FROM THE PROCESS AND INFLUENCE CHANGE?

Phase	Descriptor	Application	Current technology examples
Nine	**Data storage and analytics** The use of software tools to ensure effective storage of various data streams over time relative to individual athletes to analyse and understand long-term trends for future performance planning.	Typically includes web based storage and app developments that provide various levels of security, data entry formats and visual display methods of historical data trends.	Various data management tools including excel, Smartabase, Edge 10, Apollo, Kitman labs, Kinetic Athlete.
Ten	**Feedback and learning.** The use of visualisation methods and tools, e.g. smartphones, tablets to help others interpret and understand data from various acute and chronic assessments.	Typically includes simple ways of transmitting data in real time to inform decision making in a field based practical way; or post event methods to display data in a format that enables rapid learning and interpretation.	Various real time data feedback tools, e.g. smartwatches, Google glass and data visualisation software tools such as Chartio, Info.gr

Notes on tests and testing

All coaches equip themselves early with tests to address one or several of these purposes. Some coaches design their own; some rely on those supplied by more experienced coaches. Some move quickly into the relatively new world of information technology. That world is explored later in this chapter.

Whichever testing technique is used, the coach must build their testing resource and conduct testing sessions with care. Every testing procedure must be:

- Valid – testing what it purports to test.
- Reliable – consistency of reproduction.
- Objective – consistency of delivery, whoever conducted the test.

The following points may help to achieve this:

1. A test should measure only one capacity/ability/factor.

2. Unless technique is being assessed, the tests should not require technical competence on the part of the athlete.

3. There is little purpose in duplicating tests within the same unit (i.e. testing the same parameter with different tests) unless the purpose of the session is to validate new methods of testing.

4. Each athlete in the test situation must understand exactly what is required, what is to be measured, and why. At conclusion, the results should be interpreted for the athlete.

5. The method of conducting the test (e.g. administration, organisation, environmental requirements) should be standardised. (A set of simple instructions will help to standardise procedure on subsequent sessions. For example, in strength tests, starting and finishing joint angles must be specified and adhered to.) The standardisation of procedure should be as strict as possible (e.g. constant venue, temperature, time of day, day of menstrual cycle for girls, degree of motivation, tester, previous nutrition, time allowed for warm-up, nature of the equipment, etc.).

6. The venue, score cards, equipment, etc., should be prepared in advance.

7. The coach will find knowledge of statistics, mathematics, and presentation of data (e.g. graphs) very useful.

8. The complete evaluation process involves physiologists, physiotherapists, general practitioners, psychologists, the coach and, in some cases, parents, other coaches and athletes. The sum evaluation by this 'team' should be documented and filed, but a record of tests conducted by the coach may also be kept in the athlete's training diary.

9. The coach should establish a sense of regular routine of review, through reflective learning and appropriate testing from training unit level to competition; to training cycles to year plan and they must keep meticulous records.

10. Advances in information technology are now so significant and substantial, that it is essential for coaches to understand where we are in the incredible advantage it affords their work in athlete development. It is entirely appropriate, then, that we examine that world in more detail here. Stoll and Schubert's quotation perfectly introduces the subject:

'Data is not information, information is not knowledge, knowledge is not understanding, understanding is not wisdom.'

Moore's law predicated that computer processing power would double every two years but no one could have predicted the impact on coaching. We are in an era of big data, but it brings with it the problem that, sometimes there is too much information for a coach to handle.

The growth and development of science, medicine and technology in performance sport through the increasing commercial and government investment across all sporting domains aligned to the miniaturisation of electronics; increase in processing power; increased sophistication in end user devices, e.g. tablets, smart phones; and the availability of rapid, real time data and information through wireless networks and web based technology has fundamentally changed the performance environment within which coaches now operate. However, the fundamental principles of the coaching and athlete development process remain the same.

For the remainder of this chapter, we review the development of performance technology in modern day sport and provide some current working examples across different sports. As most technology developments are out of date as soon as purchased we will provide a framework that will ensure your ability to maximise this ever-changing space is relevant regardless of available resources.

This framework outlined in table 18.1 provides the various technical steps needed to break down a performance and how technology can support that process depending on the sport and event. To improve your capability of choosing the right tools and technology it is important to construct the performance journey by starting at the final competition and planning backwards. Performance technology provides the means by which you can describe the athlete and coach journey through this plan and improve your probability of making the right decision at the right time.

What we propose here is a short concise overview that maps to this framework based on the following steps:

- Step 1. Strategy and performance planning – a structure to maximise the use of science, medicine and performance technology.
- Step 2. Competition analysis. What will it take to win?
- Step 3. Gap analysis. Where is each athlete-coach relative to the future requirements of winning?
- Step 4. Training analysis. What are we doing in training to develop towards the winning profile?

Whereas the OPERA approach sets the basic approach to pursuit of objectives in the athlete development pathway, these steps tighten the focus at the high performance end of the pathway.

Step 1. Strategy and performance planning – a structure to maximise the use of science, medicine and performance technology

Your performance strategy is not the product of hours of careful research – it is the result of a simple and quite rough-and-ready process of thinking through what it would take to 'win' and then assessing whether it is realistic to try (Martin, 2014). It is crucial to recognise that a strategy is not the same as performance planning. Strategy has to be about using your wisdom and that of others around you to set the vision for the future and the path you want to take to get there.

Performance planning is the process by which an individual and/or team aligns all available resources (money, people, knowledge and time) to maximise the probability of an athlete(s) achieving their best performance at the right time. Planning is the process by which you determine your training process, periodisation model, training location(s), timing of training camps and competitions, interventions and projects, and then align all your costs to achieve it for each individual. This is the element that makes most people feel comfortable because it is about controlling the controllables; but strategy is where the magic happens and sets the tone for the performance journey.

There are a multitude of methods and approaches to achieving a winning strategy and plan but fundamentally there are a number of key critical questions that need consideration during the process. These include:

Strategy
- Do you know what it takes to win in your sport/event?
- Do you know where your athlete, support team and you are relative to winning?
- What risks do you need to be aware of that need consideration?
- What are you going to do differently than your competitors to get there quicker than them?

Planning and prioritisation
- What competition data do you have that informs the trends of winning performances and are there any future changes that you need to plan for, e.g. rule changes, new events?
- Using the same data driven approach how far away is the athlete, support team and coach from achieving that future performance requirement, e.g. competition analysis, people reviews, etc.?
- What are the interventions available to you to shorten that gap by the time of that major event through better training management and proactive risk management?
- What process do you have to determine which interventions you take forward, which ones you park, which ones you dismiss, which ones you adopt and apply immediately, which ones you need to systematically test and evaluate through other populations/your athlete/s?
- What's your process for measuring, managing, storing and monitoring the plan as it is executed and to ensure the strategy and plan are still relevant?

By answering these questions, developing the detail and placing your 'bets' on your performance journey you put yourself in a position of knowing where you need to apply various scientific, medical and technological methods as part of your plan, do, review process.

You cannot do this without engaging with external specialists from academia and industry because of the modern day deluge of data, information and knowledge. Technology now ensures we are not limited by the ability and rate at which we obtain information – whether subjective opinion or peer reviewed scientific articles. A word search of 'strength training and sport' on PubMed online from 1990–2000 compared to the period from 2000–2010 demonstrates nearly a tenfold increase in articles over these decades. The rate-limiting step is no longer the availability or speed at which we can obtain data and information – it is our ability to filter the right information at the right time for the right athlete for the right application.

Your performance strategy and performance plan will provide a means for effective targeting of the information you have at your disposal and by adopting a problem solving approach to engagement with specialists you can provide a context by which you can filter and apply knowledge.

Step 2. Competition analysis: what will it take to win?

The first critical stage of any performance planning process is to identify those behaviours and performance indicators which if met, are likely to improve the probability of winning in your sport and event. These can often be as crude as future winning times in some sports but can also include critical events in your sport that if increased in quantity and efficiency across the board are likely to lead to improved probability of success. For a more detailed review of the different type of performance indicators in sport see Hughes and Bartlett (2002).

The development of the field of performance analysis has played a significant role in performance sport (Hughes and Franks, 2008). Its increasing popularity in the last few years has been highlighted through practical stories whereby winning performance strategies have been fuelled by the use of performance metrics to inform and shape strategy and planning. There is no better example than *Moneyball* (Lewis, 2003). However, there has been a downside to the growth of using numbers to describe sporting performances. Anderson and Sally (2013) provide a popular science review of the growth, development and application of such performance data in professional football and the role that chance has in determining the outcome. They provide a different perspective and insight into the interpretation of performance data to inform strategy. The collection of data and its translation to information and knowledge is dependent on the reasoning and decision making of the end user (Mercier and Sperber, 2011) and needs consideration in any decision making processes around the performance strategy.

The growth and development of performance metrics has been fuelled by technology that can capture field based events and activities at a high frequency, non-invasively and in dynamic situations, for example, Prozone Sports www.prozonesports.com and Imotio tracking, www.inmotio.eu. There are also worn devices which are increasingly being used to track time, motion and biometrics data during training and competition such as global positioning systems (GPS), for example, www.gpsports.com or www.catapultsports.com which can help describe some of the winning characteristics of high performance in different sports.

Step 3. Gap analysis: where is each athlete-coach relative to the future requirements of winning?

Some of the applied methods and approaches outlined in step 2 provide the basis to give an understanding of where your athlete/team sits relative to a winning performance. However, there are numerous factors that impact and influence on how the performance plan can be executed. The most significant factor in this is the coach. Much like the challenges with measuring and understanding athletic performance in the field over a long duration, it is impossible to truly study and understand the coach–athlete relationship in laboratory based conditions. However, there are a number of technological methods now available to understand and unpick how effective a coach is in getting the best out of their athlete in training and competition. It is crucial to capture all aspects of the coaching process and interactions with athlete, support personnel, parents and colleagues including actions, language, observations and thought process.

In recent years there has been a growth in a concept called life logging – the use of miniature computers to capture as many aspects of your life as possible on a continuous basis. Examples of these include 'Get Narrative' http://getnarrative.com/, Vicon Revue http://viconrevue.com/product.html and Lifelapse (app via your iPhone) http://www.lifelapse.com/. These approaches provide a novel but practical solution to objectively capturing the coaching process. The use of these concepts has been adopted in other industries for alternative purposes, for example, by people who work in isolation to monitor efficiency in areas such as time management, process management and health and safety. – see Edesix Video Badge (www.edesix.com). The Edesix video badge is a body worn video system based on an ID holder that can record up to 8 hours of quality video and audio.

The development of these technologies provides a minimally invasive and simple method of capturing the life of the coach and using such data to quantify their role as described by time motion analysis, for example, the percentage of time spent in meetings, the percentage of time spent instructing, the percentage of time planning, etc. The technology can also reveal how the coach goes about their role, for example the approach they take with different individuals to deliver the same message; and, through further analysis a better understanding of how effective the coach is in these engagements through the interactions and communication methods used with athlete and peers. Some of the original approaches to this analysis of coaching behaviour was conducted by More and Franks (1986) using video based methods and hand notation but the development in performance technology now provides a more adherent platform to review the demands of the modern coach and their impact on the athlete's development process.

Step 4. Training analysis: what are we doing in training to develop towards the winning profile?

'No plan survives the first contact with the enemy.'
Helmuth von Moltke, German military strategist

Once a performance strategy has been developed through a probabilistic understanding of those critical determinants of successful performance; an assessment of the performance gap relative to each athlete; and the design of a performance plan to meet that gap, the task of development begins.

'It's a bad plan that admits of no modification.' (Publilius Syrus). The ability to regularly change and communicate a performance plan is crucial. No plan should stay the same – if it does, something is wrong in the process due to the individualised nature of responses to acute and chronic training stress. To manage a live performance plan, technology can play a role in capturing, recording, tracking and communicating the technical detail for athlete, coach, science and medical staff. This covers and includes a number of functions:

- Recording of individual training session content versus planned training, i.e. volumes, intensities, durations, session RPEs.
- Subjective recording of wellness, health and recovery when not training.
- Monitoring individual training sessions using the framework outlined in table 18.1.
- This includes functional measures, i.e. times, forces, power, speeds; non and minimally invasive physiological responses, i.e. heart rate, lactate.
- Laboratory and functional testing.

To manage this diverse range of potential data sources as a modern day coach there has been the emergence of all-encompassing software tools that allow rapid upload of data from many sources with multiple functionality to manage security, automated information sharing, and alerts to inform individuals of unexpected patterns, trends and responses. Increasingly these tools can allow data to be viewed on computers, tablets, smartphones and all synchronised to ensure the data remains clean for all parties.

Current examples include Smartabase (www.fusionsport.com/products), Edge 10 (www.edge10.org), and Reason Incorporated (www.reasonincorporated.com/playrpro.html). Cloud based web storage systems like Dropbox also provide a lower cost method to allow effective file storage and sharing between performance teams albeit in a less efficient way when it comes to the analysis and interpretation process.

Each of these governing software systems can be fed detailed files from a varied source of training monitoring tools to track acute and chronic responses to training over time which meet the framework in table 18.1. Examples include the use of miniature tracking devices (GPS and inertial measurement systems – see Freesense www.sensorize.it) and other 'local' measurement systems to track various mechanical measures for running based activities (see Optojump www.optojump.com). In addition, there are now effective 'power measuring systems' for the gym environment (see Gymaware www.kinetic.com.au). More details on some of the current capabilities for informing this coaching process are outlined below.

FreeSense

FreeSense is a wireless, light and compact measurement system, which measures 3D linear accelerations, 3D angular velocities and GPS coordinates. When used in wireless mode, it also provides real-time visualisations of data directly on to your PC for rapid and real time feedback. FreeSense is currently being used and tested in research labs around the world. One group in Italy at the Bioengineering Laboratory of the University of Rome, are investigating the biomechanics of sprinters. Getting insight into crucial information such as trunk inclination during the start phase, foot contact times, flight times, and acceleration profile is fundamental to improving the performance of sprinting and its contribution to horizontal jumps.

Optojump

Optojump is an optical measurement system consisting of transmitting and receiving lights. The system detects any interruptions in communication between the bars and calculates their duration. This makes it possible to measure flight and contact times during the performance of a series of jumps with an accuracy of 1/1000 of a second from anything from 2m to 100m. There are numerous applications for the device but the main function has been in running activities to measure step length, step frequency and contact times which are fundamental to understanding running speed.

GymAware

GymAware is a power monitoring training system that can be used to measure a number of key performance indicators with activity from the weights room. These variables include acceleration, power, velocity, displacement, force and work down. The basic technology behind the concept relies on some known engineering principles through the use of optical encoders. The GymAware sensors calculate all the output parameters based on first principal determination of displacement and a quartz crystal time base. From time and displacement, velocity can be calculated and then acceleration. If weight is entered, force, work and power can be calculated for that athlete. The current commercial system has been validated against known gold standard measures (www.kinetic.com.au/lang-en/products/gymaware/faqs/validation) and tested across various dynamic movement patterns.

App technology

At the other extreme of financial investment, the growth of tablets and 'app' technology has seen the emergence of lower cost methods and approaches to monitor and track aspects of training. For example 'apps', which are now readily used and can provide some form of coaching and athlete functionality, include pacing tools (PaceDJ), training monitoring tools (Training Load) and video analysis (Excelade).

PaceDJ

PaceDJ is an app that can work off your iPhone using an athlete's favourite music to help pace efforts when training. This is primarily designed and targeted at the health and fitness market but can also be used to help with training sessions to give some real time auditory feedback to help athletes with training efforts. Different music can be used to alter pace and the beats per minute (BPM) can be changed manually if not quite accurate enough.

Training Load

Training Load allows anyone to record and track the 'dose' of exercise for a single person with two common methods – Session-RPE and the Training Impulse (TRIMP). Both methods integrate training intensity and training duration into a single number representing the overall dose of training. Training Load allows you to enter the RPE, the maximal and resting heart rate, the mean heart rate for the training session and the session duration. By entering these values via the sliders it takes just a single button tap to then calculate the TRIMP and Session-RPE. Training Load graphs all individual training sessions so that you can see the daily progression in the TRIMP and Session-RPE. The weekly graph for TRIMP also displays the percentage change from the previous week. The weekly graph for Session-RPE displays the monotony, percentage change from the previous week, and strain.

Excelade

Excelade is one example of a video analysis tool that allows you to capture, share and review video clips from various training and sporting performances. It provides the basic functionality to allow rapid review of skills executed in the training environment. Excelade allows slow motion playback, playing videos simultaneously for comparison, allows editing with text and drawings, and allows sharing with others once an account has been set up. The app allows low-level entry into the video playback market and provides a simple but effective feedback tool.

SUMMARY AND FUTURE DEVELOPMENTS

This chapter has provided an insight into evaluation in principle and practice; and into the growth, development and application of performance technology in modern day coaching. Numerous examples have been provided based on current commercial availability and use by sports across the world. In five years' time expect the methods adopted to have moved on and the range and availability of tools and approaches to have decreased in cost and increased in availability. Indeed, as you read this chapter the emergence of 'quantified self' developments such as Lumo Lift (www.lumobodytech.com) or Jawbone UP (https://jawbone.com/up) will not only influence the everyday consumer but also elite sport as the processes of tracking vital signals and performance become more automated and informative through smart artificial learning software tools in this era of 'big data'.

The development and application of other web-based methods such as crowd sourcing are already being used as a tool to support talent transfer methods in elite sport, for example create.it (https://create.it/).

The one major fear expressed with this growth in performance technology is that it could one day replace the coach. That will not happen. The purpose of sport and athlete development has not changed – just the methods by which we can now generate a breadth and depth of data from the training and competition process. The ability to convert data into information – information into knowledge – knowledge into wisdom – wisdom into performance – will always be dependent on the athlete-coach relationship. The rate-limiting step will always be with the human capability.

REFLECTIVE QUESTIONS

1. How can GPS be used to help field game managers to time their substitutions of players in a game?

2. Sports science testing procedures are seldom accessible for regular sports clubs. List tests that are readily available and may be applied in a club context to measure and monitor the effectiveness of training programmes. For each test state what is measured and how the coach may use that information.

3. Compare and contrast tests for jumping power. Explain possible differences in predicting long jump from horizontal jump tests or high jump from vertical jump tests.

4. 'The only truly valid test in predicting performance is in the performance itself.' Discuss this statement.

5. Following review of current technology, prepare an evaluation of mobile phone and other applications which an athlete might use to measure and monitor their own development.

SUMMARY OF PART 4

The interpretation of fitness for an individual is unique to his lifestyle. For athlete and non-athlete it should be understood that lifestyle in the teens influences that in the 20s, and this in turn influences that in the 30s, and so on. A well-balanced daily routine which includes physical activity might be seen as a basis for a healthy life and should be established early on. Physical activity will range from walking and jogging, each of which requires little or no equipment, to those sports which are practised in recreation or sports centres or which require specialist facilities, such as in skiing and sailing.

For the athlete, part of his lifestyle is pursuit of competitive advantage and fitness must be developed accordingly. On the sound basis of general strength, endurance, and mobility, technical efficiency is developed and progressed towards the specific requirements of physical and physiological status demanded of a given sport. The broad direction of development is from general to specific, as well as from a basic technical model (or models) towards expressing that model with greater strength and speed, sometimes in the climate of endurance factors where there are such facets of a particular sport. Against the constant backcloth of a well-managed training and non-training environment, the final sophistication of development is a mature competitive attitude which permits sound performance in progressively variable situations.

Perhaps the most demanding problem for the coach is arriving at the most appropriate training plan for the development of physical and physiological status. The relative contributions of strength, speed, mobility, endurance (and their derivatives) may, in most instances, be established with the intelligent use of evaluation procedures. Nevertheless, the coach requires the full measure of his artistry to create an individually orientated programme from the expanding areas of related theory and practice.

REFERENCES FOR PART 4

Anderson, C. and Sally, D. *The Numbers Game: Why Everything You Know About Football Is Wrong.* New York: Penguin. (2013)

Ballreich R. 'Model for estimating the influence of stride length and stride frequency on time in sprinting events'. In P. V. Komi PV(ed.), *Biomechanics V-B*, 208–12. Baltimore, MD: University Park Press. (1976)

Fleishman, I. E. *The Structure and Measurement of Physical Fitness.* Upper Saddle River, NJ: Prentice Hall. (1964)

Grosser, M., *Schnelligkeitstraining.* Munchen: BLV Verlag (1991)

Harre, D. *Trainingslehre.* Berlin: Sportverlag. (1973)

Hughes, M. and Bartlett, R. B. 'The use of performance indicators in performance analysis'. *Journal of Sports Sciences* 20(10): 739–54. (2002)

Hughes, M. and Franks, I. (eds). *The Essentials of Performance Analysis.* Abingdon: Routledge. (2008)

Kraemer, W. J. and Häkkinen, K. (eds). *Strength Training for Sport.* Oxford: Blackwell Science. (2002)

Lewis, M. *Moneyball – The Art of Winning an Unfair Game.* New York: W.W. Norton & Company. (2003)

Logan, G. A. and McKinney, W. C. *Kinesiology.* Dubuque, IA: Wm. C. Brown. (1970)

MacIntosh, B. R., Gardiner, P. F. and McComas, A. J. *Skeletal Muscle Form and Function.* 2nd edn. Champaign, IL: Human Kinetics. (2006)

Mallett, C. J. 'Self-determination theory: A case study of evidence-based coaching'. *The Sport Psychologist* 19: 417–29. (2005)

Martin, R. L. 'The big lie of strategic planning'. *Harvard Business Review* January–February: 78–81. (2014)

Matveyev, L. P., *Fundamentals of Sports Training*. Moscow: Process Publishers (1981)

Mercier, H. and Sperber, B. 'Why do humans reason? Arguments for an argumentative theory'. *Behavioural and Brain Sciences* 34: 57–111. (2011)

Osolin, N. G. *Das Training Des Leichtathleten*. Berlin: Sportverlag. (1952)

Saziorski, W. M. 'Die Korperlichen Eigenschaften Des Sportlers'. *Theorie Und Praxis Der Korperkultur* 20 (Suppl.). (1971)

Sinkkonen, K. 'The programming of distance running'. Paper presented to ELLV Congress, Budapest. (1975)

Spriet, L. L. and Howlett, R. A. 'Metabolic control of energy production during physical activity'. In D. R. Lamb and R. Murray (eds), *Perspectives in Exercise Science and Sports Medicine, Vol 12: The Metabolic Bases of Performance in Sport and Exercise*, 1–44. Carmel, IN: Cooper Publishing Group. (1999)

Stein, M., 'Speed Training in Sport' in Elliot, B. and Mester, J., (consulting editor) *Training in Sport – Applying Sport Science*. Chichester, UK: Wiley & Sons (1998)

Stoll, C. and Schubert, G. in Keeler, Mark R., *Nothing to Hide: Privacy in the 21st century*. New York: iUniverse (2006)

Upton, A. R. M. and Radford, P. F. 'Trends in speed of alternated limb movement during development and amongst elite sprinters'. *Proceedings of Vth International Congress of Biomechanics, Jyväskylä, Finland*. (1975)

Van Loon, L. J. C., Greenhaff, P. L., Constantin-Teodosiu, C., Saris, W. H. M. and Wagenmakers, A. J. M. 'The effects of increasing exercise intensity on muscle fuel utilization in humans'. *Journal of Applied Physiology* 536: 295–304. (2001)

Viru, A. A., Urgenstein, Y. U. and Pisuke, A. P. 'Influence of training methods on endurance'. *Track Technique* 47. (1972)

Ward, P. E. and Ward, R. D. *Encyclopedia of Weight Training*. 2nd edn. Laguna Hills, CA: QPT Publications. (1997)

BIBLIOGRAPHY

Arthur, R. 'What swimmers can teach to runners'. *Modern Athlete and Coach* 1: 3. (May 1973)

Bloomfield, J. Ackland, T. R. and Elliot, B. C. (eds). *Applied Anatomy and Biomechanics In Sport*. Carlton: Blackwell Scientific Publications. (1994)

Brunner, J. A. 'Untersuchungen über Statisches (Isometrisches) und Dynamisches (Isotonisches) Muskelwaining'. *Körperererziehung* 5. (1967)

Bührle, M. *Prinzipen des Krafttrainings*. Die Lehre Der Leichtathletik. (1971)

Clarke, H. H. *Application of Measurement to Health and Physical Education*. 4th edn. Upper Saddle River, NJ: Prentice Hall. (1967)

Counsilman, J. G. *The Science of Swimming*. London: Pelham Books. (1970)

Dyatchkov, V. M. 'High jumping'. *Track Technique* 36. (1969)

Elliott, B. *Training in Sport*. Chichester: John Wiley. (1999)

Endemann, F. 'Learning practices in throws'. *6th Coaches' Convention Report*. (1975)

Gambetta, V. A. *Athletic Development – The Art and Science of Functional Sports Conditioning*. Champaign, IL: Human Kinetics. (2007)

Gundlach, H. 'Zur Trainierberkeit Der Kraft–Und Schnellkeitsfahigkeiten Im Prozess Der Korperlichen Vervollkommnug'. *Theorie Und Praxis Der Korperkultur* 17 (Suppl. 11): 167. (1968)

Hettinger, T. H. 'Muscle trainability of men and women'. *Modern Athlete and Coach* 13(4). (1975)

Hettinger, T. and Muller, E. A. 'Muskelleistung Und Muskeltraining'. *Arbeitsphysiologie* 15: 111–26. (1953)

Hogg, J. M. *Land Conditioning for Competitive Swimming*. Wakefield: E. P. Publishing. (1972)

Ivanova, L. S. *Die Korperliche Vorbereitung Der Sportler Hoherer Leistungsklassen: Entwicklung Der Kraft*. Moscow: Fiskultura i Sport. (1967)

Jäger, K. and Oelschlägel, G. *Kleine Trainingslehre*. 2nd edn. Berlin: Sportverlag. (1974)

Jensen, C. R. and Fisher, A. G. Scientific Basis of Athletic Conditioning. Philadelphia, PA: Lea & Febiger. (1972)

Jesse, J. P. 'Young athletes and weight training'. *Modern Athlete and Coach* 14(1). (1976)

Karvonen, M. J., Kentala, E. and Mustala, O. 'The effect of training on heart rate'. *Annales Medicinae Experimentalis et Biologae Fenniae* 35. (1957)

Kendrick, D. 'Activity and ageing'. *New Behaviour* 1(6). (1975)

Keul, J. *Limiting Factors of Physical Performance*. Stuttgart: Thieme. (1973)

Koslov, V. 'Application of maximum power in throwing'. *Modern Athlete and Coach* 8(4). (1970)

Kusnetov, V. V. *Kraftvorbereitung–Theoretische Grundlagen Der Muskelkraftenwicklung*. 2nd edn. Berlin: Sportverlag. (1975)

Lay, P. 'Fundamentals of weight training'. *Athletics Weekly* 13 December; 10 January; 7 February; 28 February; 11 April; 16 May. (1969–70)

McCardle, W. D., Katch, F. I. and Katch, V. L. *Exercise Physiology: Nutrition, Energy and Human Performance*. Baltimore, MD: Lippincott Williams & Wilkins. (2009)

Margaria, R. *Biomechanics and Energetics of Muscular Exercise*. Oxford: Clarendon Press. (1976)

More, K. G. and Franks, I. M. 'Analysis and modification of verbal coaching behaviour: The usefulness of a data-driven intervention strategy'. *Journal of Sports Sciences* 14(6): 523–43. (1996)

Murase, Y., Hoshikawa, T., Yasuda, N., Ikegami, Y. and Matsui, H. 'A study of analysis of the changes in progressive speed of 100m from the points of view of anaerobic energy output and running patterns'. *Proceedings of Vth International Congress of Biomechanics, Jyväskylä, Finland*. (1975)

Osolin, N. G. 'Speed endurance'. *Modern Athlete and Coach* 11(1). (1973)

Pahud, J. F. and Gobbeler, C. 'Training at altitude: General principles and personal experience'. *New Studies in Athletics* September. (1986)

Petrovski, V. and Verhoshansky, J. 'Aspects of sprint training'. *Modern Athlete and Coach* 13(4). (1975)

Pickering, R. J. *Strength Training for Athletics*. 2nd edn. London: BAAB. (1968)

Pohlitz, L. 'Practical experiences of altitude training with female middle distance runners'. *Leichtathletik* 3. (1986)

Polunin, A. 'Training in middle and high mountains'. EACA Workshop Paper, Belmekan. (1994)

Radcliffe, J. C. and Farentinos, R. C. *High-Powered Plyometrics*. Champaign, IL: Human Kinetics. (1999)

Ritzdorf, W. 'Strength and power training in sport'. In B. Elliot (ed.), *Training In Sport: Applying Sport Science*. Chichester: John Wiley. (1998)

Schmolinsky, G. *Leichtathletik*. 7th edn. Berlin: Sportverlag. (1974)

Scholich, M. *Circuit Training*. Berlin: Sportverlag (1986)

Schon, R. 'Recommendations based on experience of altitude training with young athletes'. EACA Workshop Paper, Belmekan. (1994)

Shephard, R. J. *Endurance Training*. Toronto: University of Toronto Press. (1969)

Skaset, H. B. *Trainingslaere*. Oslo: Norges Idrettsforbund. (1970)

Stone, M. H., Stone, M. and Sands, W. A. *Principles and Practice of Resistance Training*. Champaign, IL: Human Kinetics. (2007)

Taylor, A. W. *Training: Scientific Basis and Application*. Springfield, IL: Charles C. Thomas. (1972)

Tegtbur, U., Bussg, N. and Braumann, K. M. 'Estimation of an individual equilibrium between lactate production and catabolism during exercise'. *Medicine and Science in Sports and Exercise* 25: 620–27. (1993)

Van der Woude, L. H. V., Veeger, H. E. J. and Dallmeijer, A. J. 'The ergonomics of wheelchair sports'. In G. Atkinson and J. Reilly (eds), *Sport, Leisure and Ergonomics*, 3–12. London: E. & F. N. Spon. (1995)

Verhoshansky, J. W. 'Grundlagen Des Speziellen Krafttrainings Im Sport'. in *Theorie Und Praxis Der Korperkultur* 20. (1971)

Wagner, P. 'Male–female differences in middle distance training and competitions'. *7th Coaches' Convention Report*. (1976)

Wasserman, K. 'The anaerobic threshold: definition physiological significance and identification'. *Advances in Cardiology* 35: 1–23. (1986)

Whitehead, N. *Conditioning for Sport*. London: A. & C. Black. (1988)

Williams, C. 'Special forms and effects of endurance training'. *5th Coaches' Convention Report*. (1974)

Young, W. 'Laboratory strength assessment of athletes'. *HSA* 10–11: 89–96. (1995)

Zatsiorsky, V. M. *Science and Practice of Strength Training*. Champaign, IL: Human Kinetics. (1995)

PART 5
PLANNING THE PROGRAMME

Without knowing our destination, we cannot plan our journey. Our destination in sport is the competition objective or goal. It is performance and/or result related. It might be to win a league competition, a cup tournament, an Olympic medal, a place in the national championships, a qualifying performance for team selection, or a lifetime best performance in a particular competition. It should stretch the athlete or team to go beyond present achievement limits. It must be 'beyond the probable', yet realistically believed in, as agreed by coach and performer(s). Our journey is the preparation programme planned to help reach the objective or goal; it is quantifiable and has a timescale.

The structure of that plan and its details must, however, be sufficiently flexible to move and adapt to the dynamics of athlete, coach and situation. The destination is not a terminus, but a milestone in a performance development journey. The programme must be capable of adjustment on the way to that milestone, and for progressing beyond it.

We must, however, start with some kind of 'route map'. The division of the training year into periods of varying duration, characterised by their progressive contribution to reaching the 'destination', is such a 'route map'.

For summer sports, it grew from such origins as:

Period 1	*Autumn and winter*	*Training for and competing in winter field games*
Period 2	*Spring*	*Training for a summer sport*

Period 3   *Summer*   *Lighter training and competing in a summer sport*

to:

Period 1   *Winter training*
Period 2   *Pre-competition training*
Period 3   *Competition training*

to current systems of periodisation.

This evolution of how the year is planned might be thought of as a progressive shift towards considering training as a cyclical year-round process, which is part of a total development of training and performance over several years.

In part 5, in order to explain the underlying principles of designing a year-round programme, it is expedient to illustrate the process with reference mainly to a summer season sport – athletics. Here, the preparation portion of the year is long – and the competition portion(s) short. This makes things very simple. However, in long competition season sports such as winter games (e.g. the several football codes, ice/snow sports, basketball), or year-round sports (e.g. tennis, golf), life is rather more complicated and both preparation/conditioning and competition objectives must be pursued simultaneously on the foundation of a very brief (1–2 month) preparation/conditioning base. This is achieved through thoughtful design and delivery of short cycles which must balance raising fitness and performance levels, stabilising gains and recovery.

Part 5 sets out the athletics training year and, where relevant, reference is made to the application of training principles in practice in long season/year-round sports.

19 PERIODISING THE YEAR

Periodisation may be described as an organised division of the training year in pursuit of three basic objectives:

- To prepare the athlete for the achievement of an optimal improvement in their performance.
- To prepare the athlete for a definite climax to the competition season (e.g. Olympic Games, national age group championships, etc).
- To prepare the athlete for the main competitions associated with that climax (e.g. trials or qualifying competitions for the Olympic Games; national age group championships, league matches, rounds of a cup competition, etc.).

Occasionally, annual objectives are not embraced by the three stated. These may be considered under two separate headings:

- To aid recovery from injury, illness or a particularly stressful training year (e.g. regeneration post-Olympic season).
- To prepare the athlete for meeting the above objectives in subsequent years, by increasing special training status, stabilising technique or performance, and so on, over the period of one or more years (e.g. one to two seasons pre-Olympic season).

Special programmes are required to meet the last two objectives and, although they are not dealt with in detail here, the terminology and broad principles of programme construction still apply.

Modern theory of periodisation was originally advanced by L. P. Matveyev (USSR), in 1965, as an updating of work which he first introduced in 1962.

month	Oct	Nov	Dec	Jan	Feb	Mar	Apr	May	Jun	Jul	Aug	September
macro	← preparation ————————————————→							← competition ————→			← transition →
meso	1					2	3			4	5	6

FIGURE 19.1 The division of the training year will obviously be influenced by the 'competition calendar'. The division shown here was used by the USSR in preparation for the Munich Olympics in 1972, where athletes used a 'single periodised year' (from Osolin and Markov, 1972).

double		1	2		3 1	1	2		3 2	4	5	6
single			1			2	3		4	5		6
month	Nov	Dec	Jan	Feb	Mar	Apr	May	Jun	Jul	Aug	Sep	Oct

FIGURE 19.2 Single and double periodised years

From early ideas of preparing an athlete for a competitive programme distributed throughout a season, he looked towards a specific competition climax or peak (e.g. Olympic Games, national age group championships, etc.), for which not only training periods, but also a selected competition programme was a totality of preparation. Matveyev suggested that the year be divided into three periods: preparation, competition, and transition. These are referred to here as macrocycles, and they describe the cyclic performance development model of *preparation* (*adaptation*) – *competition* (*application*) – *transition* (*regeneration*). He subdivided these into shorter training phases, which are referred to here as mesocycles (figure 19.1). These in turn are divided into microcycles (see chapter 21). It is important to understand:

- Each cycle builds on the cumulative effect of the previous and prepares for those to follow.
- The outcome of the process is that the athlete and/or team is prepared to deliver desired performance 'on the day' whatever the conditions or circumstances.
- The periodised year for summer season sports as described here allows for big blocks of training to achieve training objectives. The long season sports and those sports which are virtually year round must still address the same training objectives. Long term objectives cannot be achieved without doing so.
  A closer look at these mesocycles will help identify their individual character.

PREPARATION MACROCYCLE
Mesocycle 1

This is the longest phase in the annual cycle and should occupy one third of that cycle. Thus, in the single periodised year (figure 19.2), it occupies four months (3 × 6 weeks) while in the double periodised year (figure 19.2) it occupies 8–10 weeks, to be reintroduced after the first competition macrocycle (31) for a further 6–8 weeks.

The main aim is to increase the athlete's ability to accept a high intensity (quality) of loading in mesocycle 2 by increasing the extent (quantity) of loading during mesocycle 1. The high volume of work involved necessitates a very gradual increase in intensity during this mesocycle, but this increase is essential to progress in mesocycle 2 and to the stabilisation of performance in the competition macrocycle. Training is more general in nature, and during this mesocycle the athlete is working at the endurance end of his event development. However, in the interest of continuous development of performance, it is also necessary to pursue related training and specific training. A mixed programme is required, which must take into account the particular event and the athlete's stage of development when establishing a ratio of general:related:specific training. It may be useful to describe these broad areas of training.

- **General training:** This training establishes and maintains the platform of physical competencies on which the annual training programme is built. So aerobic training provides endurance to accept and recover from the progressive training loads of the programme; all round, balanced strength and mobility ensures that techniques may be learned free from compensations and compromises to sound and robust basic technical models for a given sport.
- **Related training:** This is training to perfect the individual components of sports techniques and specific fitness. So, for example, this will include the specifics of strength as they relate to joint actions and movement dynamics of a technique; or the specifics of endurance as they relate to the energy system demands of a sport or discipline; or the specifics of speed as they relate to the synchronising of joint action compo-

nents within a technique, reaction or response speed, sprinting speed, etc.; or mobility specifics as they relate to a range of movement necessary to efficient and effective technique.

- **Specific training:** this is training where technique is completely rehearsed and, more importantly, in progressive intensity and competitive situations. This area has variations from specialised exercise routines to rehearsal of competition sequences to actual competition. It embraces technique, tactics, etc. It plays a much smaller part in the total extent of training than general or related training.

At the risk of being over repetitive, all three areas are covered throughout the year, but their contribution will vary from mesocycle to mesocycle. At the end of mesocycle 1, the basic components of fitness for a specific event must have reached the level necessary to ensure a planned increase in performance. Tests should be used to check this. For example, a long jumper working towards 8m from a 20-stride approach should jump 7m from 10 strides.

This mesocycle establishes the platform for technical and fitness progression consistent with a sport's related athletic fitness and technical training demands.

Once again, however, it is important to understand that each cycle builds upon the cumulative foundation of those that have gone before – microcycle on microcycles, mesocycle on mesocycles, macrocycle on macrocycles, annual cycles on annual cycles.

Mesocycle 2

This mesocycle, according to Matveyev (1965), lasts eight weeks when single periodisation is used and six weeks in double periodisation. However, it is possible to stretch this to 8 or 12 weeks, and four weeks plus four weeks respectively, if the annual cycle is extended slightly beyond 52 weeks. There are many advantages to such stretching, but most important is that the increase of load intensity will be gentler. There is no doubt, however, that this is the hardest working mesocycle in the year. It represents a major test of a coach's judgement in adjusting the overall balance of training load extent and intensity – the 'structure of loading' (see page 330) across the mesocycle.

Mesocycle 2 runs directly into the competition period. Its aims are to unite the component parts or foundations of training into a harmonious whole (i.e. training moves from workshop to assembly line). While the character of this mesocycle is that of increasing specialisation, the areas of training in the first mesocycle are continued. The training ratio decreases in the general area and, while the total extent of work remains the same or is gently reduced, the intensity of loading in related and specific training increases sharply. Technique must be schooled and stabilised as the athlete learns to use increased strength, speed, etc. It is absolutely essential that technical development and development of strength, speed, and so forth, are advanced together. A season can be completely lost if they are 'out of step'.

Towards the end of this mesocycle, the athlete must be exposed to more open conditions and situations in training and increasingly in a climate of competition. These conditions and situations may include adverse weather or distractions such as noise, interruptions, time of day, floodlights, etc. Should training progress successfully, the young athlete will (according to Harre, 1973) improve on previous best performance after three competitions. The experienced athlete should at least equal his previous best. It would appear from personal observation that if the young athlete is within 2.5 per cent of his best performance in a technical event after three competitions (spaced over 2–4 weeks), it is reasonable to assume that progress is 'on schedule'. By increasing load intensity, particularly via competitions, he will improve performance still further. If no improvements follow, it is frequently a result of the intensity having been raised too rapidly in the second mesocycle, or the extent of competition loading being too great, or the total extent of loading at the end of the preparation macrocycle having been excessively reduced.

This mesocycle establishes the platform for effective delivery of competitive performance objectives.

COMPETITION MACROCYCLE

Although mesocycles 3, 4 and 5 have their own characteristics and objectives, there is a sense of a single process. The annual cycle of course, is about raising performance. Given a well thought out and delivered preparation macrocycle, that objective will be achieved. But the harder edge of effective coaching is ensuring that on the day of the major or most important competition(s) of the year, the athlete delivers their best performance of the year. To achieve a season's best performance in mesocycle 3 and not at the major competition in mesocycle 5 suggests a review of the relationship between mesocycles 2, 3, 4 and 5.

Mesocycle 3

The main task of this mesocycle of the competition macrocycle is to develop and stabilise competition performance as fully as possible (see also chapter 24). The athlete will then be able to produce optimal performance in key competitions. The blending of new levels of specific sport or event fitness, which has been developed throughout the preparation macrocycle, must be continued in order to produce high-level performance. Moreover, these new levels of fitness must be maintained via specific loadings and competitions themselves. Consequently, the loadings in this area are increased, while those in the general and related areas are reduced. The total extent of training is therefore decreased as the intensity rises. The reduction of extent is very steep where sports demand maximum or elastic strength or speed (e.g. jumps, throws, weightlifting, games), but only slight in endurance sports in the interest of maintaining aerobic fitness. General training should be seen primarily as a means of active recovery in the non-endurance sports.

It is important not to neglect the status of basic fitness components such as strength, speed, mobility, etc., in favour of technical development. Strength losses, for example, can be considerable, even over 2–3 weeks and such losses, if continued, will be reflected in performance. Consequently, the strength programme has its place in the competition macrocycle (figure 19.3).

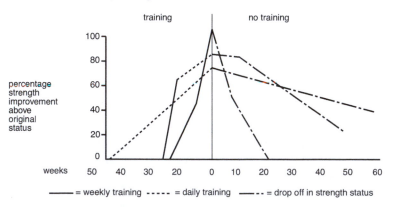

FIGURE 19.3 An outline of work conducted by Hettinger, illustrating not only different effects of daily and weekly training, but how strength training loses its effect once stopped (from Hettinger, 1968).

The frequency of competitions depends on the individual athlete's capacity for the emotional and physical stress of competition loading. It is very difficult to establish ideal numbers of competitions and this topic is discussed more fully below. At one end of the scale, an elite athlete might feel that two major marathons in one year is acceptable but, at the other, a 13-year-old may be happy to spend all year competing twice a week in several sports.

Competition frequency and the amount of specific loading determine development of performance in the competition macrocycle. An optimal balance can only be arrived at individually, but, once known, the athlete can expect to record best performances 6–8 weeks from the start of this mesocycle (i.e. mesocycle 3 single periodisation, and mesocycles 3_1 and 3_2 double periodisation). Thus, after three competitions (4–6 weeks from start of mesocycle 3), the athlete will be within 2.5 per cent of lifetime best and by 6–8 weeks will have improved upon lifetime best. Trials and qualifying competitions, and most of the main contests for young athletes, should therefore fall within mesocycle 3 (single) and mesocycle 3_2 (double).

This mesocycle establishes a platform of raised performance quality consistency in preparation for the best performance(s) of the season in mesocycle 5.

Mesocycle 4

Even if the mesocycles to date have not led to qualifying the athlete for the target major competition(s) of the year, coaches should follow through as if the athlete has done so. This affords opportunity to leverage the learning experience for both coach and athlete. It may be necessary to create appropriate competition(s) for this purpose.

As competition continues beyond mesocycles 3 and 3_2, it is advisable to introduce a mesocycle of 4–6 weeks in which the proportion of specific training is reduced, competitions are eliminated, and general and related training are increased. The value of general training should be noted here, as it serves an important role in active recovery from the emotional and physical stresses of competition.

If the athlete has not been brought to peak performance in the previous 6–8 weeks, a longer period may be necessary, and mesocycle 4 may be omitted and the training ratio left unchanged. If the athlete has achieved peak performance, mesocycle 4 aids recovery, protects from injury, and prepares for mesocycle 5. The latter is most important in a major season (e.g. Olympic Games) as this mesocycle will be seen as a special preparation macrocycle. This mesocycle raises the game for delivery of the season's best performance in mesocycle 5.

Mesocycle 5

Again, by evolving an optimal blend of competitions and specific training, further improvement in performance may be expected within 3–4 weeks. Ideally, the major event of the athletic calendar will fall within this mesocycle (Olympic Games, national championships, etc.).

This mesocycle is what all mesocycles this year and in previous years were in preparation for.

TRANSITION MACROCYCLE
Mesocycle 6

Just as restful sleep must follow a hard day's work, so a period of regeneration must follow a hard year's training and competition. This period of regeneration must bring the athlete to the commencement of the next training year totally prepared for training; from positive motivational profile through to fully 'recharged energy batteries'.

If the season has been 'low key', little wear and tear on the organism might be expected and, following a medical and physiotherapy check-up, the athlete will go straight into general activity for basic strength, mobility and aerobic endurance after mesocycle 5. In effect, it is a build into preparation mesocycle 1. This would mean a rapid increase in the extent of training and a drop in intensity. If, on the other hand, the season has been 'high key', 3–6 weeks active recovery must precede the next preparation macrocycle. The athlete should not start the new preparation macrocycle without a full recovery from the previous competition season, otherwise the effect of future loading will be extremely limited, adaptation problems will quickly arise, a risk of injury will occur, and the disappointment of poor progress in training may have effects reaching into the next competition macrocycle.

The transition macrocycle sees the gentle reduction of all loadings, with general training assuming the leading role in the training ratio. While technical schooling may now be introduced, the emphasis should be on physical, emotional and intellectual regeneration involving leisure pursuits. On no account should this macrocycle be passive. This mesocycle is well thought out rest, recovery and regeneration.

YEAR-ROUND ADAPTATIONS

The mesocycles 1–6 represent interpretation of 'Preparation (Adaptation) – Competition (Application) – Transition (Recovery)' on a large block timescale. Long season sports and year round sports do not have that luxury, yet must address this cycle of things. To do so, it is fundamental to the concept that in their early development years an all-round foundation of general fitness in endurance, strength and mobility is established to permit shorter timescales to be used to advantage.

In broad terms, it is possible to establish a 'competition' macrocycle which constitutes priority competitions and another 'preparation' macrocycle where there are no competitions or very low priority ones. For example, soccer's competition season may spread over 40 weeks. This leaves approximately 12 weeks for the preparation macrocycle during which the regeneration objectives of mesocycle 6 and the objectives of mesocycles 2 and 4 are pursued. The loose guide to training unit distribution here is general:related:specific – 50%:30%:20%. Through the competition season it is a matter of ensuring that microcycles of seven days, variously having one or two or even three competitions, are designed to regenerate; to produce competition sharpness; and to maintain general:related:specific conditioning status. A possible unit distribution to achieve this would be 20%:30%:50%, bearing in mind that competitions themselves are included in the 50 per cent specific.

This said, the programme should be sufficiently flexible to return to the preparation macrocycle distribution should the opportunity arise. In some sports and countries, such an opportunity is afforded by a mid-season break. In international tennis, players must create blocks of time to regenerate and build a conditioning base by prioritising their tournaments through what can amount to a 12 month 'season'!

SUMMARY

Periodisation is an organised division of the training year in pursuit of basic objectives of training. The divisions are, in the first instance, those of preparation, competition and transition. These are referred to as macrocycles, which are further subdivided into mesocycles. Mesocycles 1, 2 and 4 are planned according to specific objectives of preparation, while mesocycles 3 and 5 are planned in pursuit of specific objectives of competition. Mesocycle 6 coincides with the transition macrocycle. The principles of the cyclic process of preparation (adaptation)–competition (application)–transition (recovery) may be adapted to short term cycles of long season and year round sport.

REFLECTIVE QUESTIONS

1. Design or access a blank proforma for a year plan in the sport of your choice. Discuss the factors which influence the division of the year into macrocycles and mesocycles.

2. Major international championships and games are held mostly in the northern hemisphere, while in sports such as athletics, the European outdoor season features the majority of top class international meetings. So for southern hemisphere countries such as Australia, their own domestic season runs directly into the major competitions of their athletes' year. Discuss the advantages and disadvantages of this situation.

3. 'There comes a point in the arena when you alone must decide what to do. It's at the very edge of risk when you learn things no one can teach you.' Outline how you would prepare yourself and the athlete to whom you give this advice and ownership, for the arena and at that point.

4. Although possible, it is seldom the case that an athlete or team can win back to back annual major championships or titles. Discuss the case for seeing preparation as a two or more year process rather than one year at a time. How would you propose designing what is, in effect, periodisation over two or more years rather than annually?

5. In designing training content for an athlete's or team's year ahead, you must have a performance goal for athlete or team and knowledge of their current status. Discuss the variables you must consider in pursuit of those changes that will bridge the gap from current status to desired goal.

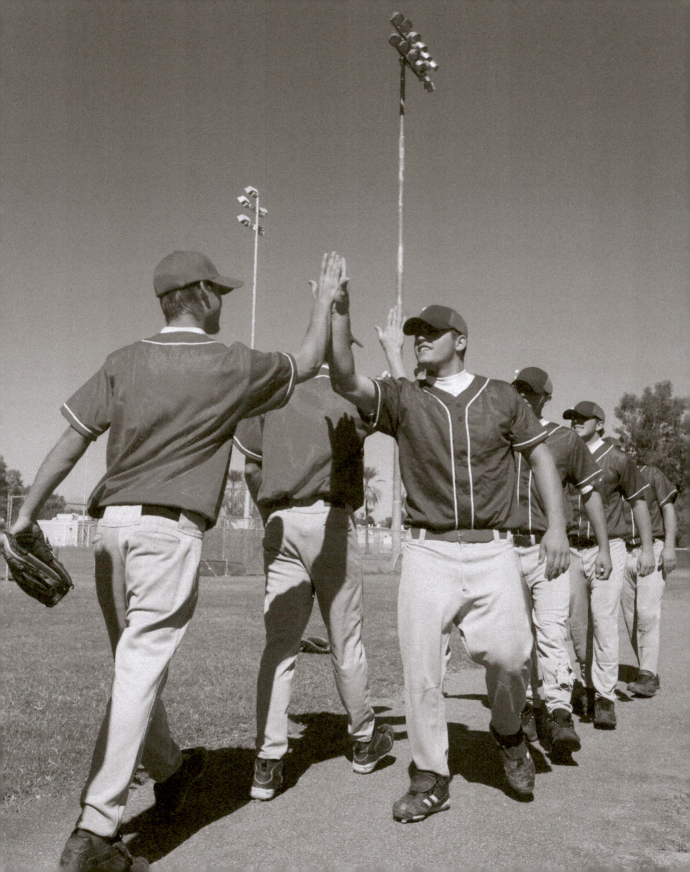

20 REFLECTIONS ON PERIODISATION

Preparation for fulfilling an athlete's lifetime competitive goal of achievement be that at national, continental, world or Olympic levels etc., commences with his earliest experience of sport and is brought to fruition sometime during the athlete's peak performance years in his chosen sport. This is a process described as the 'athlete's long term development and performance pathway'. It might be depicted as in figure 20.1:

EXCITE TO PARTICIPATE	PARTICIPATE TO PRACTICE	PRACTICE TO PREPARE	PREPARE TO PERFORM	PERFORM TO COMPETE	COMPETE TO LEARN	LEARN TO WIN

FIGURE 20.1 The athlete's long term development and performance pathway

Excite to participate

While it is very natural for children to be physically active, not all commit to regular participation in physical activity. We each are motivated in different ways to build things into our lives. Moreover it cannot be assumed that each generation will pursue physical activity for the same reasons as the previous generation. So we must be careful to work out what motivational climate will excite children and young people to participate in physical activity – hopefully for life.

Participate to practice

Certainly in the early stages of athlete development, physical activity in general and participation in sport in particular, must be enjoyable and engaging. Making it 'fun' or 'sugaring the pill' is key to encouraging that level of practice which lays the foundations of physical fitness and motor coordination that are preparation for a healthful and purposeful active life.

Practice to prepare

Once physical activity and sport is built into lifestyle, there is a motivational climate for creating training programmes and discipline. This may be enhanced when athletes work together, hence the value of squads, clubs and team activities in early years, even in individual sports.

Prepare to perform

Now the periodised annual programme is created, its variations linking units and microcycles to major competitions. The coach is in the serious world of designing and delivering on performance targets through effective plans, strategies and programmes.

Perform to compete

Delivering planned personal performance in a climate of competition with others is the next step. It must be carefully managed by selecting the right level of competition to stretch athletes and teams to raise their performance. Even if results are not the ones the athlete wants, the performance must be. This stage is learning how to raise the athlete's game under pressure.

Compete to learn

There is a stage – often over 2–3 years when athletes, having made their way through to the top of their age group progressions to senior level, are in a very different level of competition. The opposition has years of experience in their favour. Here the athlete is using each competition to learn about competing at the highest level, bridging the experience gap but most importantly to learn about himself. This is in part about addressing the strength of his commitment to go the distance to the top but also about simply understanding how to turn each moment in the arena, and in preparation for it, to their advantage.

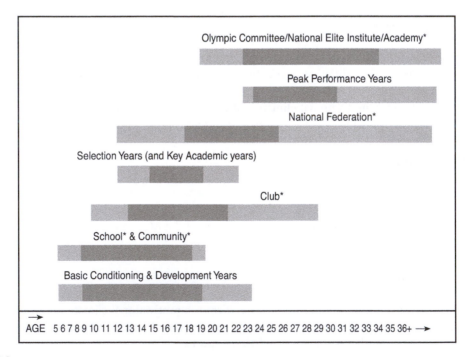

FIGURE 20.2 Management of the athlete's development progress requires a commitment to partnership as the athlete moves through the process. Possible 'partners' are indicated with an asterisk.

Learn to win

The athlete is now in the peak performance years of his sport. Everything to date is preparation for this. The athlete is now at that point where fractions of a percentage separate victory from defeat. Managing those fractions physically, mentally and emotionally is learning what to do and how to do it inside and outside the arena, to win persistently when it matters.

Although the seven stages of the pathway do not necessarily fall into comfortable age groups, developmental emphases shift as the athlete progresses from the earliest involvement to the peak performance years (table 20.1). In broad terms, 4–11/12 years old may be *excite – participate – practice*; 12/13–18/19 years old: *practice – prepare – perform*; 19/20–22/23 years old: *perform – compete – learn*; 22/23–35+ years old: *learn – win*. Management of the pathway process through the several years should be considered shared 'partnership' responsibility, something along the lines of figure 20.2.

Approximate age range	Development emphases
4–11/12 years	• General all-joint mobility • General all-round strength • Basic health • Positive attitude to exercise and sport • Wide range of sound basic technical models and complex model components • Competitive attitude – challenge/ performance
12/13–18/19 years	• General/related/specific strength • General/related/specific endurance • Specific technical models • Participation/competition opportunity in range of sports • Speed of technical execution • Competitive attitude – performance/results
19/20–22/23 years	• Progressive competition experience • Performance goals acceleration • Dedicated specific training programmes • Long-/medium-/short-term goals preparation • Competitive attitude – results performance
22/23–35+ years	• Pursuit of critical career best performance • Refinements of specific training programmes • Long-/medium-/short-term goals delivery • 'Full-time' approach • Competitive attitude – results
35+ – Life	• 'Detraining' = fitness programme for life wellness

TABLE 20.1 An athlete's development from the earliest years of exercise/sport involvement through the post-competition years requires a strategic approach to addressing development objectives/emphases

Each year of development must be carefully structured to build on previous years' development and as preparation for those to follow. They are each quite different. Here, a close examination is made of the 12-month cycle of an athlete committed to high-level achievement in sport.

SETTING OUT THE TIMESCALE

The start of the competition macrocycle(s) is dictated by (1) the number of competitions necessary for the athlete to reach and stabilise best performance, (2) the dates of the major competition and main competitions, (3) the recovery period required by the athlete between competitions, and (4) the period required for preparation for the major competition (this period must take into account possible acclimatisation to a new environment – time adjustment in east/west shift, altitude adjustment, etc.). These conditions are worth further explanation.

1. **Number of necessary competitions.** Although Harre (1973) suggested 6–8 weeks, other authorities have advanced 6–10 weeks as a reasonable range of time for athletes to reach and stabilise their best performances in mesocycle 3. Harre's (1973) suggestion is more acceptable for mesocycle 3_2 if double periodised. Some athletes commence the competition macrocycle with low-key, non-pressure competitions which are virtually an extension of training time trials. These constitute a type of 'competition control', reintroducing the disciplines of competition warm-up and reporting procedures. Moreover, irrespective of the athlete's level of performance, he has an opportunity to 'get the adrenaline moving' without the stressors of pressure which will come later in the season. Once this stage is completed, the athlete then decides with his coach, the venues, levels of competition and frequency of competition which are required to produce his best performance, his springboard for the main business of the season.

   The coach should be aware of the influence which early good performances by opponents have on an athlete. The season's objectives and the week by week objectives must be understood by athlete and coach. The athlete's early season performances should not be so far adrift from those of the opposition that the athlete feels pressure. Consequently, coaches should introduce the athlete to competitions only when the athlete is ready and only when the objective is understood and attainable.

2. **Dates of competitions.** The important qualifying rounds should be found in the latter 2–4 weeks of the suggested range, thus giving up to six weeks of preparatory contests and up to four weeks of main contests. The major competitions will be, as it were, the 'fixed point' of the season. Thus, if the athlete views the national championships as the major competition, mesocycles 3 or 3_2 and 4 are worked from that date. The coach has the problem of providing the relevant mesocycle 3 (3_2) levels of competition for the athlete over the time-span dictated by the national championships date. On the other hand, the major competition may be an Olympic Games. It would then be in the interest of the Olympic athletes for trials and competitions, designed to produce qualifying marks, to be timetabled for a relevant mesocycle 3 or 3_2. Moreover, as Olympic Games and other major championships constitute a tournament rather than one-off competitions, the athlete must be afforded the opportunity to rehearse the sequence of qualifying rounds/heats and finals in the period leading up to the final selection dates or in the course of the final selection dates.

3. **Recovery period.** This will vary from athlete to athlete according to event, age, experience and standard of competitions. The young athlete, whose ability to produce performances near the limit of his capacity is as yet undeveloped, will compete very regularly – as often as twice to three times per week in inter-club, intra-club, league or open meetings, etc. Although competitions are meaningful to such an athlete, times, distances and heights are a long way from being an ultimate expression of ability. On mounting the club/district/regional/national/ international record ladder, however, the athlete begins to take a more serious view of success and failure. With this change of approach from 'playing' to commitment, both physical and psychological stressors mean more time to prepare for and recover from competitions. It is not unusual, then, to find an athlete at this stage competing only once a week, or every other week. Again, the idea might be extended so that there are only two or three competitions in the season (specific competition climaxes or peaks), while a few other competitions are entered to test fitness or for practice.

Matveyev (1965) suggests that in explosive sports, where the technical component is high (e.g. field events, tennis, gymnastics, team games), several peaks may be pursued. However, where the technical component is lower (e.g. sprints, hurdles), three peaks per season at most can be worked for. This argument can only be defended if, by 'peak', we consider a block of time rather than a particular time on a particular day. On this basis, it is suggested that most athletes cannot sustain maximum performance levels beyond 21 days, and even then such performances are not being repeated at high frequency within these 21 days. The main problem here is as much a psychological/emotional one as it is physiological/physical. Clear understanding and application of the concept of regeneration is essential to ensuring that peak 'blocks of time' can be repeated not only within a given season, but also over several seasons.

In endurance events, where complex training has been used, only two peaks can be expected. The first of these peaks might be considered a 'performance peak' where the athlete pursues a performance objective such as a record, or a performance control on which to base achievement targets for the main competition focus. The second is a 'competition peak' where the athlete builds on what has been achieved in pursuit of the first peak through tournament planning and tactics, to reach for success in the season's major championships. Endurance athletes using the Lydiard method normally aim for one peak in the season. This peak embraces pursuit both of performance and competition objectives and is sustained over a period of up to six weeks during which time competitions are judiciously spaced to have both objectives coincide with the major championships.

It is clear that the process of planning an athlete's season up to a selection date is unique to a given athlete. Ideally, the programme of local, area, national and international competitions made available to athletes is such that the athlete can select those competitions which best suit his programme of preparation. This means that athletes must occasionally make value judgements on whether or not to compete on occasions which have high priority for those organising the competitions, but low priority for the athlete. The objectives of periodising the year were set out at the start of chapter 19. The athlete's value judgements must be made within the framework of these objectives if he is to produce optimal performance at the major championships.

4. **Preparation period.** This period is really mesocycles 4 and 5 looked upon as a whole, with mesocycle 4 lasting 4–6 weeks and mesocycle 5 lasting 3–4 weeks. The content of mesocycle 4 will, of course, be altered considerably from that just described in that it represents a specific programme of preparation for a specific competition. For the young and developing athlete, there seems little justification for imposing a rigid structure of competition in the competition macrocycle. For the mature national and international athlete, however, it is essential. Top-level athletes cannot be expected to produce maximum performance

on every outing. To avoid pressure to do so they may choose to be selective in when to compete against key opposition. In commercially orientated sport, the pressure is great to meet various contractual obligations. Decisions must be made early when planning the year's programme to strike a balance which will avoid compromise to the pursuit of performance and competition objectives, yet will satisfy the sport's commercial sector. When an athlete is preparing to meet the best in the world, both preparation and competition represent intense mental, emotional and physical efforts and cannot be entered into at short intervals. Failure to accept this will lead to an athlete 'burning himself out', and can set the scene for falling short at the major championships. In long, persistent season sports like soccer, managers must rotate players over approximately 6–8-week cycles to avoid similar burn-out. That means that players in squads are operating through different training cycles so that they are at different levels of performance capacity. The cycles are monitored by the manager and his coaching and performance staff. This ensures a generally consistent high quality team output while allowing regeneration and learning opportunity across the squad of players.

According to Harre (1973) the total process of the main competition period spans 12 weeks. Personal experience suggests that this can be 16 weeks in a single periodised year. Young and developing athletes should not go beyond 12 weeks; developing athletes may reach 16 weeks due to the more general nature of their training; and top-level athletes will operate between 10 and 16 according to how they have periodised the year, and how they may have organised the progression of competitions and the competition peaks within the season. Several countries arrange their fixture lists in such a way that a periodised competition season may be followed.

SINGLE AND DOUBLE PERIODISATION

Several attempts have been made to accelerate performance improvement by establishing two competition seasons. The concept of two competition seasons is referred to as double periodisation, while one competition season is single periodisation. The double periodised year has been successfully applied to swimming and track and field. Matveyev (1965) has demonstrated that by this method it is possible to achieve a greater increase per year in those events where maximum and elastic strength are key characteristics (table 20.2).

Event	Double periodisation	Single periodisation
100m	1.55%	0.96%
Long jump	1.46%	1.35%
High jump	5.05%	2.40%
Shot	3.85%	2.58%
Discus	3.87%	3.11%

TABLE 20.2 Percentage annual improvement in performance comparing double and single periodisation (from Matveyev, 1965)

Matveyev's explanation is that the more rapid sequence of competition periods prevents an undue fall-off of competition performance and contributes to the stabilisation of technical performance. By stabilisation it is presumed he is referring to the continued integration of technique and conditioning of one keeping in step with the other. However, this implies a certain status in technical development. It should be emphasised, then, that where long periods of consolidation and development are needed (e.g. basic strength, speed, etc.), and in technique as in the young and developing athlete, double periodisation does not have a strong case. To sub-divide the year into short periods of preparation will only result in incomplete mastery of technique, unstable performance, and a reduced rate of development in the foundations of fitness. The stressor of competition in these circumstances will exaggerate those faults which accompany the pursuit of immediate wins, as opposed to an ultimate optimal improvement in performance. This said, any discussion of single or double periodised years should assume that the athlete has a training maturity of several seasons. The young and developing athlete should therefore use any second season as an adjunct to training rather than a deliberate competition climax (e.g. other games, cross-country, etc.).

Since this discussion implies mature athletes, the main competition period is long both for single and double periodisation. This period is subdivided for both systems into mesocycles 3, 4, 5 or 3_2, 4, 5. So the fundamental difference between single and double periodisation, then, is the existence of a second season. Despite Matveyev's evidence to support the double season, it is not without its antagonists. Although, their criticisms are more requests for caution than rejections, and should be noted, it was always made clear by Matveyev and interpreters of his work that the notion of double periodisation was not generally suited to endurance sports. Of course, there are exceptions where athletes have won world indoors or cross-country titles, then achieved World or Olympic titles in the summer season. However, the breaking up of the preparation period necessary for endurance excellence does not lend itself to continuing endurance sport competition achievement.

It is worth reflecting that the principle of 'double periodisation' has been part of normal sporting life for southern hemisphere sports. These countries' athletes, when it comes to major international championships and games have routinely been exposed to having to deliver high performance through their own season and through the northern hemisphere season.

Implications for the long season sports

Simply playing a team game, as opposed to an individual sport, does not make players different in their capacity to produce peak performance. It becomes essential, then, for team managers in sports such as rugby, ice hockey, basketball, etc. to establish some form of rotation of players as suggested. The biggest competitions for the team in a season will demand that the best players are at their best. These players' preparation plans should be woven around dates of those competitions. If players are also to be able to peak for international team duties, these dates must also be in the equation. If international tournaments such as World or European cups extend the season to the point where the transition cycle is substantially eroded, it is essential to the players' wellbeing that additional weeks are made available for regeneration.

So, many peaks, by definition, means a well-planned regeneration programme and the cyclic reintroduction of general and related training units. In those sports with high and multiple technical demands and conditioning demands, there is a year-round requirement for technical and conditioning work. Cycles of general:related:specific work cannot be compromised to meet the demands of ranking systems. Short-term objectives must be consistent with long-term objectives, and not ends in themselves. The key is to ensure the unbroken competition period is not so long as to erode the general/related conditioning base.

The twenty-first century has seen increasing application of player monitoring (see p. 301) in team games during competition to help make decisions on when to replace players. This is not to be confused with tactical substitutions. It is an acknowledgement that players live on the very edge of these fitness parameters in high performance sport and the slightest impact of fatigue on their efficiency has consequences for the team and the player.

SUMMARY

Designing the periodised year requires thoughtful interpretation of periodisation principles and an understanding of the athlete long term development pathway. A double competition season provides a greater potential for increase in annual performance in most disciplines, but probably not endurance. The advantage gained by expanding the time available for competition opportunity must be weighed against the loss to preparation time. Consequently, when applying double periodisation, careful thought must be given to the phasing of the preparation period within the annual cycle. Moreover, in the athlete's competitive 'life', sound judgement is required in the distribution of double periodised years.

REFLECTIVE QUESTIONS

1. Discuss the value of an athlete tracking programme designed to manage the athlete's development progress to a coach who only works with beginners. What information would you want him to provide as part of the programme? What value would such information be in the short term for the athlete and in the long term for the programme?

2. With reference to table 20.1 outline how you might address the development emphases for the 12/13–18/19 year age ranges over a periodised year.

3. In professional rugby, the less wealthy clubs have a more limited pool of high quality players than the less economically challenged. Consequently the club's best players become essential selections every game to address the bigger teams. Outline your strategy to cope effectively with this situation within the framework of a periodised year with 7–8 months of competition and the cycle of adaptation-application-regeneration.

4. What explanation would you propose for the phenomenon where athletes deliver their best performance of the year in the period up to selection and deliver a lower performance in the championships or games they have been selected for? How would you suggest changing this?

5. Double periodisation has enjoyed some success for summer sports but there is little evidence that it has been applied successfully to the Nordic and Alpine winter sports. Discuss the pros and cons of such a programme and outline a plan to deliver it.

21 UNITS, MICROCYCLES, MESOCYCLES AND MACROCYCLES

The world of 'schedules and sessions' is now examined, although these expressions are losing their popularity. Consequently some of the expressions used here may be new and it may therefore be useful to define them.

THE TRAINING UNIT

The training unit is a single practice session in pursuit of a training objective. For example, the objective may be to develop sprinting speed so the unit might then be $3 \times 4 \times 30$m rolling start sprints, four minutes between repetitions, 7–10 minutes between sets. The objective may be development of aerobic endurance so the unit might be a 20km steady run, or the objective might be active recovery so the unit could be 20–30 minutes football or tennis, and so on.

An athlete's visit to a training venue may, in fact, allow him to work on one or several training units. For instance, a female basketball player may work through three units in one visit to the gym. At 13.00 hours she begins the first unit (mobility exercises) to develop mobility. At 14.00 hours she practises shooting drills to develop accuracy. At 15.00 hours she begins the third unit of $3 \times 3 \times 3$ lengths turnabout court sprints in 15 seconds, with 60 seconds easy run between reps and two minutes between sets, to develop running speed endurance. On the other hand, an evening or lunchtime session may only allow time for one unit. So, simply referring to both situations (i.e. three units in one day, and one unit in one day) as two 'sessions' might cause confusion. This would certainly be the case if one were discussing the number of units per week. To say 'six sessions per week' might mean anything from six to eighteen units!

THE MICROCYCLE

The microcycle is a group of units organised in such a way that optimal training value can be obtained from each unit. Moreover, the microcycle may be repeated several times in pursuit of the overall objectives of a mesocycle or macrocycle.

It is expedient to plan microcycles for a period of one week (table 21.1) as this helps to fit training units into the general framework of social routine. However, it is clear that for many younger athletes the unit ratio of work to rest, even on a one unit per day basis, can lose its training value at 6:1.

A regular cycle of 3:1 may suit this athlete's development better, but the training cycle will fall out of synchronisation with the calendar cycle of one week. If this causes problems, the units might be rearranged. For example, one unit on Saturday, two on Sunday, none Monday, one each on Tuesday, Wednesday and Thursday, and none on Friday. Naturally, the units on Sunday would require careful selection. The ratio of the number of training units to the number of recovery units within a microcycle is the inter-unit training ratio.

Several points are worth noting on the construction of a microcycle:

1. The profile of extent of loading and intensity of loading must be given careful consideration. This profile is often referred to as 'the structure of loading'. Both extent and intensity of loading will be dealt with in greater detail in chapter 22.

2. The demands made on the athlete vary in individual training units in terms of the intra-unit training ratio. This is the relationship of stimulus:recovery within a unit. Thus, the training load represented by each unit has anything from a very high to a slight demand upon the athlete. The athlete must not be exposed to very high demands upon his system in successive units (table 21.1). Although assessments of demand are mainly subjective on the part of the athlete, the observant coach should read the effect of units upon the athlete with whom he is working. Athlete and coach share responsibility for value judgements on the effect of training, and apply their collective input to programme planning as a consequence.

3. Each unit is in pursuit of a specific objective and should vary within a day, and from day to day. Programme planning should then have not only an inbuilt variety of general, related and specific units according to

Day	Objective	Unit	Demand*
Sunday	general conditioning and mobility	Fartlek and woodland conditioning circuit	Medium
Monday	Elastic and maximum strength	maximum and sub-maximum weights	High
Tuesday	special development	throws in weighted jacket with heavy implements	medium–high
Wednesday	elastic strength	combined submaximum weights and jumps	High
Thursday	maximum strength	maximum weights	very high
Friday	general throwing	other throws, jumps, hurdles, special exercises	medium
Saturday	technique development and strength testing	throws and tests	High

*Note varying demands of each unit. Classification was made according to athlete's own impressions in working through programme.

TABLE 21.1 Mesocycle 1 microcycle of a male discus thrower

athlete, sport and place of training, but also variations in unit detail in pursuit of a specific objective. Notwithstanding the need for variety, athletes also require a sense of routine in the programme. The values here range from a basis for comparison to monitor progress, through to the 'comfort' of an established microcycle design. Part of the coach's art is to arrange microcycles in such a way that variety is a key feature within a flexible framework of routine.

4. In order to avoid over-exertion, the interval between two training units should be long enough to allow the athlete to recover sufficiently to gain maximum training effect from the next unit.

5. Recovery is accelerated if units of active recovery, or 'regeneration' units are introduced into the microcycle (see chapter 23).

6. When training units with different objectives and varying demands follow each other, it may not be necessary to await complete recovery. This is the case when different systems are being stressed. This also helps protect the athlete from 'overuse' types of injury.

7. Microcycles also permit concentration on one particular objective in individual units, allowing some optimal period of time when the athlete can be exposed to the desired stimulus. This helps adaptation to develop in a particular area. Poor organisation may bring conflicting objectives into badly grouped units (e.g. when speed loading and endurance loading are brought together some contribution is made to speed and endurance, but the maximal development of either is impossible). Similarly, when an athlete rushes intervals between repetitions of set pieces in games, development of technique is impaired and very little contribution to speed or endurance is made.

8. Microcycles reduce monotony in training despite the high frequency of training units. Failure to use these cycles may mean a standard unit or variation on a unit being used ad nauseam, the result of which would be a stereotyped reaction to the exercise stimulus and an ultimate stagnation of performance, as there is no adaptation challenge.

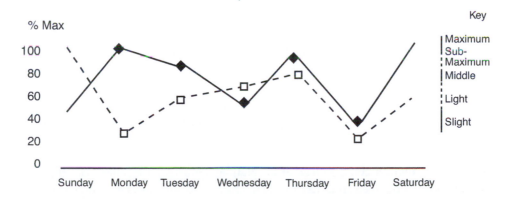

FIGURE 21.1 Alterations in intensity:extent ratio in the course of a microcycle in Mesocycle II. The subject is a female long jumper, and the scale of intensity (maximum, submaximum, etc.) is read against percentage of maximum (vertical scale). The scale of intensity is as suggested by Carl when he advanced the concept as 'spheres of intensity' for weightlifting (from Carl, 1967).

9. Demands on speed or elastic strength or maximum strength should be carried out on days of optimal capacity and never following days of high demand, especially if this involves lactic-anaerobic endurance training. A similar rule will apply when several units are being worked in the course of one day. So the following order of events should be pursued:

Several units in one day:

- warm-up and/or mobility
- neuromuscular work (e.g. technique, speed, elastic strength, maximum strength)
- energy systems work (all endurance – heart, speed, strength)
- aerobic warm-down.

From day to day:

- aerobic/general/recovery
- neuromuscular
- anaerobic endurance.

In the events carried out for maximum strength training the day-to-day pattern alters by intensity and/or exercises.

10. As a rule, 48 hours minimum are required to recover from maximum loadings which will, of course, include competitions. Consequently the loading in the competition period must be so placed that the competition can be carried out in the phase of accentuated capacity (or overcompensation) brought about by optimal loading two to three days beforehand (figures 21.2 and 21.3). Although discussed further in chapter 23, it is worth emphasising here, that adaptation occurs during the recovery phase, so it is important to understand the timescales (b) and (c) in figure 21.2, and the regeneration process.

Adaptable microcycles

For some sports, there are occasions where microcycle design cannot be fixed for any length of time. For example, where players are 'on the road' in constant national or international travel, changing time zones, training and competition venues; or where what happens in terms of tournament progression dictates subsequent training time, availability and location. This is very much the situation for the full-time professional athlete or player.

In these cases, against the background of the foregoing points on microcycle construction, and on the understanding that there is a sound conditioning base, the following notes may help meet the player's or athlete's training needs.

1. In the main, try to follow a cyclic pattern of adaptation; application; regeneration; through training units, with full recovery between units. Extent and intensity of loading in adaptation units should be low to medium, while loading in application units should be low to medium in extent, but high to very high in intensity.

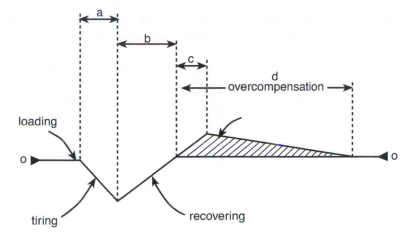

FIGURE 21.2 Cycle of over-compensation (from Yakovlev, 1977). a–d represent periods of time; o represents original status of capacity being trained. a = catabolic effect of training; c = anabolic effect of training.

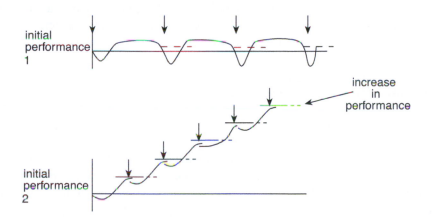

FIGURE 21.3 This illustrates the cumulative effects of training. Since the period of overcompensation, or improved performance, gradually diminishes, there is less increase in performance with longer intervals (1) than with shorter intervals (2). The optimal improvement in performance is achieved when the new loading is presented at the highest point in the overcompensation phase (from Harre, 1973).

2. Create for the athlete/player a selection of those microcycle structures which may be called for, given certain situations. For example there should be a structure provided for one, two, three, four, or five days training opportunity. Where there are more days, either the basic microcycle for that mesocycle in the year, or a special training camp microcycle will apply.

3. Provide a selection of training units from which the athlete will choose the best suited to a given training situation. For example, a player's training microcycle has 'aerobic run' as a unit. The selection on the programme is either 45 minutes easy run (heart rate 155–165) or 30 minutes hard Fartlek on undulating terrain (heart rate should vary between 140 and 180) or 30 minutes steady aqua jogging (heart rate

155–165) or steady mountain bike ride for 75 minutes (heart rate 150–160) or 20 x interval runs using the diagonal of a soccer pitch for the fast run (heart rate 180), jogging the length of the side line as recovery (heart rate 135–145 in 60 seconds).

If the player is in a hotel in the centre of a city which has a swimming pool, the player is able to aqua jog. The next day, the player may travel at midday and will not arrive at his destination until late at night. The training unit for that day is 'general strength' for which the selection on the programme is either personal weight training programme (60 minutes) or personal strength machine programme (45 minutes) or personal body circuit (30 minutes).

Time and limited equipment suggest the latter programme. In other words, the coach must prepare a series of options in advance.

4. Encourage the player/athlete to keep a record of what is done so that this information can be considered in designing the next basic microcycle.

5. Regeneration units should also be on the basis of a selection to choose from.

The player/athlete will, then, develop an involvement in establishing his cyclic training process as part of a lifestyle of continuous travel and competition which can become stressful. Regeneration units are very important inclusions in the 'adaptable microcycle' as a contribution to stress management.

MACROCYCLES AND MESOCYCLES

The macrocycle, and smaller mesocycle, is the sum of all units required to bring the status of training to that level required to meet the macrocycle objectives which relate to preparation (adaptation), competition (application) and transition (regeneration) within the annual cycle. To achieve those objectives, the coach designs and manages the content and duration of mesocycles. The mesocycle then becomes the vehicle for adjusting and adapting macrocycles to address the variance of annual objective within the overall purpose of Olympic or longer cycles. The mesocycle affords capacity for a quick and flexible response in the continuous process of reviewing, learning and changing to make macrocycles effective in their function.

A mesocycle is the sum of all units required to bring the status of training to that level required to meet its objectives. They exist to characterise progress of intensity and extent of loading, and are required to make the rhythmic changes from periods of high average loading to shorter periods of reducing loading.

Clearly they are regulated by the competition macrocycle(s). Although some mesocycles may be stretched to eight weeks, extending beyond six weeks can dull the athlete's motivation and capacity to work beyond the limits of present adaptation levels.

The shape of loading in the preparation macrocycle arises from the basic principle that within each macrocycle one establishes an optimal intensity consistent with a sound technical model, an increase in extent of loading is achieved, then the intensity in each unit is raised. The Oregon method of endurance training associated with Bill Bowerman classically illustrates this principle (see pp. 280–81). Ter-Ovanesyan (1965) describes extension of the principle to competition preparation, where, over a five week mesocycle, the total extent of loadings were increased over weeks 1–3, and then reduced, while intensity continued to increase to the competition itself.

In meeting macrocycle objectives, the coach must have collected the following information:

- The number of units of training available in the mesocycle(s). For example, in the months of November/December, the athlete may be able to programme nine units per week – approximately 70 units in total.
- The percentage distribution of general, related and specific training.
- The inter-unit training ratio.
- The structure of loading for the mesocycle.
- The structure of loading and intra-unit training ratio relevant to each type of training in microcycles.
- The manner of increasing extent and intensity within the macrocycle.
- The athlete's evaluation of the effects of training at unit, microcycle, mesocycle and macrocycle levels.

Training area	Classification	% units
aerobic endurance	general	11
speed endurance	special	11
strength endurance	general	11
speed	competition specific	5.5
elastic strength	special	11
maximum strength	special	5.5
mobility	general	11
sprint technique	competition specific	11
active recovery	general	23

TABLE 21.2 Possible breakdown of units for a 17-year-old girl sprinter – mesocycle 1

For example, in table 21.2 we have a suggested breakdown of units for a 17-year-old girl sprinter in mesocycle 1. This represents 10 units per week for five weeks. In each microcycle of one week, the athlete has a programme which is set out below:

Saturday	2
Sunday	2
Monday	1
Tuesday	2
Wednesday	1
Thursday	2
Friday	0

The next step will be to detail the objective of each unit indicated on the weekly microcycle, over all five weeks of the mesocycle. This might be done as shown in table 21.3. Obviously, the final interpretation of the percentages is flexible, but they have been kept, in the main, close to the original suggestion.

Day		Week 1	Week 2	Week 3	Week 4	Week 5
Saturday	A	sprint technique	sprint technique	sprint technique	sprint technique	sprint technique
	B	aerobic	aerobic	aerobic	aerobic	aerobic
Sunday	A	max strength	elastic strength	max strength	elastic strength	max strength
	B	speed/ endurance	speed/ endurance	speed/ endurance	speed/ endurance	speed/ endurance
Monday	A	active recovery	active recovery	active recovery	active recovery	active recovery
Tuesday	A	speed	sprint tech	speed	sprint tech	speed
	B	mobility	mobility	mobility	mobility	mobility
Wednesday	A	active recovery	active recovery	active recovery	active recovery	active recovery
Thursday	A	elastic strength	elastic strength	elastic strength	elastic strength	elastic strength
	B	strength endurance	strength endurance	strength endurance	strength endurance	strength endurance
Friday	A	0	0	0	0	0

TABLE 21.3 Approximate distribution of training objectives against the suggested percentages

When working with an experienced athlete, the coach weighs all such considerations in setting out mesocycles as building blocks through the 52 weeks of the annual cycle.

The following is an example of a mesocycle breakdown for an experienced sprint athlete over the year.

Mesocycle 1_1	2 weeks	General training – strength, endurance, mobility (if required, some compensatory focus for reinforcing rehabilitation, etc., post previous season).
Mesocycle 1_2	6 weeks	Core training to provide very strong foundation for the more specific work to follow
Mesocycle 1_3	5 weeks	Discipline – specific training focus.
Mesocycle 2_1	4 weeks	Competition preparation including training competitions.
Mesocycle 3_1	4 weeks	Competition (indoor athletics season).
Mesocycle 4_1	1 week	Regeneration, review, refocus.

Mesocycle 1_4	4 weeks	Core training 'top-up'.
Mesocycle 1_5	6 weeks	High-intensity discipline – specific training.
Mesocycle 2_2	4 weeks	Competition preparation including training competitions.
Mesocycle 3_2	6 weeks	Main competition season including key championships qualifying competitions.
Mesocycle 4_2	2 weeks	Regeneration, review, refocus (including competition preparation units).
Mesocycle 5	4 weeks	Major Championships goal.
Mesocycle 6	4 weeks	Regeneration.

Fitness and medical controls relate to key performance development milestones throughout the annual cycle.

Next, the detail of each training unit in terms of the number of repetitions, sets, distances, intervals, kilos, exercises, etc., would be listed. Finally, the progression of extent and intensity would be established. For example, numbers of repetitions and/or sets will be increased in weeks 1–3, while in weeks 4–5 repetitions and sets will return to those of week one, but runs will be faster, loads heavier, or intervals shorter.

As a guide to training ratios, table 21.4 is offered as suggested percentages on which to work for track and field. It will be noted that columns are headed G (general), R (related) and S (specific). Osolin and Markov (1972) suggest statistics for the three periods and their figures have been used in compiling the percentages listed here.

	Percentage of training units																	
	I			**II**			**III**			**IV**			**V**			**VI**		
Beginners and developing athletes	G	R	S	G	R	S	G	R	S	G	R	S	G	R	S	G	R	S
10–14 yrs	70	10	20	60	20	20	50	20	30	60	20	20	50	20	30	80	10	10
15–17 yrs	60	20	20	50	25	25	50	20	30	50	25	25	50	20	30	70	20	10
18–19 yrs	50	25	25	40	25	35	25	25	50	45	30	25	15	25	60	75	15	10
novice seniors	50	25	25	40	25	35	25	25	50	45	30	25	25	25	50	75	15	10
Experienced athletes																		
sprints, long and triple	25	55	20	15	60	25	10	55	35	25	55	20	10	60	30	80	10	10
middle distance and walkers	20	75	5	20	70	10	10	70	20	10	85	5	10	80	10	55	40	5
long distance and marathon	10	85	5	10	85	5	5	90	5	10	85	5	5	90	5	45	50	5
hurdles, high, pole vault	35	35	30	25	35	40	10	40	50	20	40	40	10	40	50	80	10	10
throws	25	35	40	15	45	40	10	40	50	20	40	40	10	40	50	80	10	10

TABLE 21.4 Percentage distribution of general (G), related (R), and specific (S) training units according to the phase of the periodised year

SUMMARY

The pattern of the training plan should be seen in relation to that of all other natural phenomena. Just as the seasons follow a cycle, and our various physiological systems follow the laws of chronobiology, so training must follow a cyclical pattern. The broad areas of the cycle may be summarised as preparation (adaptation), competition (application), and transition (regeneration). These are the macrocycles of the annual cycle. The areas are reflected at all levels from unit to annual cycle to the athlete's competitive 'life'. To progress the athlete's pursuit of competitive advantage, training units that represent specific structures of loadings are organised for optimal effect by applying correct training ratios into microcycles. These are repeated with progressions to form mesocycles, which are designed to achieve the purpose of the macrocycle to which they belong. By careful emphasis on distribution of general, related and specific training, the phases are structured to meet objectives relative to progression through the periods of the annual cycle. Finally, each annual cycle has a unique character in terms of its contribution to the athlete's ultimate sporting objective.

REFLECTIVE QUESTIONS

1. Design three training units each for four of the following so they may apply to the discipline indicated:

   a. Speed   Female Rugby union
   b. Aerobic endurance   America's Cup sailor
   c. Lactic anaerobic endurance   200m medley swimmer
   d. Creatine phosphate (CrP) energy system   Male sprint cyclist
   e. Leg power   Female triple jumper
   f. Upper body mobility   Male basketball player
   g. Speed endurance   Wheelchair paralympian 200m track
   h. Strength endurance   Long track speed skater

2. Outline a microcycle for a core training mesocycle with three units per day possible given athlete daily routine, for one of the following:

   a. A female national level gymnast – 16 years
   b. A male kayak slalom, K-1 – 24 years
   c. A heptathlete – 21 years
   d. Men's 20km biathlon – 28 years
   e. A male soccer goalkeeper –30 years
   f. A netball centre – 18 years

3. Discuss the possible bases of your decision making in changing the various microcycle units for a more discipline specific subsequent mesocycle.

4. In the first week of mesocycle 2 of a 20 year old female hurdler's year plan, she is at a warm weather training camp. The objective of the camp is pre-competition preparation, with the season starting in six weeks. The athlete has tightness in her left hamstring and right adductor. The physio's opinion is that the tightness is actually coming from tension in the lower back. Her economics from national funds is directly related to her achieving performance standards and results. Discuss how you would proceed to address this issue, including who you might consult in forming a plan of action for this mesocycle and the next.

5. In the team you are coaching, two athletes have found coaches via social media who have different views on the design of the current mesocycle you have prepared. The differences relate to technique units. Discuss how you would guide a discussion on this issue towards a constructive approach to review of the mesocycle content.

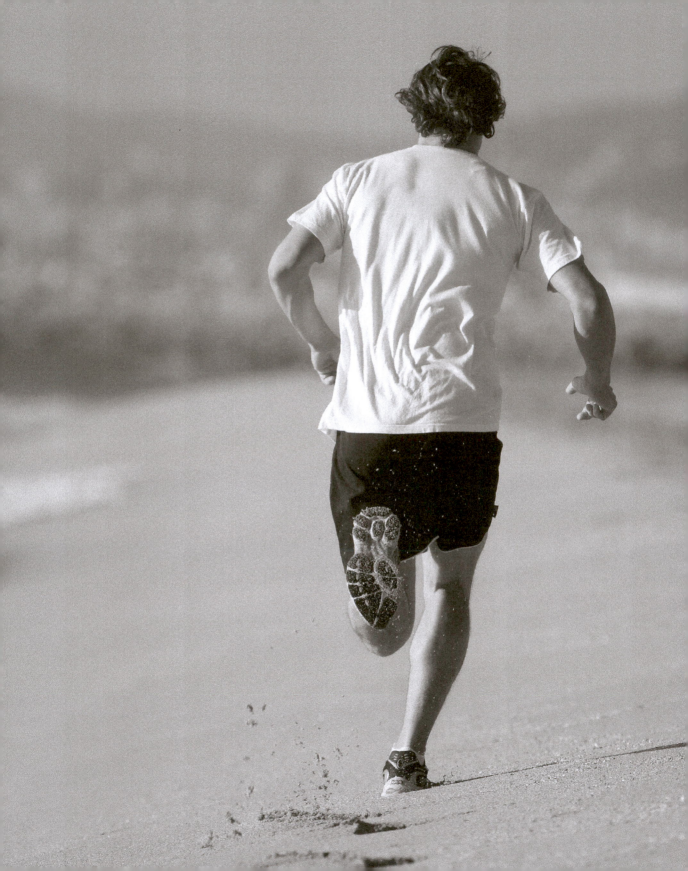

22 ADAPTATION TO LOADING

Adaptation is the raising of the athlete's functioning capacity due to external loading and/or adjustment to specific environmental conditions. Physical, intellectual and emotional adaptation must be seen as one process.

We adapt to a stressor by 'learning' to cope with it. The 'learning' follows a stress response where adaptation energy is applied to accommodate the threat to normal functions capacity represented by the stressor. Whether the stressor is physical, intellectual or emotional, it's the same general adaptation energy source which is accessed. We seldom have single stressors to cope with, rather, they are multiple and their energy requirement cumulative (figure 13.4, p. 220). So, although the adaptation focus may be, say, strength in a training unit, other stressors vie for adaptation energy. Because the total amount of adaptation energy is finite, the total stressor picture must be understood to ensure a positive, rather than negative, effect of training.

DEFINITION

Training offers the athlete external loading and it is quite obvious that there is a relationship between loading and adaptation. The three laws of training (specificity, overload and reversibility) qualify and quantify loading. However, while these laws are fairly explicit, there are some points which should be emphasised.

1. A high extent of load without the necessary minimum intensity fails to produce adaptation just as much as high intensity with too little extent.

2. The more the amounts of loading approach an optimal value relative to the athlete's capacity at the moment of loading, the more rapidly adaptation takes place. Conversely, the greater the departure from that value (either over or under-loading) the less the adaptation.

3. If the demands of loading exceed the athlete's capacity, or if the structure of loading is wrong, then the athlete's capacity to adapt is compromised and performance will stagnate or even be reduced.

4. The relationship between loading and recovery is critical and they should be seen as a whole (figure 21.2, p. 333). This will be discussed in greater detail in chapter 23.

5. While 'overcompensation' is quickly transformed to a higher level of performance in the young and developing athlete, this process may take weeks or months with the mature athlete. Each loading close to the optimum will leave behind it a trace of overcompensation, but for the mature athlete it is only due to the cumulative effect of training that improvements come at intervals, and not necessarily regular intervals. Matveyev (1965) refers to this as 'delayed transformation': '[it] prevents the continuous flow of infor-

mation on the effect of loading on training that is necessary for the optimal regulation of the training process'. Progressive adaptation is not therefore easily apparent and only the results of competition or tests at the end of mesocycle 2 or at the start of mesocycle 3 show whether or not loading has been effective. Periodic checks and test procedures geared to accurate prediction are therefore vital throughout mesocycles 1 and 2. It is feasible that the introduction of mesocycle 3_2, in double periodisation, may provide a most relevant testing procedure.

6. Loading must be systematically and progressively increased. Loadings that remain unchanged are more easily overcome in time and cause less disruption of the body's systems, but their effect diminishes until they simply maintain a stationary state of adaptation. The organism will adapt only if it is challenged to do so. The challenge of a well-designed mesocycle is optimal between six and eight weeks.

7. The rate at which capacity reduces on reduction or cessation of loading is critical to the athlete. Illness, travel during the competition season, examinations, injury, etc., all imply disruption of the systematic increase of loadings. Moreover, during the competition season, loadings are frequently reduced in extent (and even intensity by some coaches). Again, this represents a break in continuity of the adaptation process. The more recent the level of adaptation, the more quickly it will be affected by reduced loading. Long periods of gradual development are therefore indicated. Lengthy transitional periods without training loading are to be avoided and, if the interval between training units is too long, the effect of loadings is lost. Finally, attention is drawn again to the relevance of a 'polyvalent' or mixed approach and to pursuing a changing training ratio throughout the year.

8. The rate of return from the catabolic through to the anabolic peak in overcompensation is also critical to the athlete. The shorter the interval, the more training may be performed per unit of time. That interval will have an optimal duration for the athlete and specific training focus to accommodate frequency of training stimulus while avoiding the energy sapping effect of cumulative stressors.

9. Loadings of great extent and slight to medium intensity primarily develop endurance capacity. Those of less extent, but sub-maximum to maximum intensity, mainly develop maximum strength, elastic strength and speed. While this may be accurate for the mature athlete, the young and developing athlete is affected by loadings in a far more complex way. Consequently, as Harre has noted (1973), the bulk of his work which is low to middle intensity, also develops strength and speed, to a certain extent. But what exactly do expressions like 'middle intensity' mean? To arrive at an explanation, one must first examine the expression 'intensity'.

Intensity of loading

The intensity of loading is characterised by the strength of the stimulus, or by the concentration of work executed per unit of time within a series of stimuli. Intensity for endurance or speed is calculated according to the speed in m/second or the frequency of movement, for example cadence in sprinting. For strength exercises the amount of resistance is measured, and for jumping or throwing, the height or distance (loaded and/or unloaded) is used. Since intensity varies in exercise it is useful to distinguish between 'spheres of intensity', as Carl (1967) has called them. In order to compare the loading of athletes, these spheres should be established with reference to a fixed point and should be clearly delineated. For exercises to develop maximum strength, speed, elastic strength, etc., the highest possible individual intensity of stimulation is taken as the point of reference, maximum loading being equal to 100 per cent (tables 22.1, 22.2 and 22.3). In the growing years, with strength development, '10 reps maximum' should be used as the reference point for 100 per cent.

A standard scale of intensity would be most useful. It would establish a basic frame of reference and help in the evaluation of training theory. It is, after all, at the comparative level that the real meaning of loading becomes apparent. For too long there has been no marketplace to exchange the various currencies in which each coach transacts the business of relating unit to athlete. Table 22.1 is offered as a basis for such an intensity scale.

Best 150m					Percentage of best time					
(100%)	65%	66.7%	73%	75%	80%	83%	87.5%	90%	95%	97%
18.3	27.9	–	25.0	–	–	22.1	20.8	20.1	19.2	18.8
18.5	–	27.4	25.1	24.6	23.1	22.4	21.1	20.5	19.5	18.9
18.8	28.4	27.9	25.57	25.0	23.4	22.7	21.4	20.8	19.7	19.2
18.9	28.9	–	–	25.1	23.8	–	21.7	21.1	20.0	19.5
19.2	–	28.4	26.0	–	24.2	23.1	22.1	21.4	20.3	19.7
19.5	30.0	28.9	26.4	25.5	–	23.4	22.3.	21.7	20.5	20.0
19.7	30.6	–	26.9	26.0	24.6	23.8	22.7	22.1	20.8	20.1
20.0	–	30.0	–	26.4	25.0	24.2	–	–	21.1	20.5
20.3	31.3	30.6	27.4	–	25.4	24.6	23.1	22.4	21.4	20.8
20.5	31.9	–	27.9	26.9	25.9	–	23.4	22.7	21.7	21.1
20.8	–	31.3	–	27.4	–	25.0	23.8	23.1	22.1	21.4
21.1	32.6	31.9	28.4	27.9	26.3	25.1	24.2	23.4	22.4	21.7
Best 200m										
20.0	30.7	29.4	27.3	26.6	25.0	24.0	22.7	22.2	21.0	20.6
20.2	31.2	30.3	27.7	27.0	25.3	24.3	22.9	22.4	21.2	20.8
20.4	–	30.7	–	–	–	24.6	23.2	22.7	21.5	21.0
20.6	31.7	–	28.1	27.3	25.6	–	23.5	22.9	21.7	21.2
20.8	32.2	31.2	28.5	27.7	25.9	25.0	23.8	23.2	21.9	21.5
21.0	–	31.7	28.9	28.1	26.3	25.3	24.0	23.4	22.2	21.7
21.2	32.7	–	–	–	26.6	25.6	24.3	23.6	22.4	21.9
21.5	33.3	32.2	29.4	28.5	27.0	25.9	24.6	23.8	22.7	22.2
21.7	–	32.7	29.9	28.9	–	26.3	–	24.0	22.9	22.4
21.9	33.8	–	30.3	29.4	27.3	–	25.0	24.3	23.2	22.7
22.2	–	33.3	–	–	27.7	26.6	25.3	24.6	–	22.9
22.4	34.4	33.8	30.7	29.8	28.1	27.0	25.6	25.0	23.5	23.2
22.7	35.0	–	31.2	30.3	28.5	27.3	25.9	25.3	23.8	23.5

TABLE 22.1 Example of possible table for percentage intensity to be used for track running. The spheres of intensity are then derived from this. A problem arises where authorities offer varying spheres of intensity (see table 22.2).

Dick	designation of intensity	Carl (1967)*
	slight	30–50%
	light	50–70%
65–73%	middle	70–80%
75–83%	high	
87.5–97%	submaximum	80–90%
	maximum	90–100%

* Suggested spheres of intensity in weight training

TABLE 22.2 Comparison of terms used in describing loading as % max. intensity

Scale of intensity	Percentage of maximum
low	30–49%
light	50–64%
medium	65–74%
high	75–84%
submaximum	85–94%
maximum	95–100%

TABLE 22.3 Suggested standard intensity scale

When training for endurance events, intensity is ideally evaluated against the best performances over the training distance, or against the average competition speed at the moment. However, in passing, it should be noted that since training at given intensities of VO_2 maximum have great relevance to the energy system involved, the measure of intensity may well be 'read' from the working heart rate and against the percentage of VO_2 maximum (table 5.4, p. 98).

Density in loading

The density or frequency of stimulus in loading is determined by the objective of the unit, the stimulus being controlled both by its intensity and duration. Knowing this, an optimal density can be established which will allow an evaluation of the number of consecutive occasions per unit when the athlete is exposed to the stimulus, and also the amount of time between these occasions. In pursuit of specificity of loading effect, numbers of repetitions and sets are married to the interval of time between them to create an optimal density. From these precepts, crude formulae have evolved for the development of specific endurance capacities (table 22.4).

In strength and speed work at sub-maximum to maximum intensities, 2–5 minutes are necessary between successive loadings.

Characteristic	Loading:recovery	Intensity
heart endurance	continuous	light
heart endurance	2:1–1:1	high
speed endurance	1:3–1:6	submaximum

TABLE 22.4 Suggested intra-unit training ratios according to endurance characteristic to be developed

Duration of stimulus in loading

The duration of stimulus is the period of influence of a single stimulus. A difference then exists between this, the relative intensity, and the highest intensity recorded in a particular unit, or cycle. In this case, the value is known as absolute intensity, the distance covered in a repetition, or the total time to complete all loading in a unit. Just as there appear to be thresholds of intensity, so also for duration. Thus, Gundlach (1968) suggests at least 20–30 per cent of maximum holding time is essential for the improvement of isometric strength. Endemann (1973) used this information in his 'auxotonic training' where resistances were consciously controlled in their speed of movement (e.g. five seconds lowering, five seconds raising bar in bench press). Hollmann and Venrath (1962) determined that at least 30 minutes duration of stimulus was required at a given intensity for significant improvement in aerobic endurance. Moreover, it seems clear from figure 6.2, p. 106, that a minimum of two minutes duration at a relatively high intensity of stimulus is necessary to adapt the athlete to the acid base imbalance of competition in short and medium duration endurance disciplines. Obviously, the duration of work in maximum and elastic strength, mobility and speed development must not be so long that fatigue reduces the ability to perform efficiently.

Finally, in pursuit of strength endurance, the duration of loading must be such that considerable effort of will is required to complete the unit.

Extent of loading

The extent of loading is the sum of duration (time or distance) and the repetitions of all stimuli in a training unit. Consequently it will be expressed in kilometres in endurance training, in kilograms in strength training (the sum of loadings), and in the number of repetitions in strength endurance, etc. It is necessary, of course, to divide the extent of loadings into various spheres of intensity, or, if it is agreed, to divide the loadings according to the suggested scale in table 22.3.

The unit, then, is a complex of intensity, extent, duration and density of loading. For optimal value to be derived from each unit, no athlete should arrive at the start of one unit while still fatigued from the previous unit unless performance in a climate of progressive fatigue is the training objective. A full understanding of the unit complex, and the effect each unit has upon the athlete, is essential to the coach. From here the microcycle begins to evolve with an understanding of what should constitute a unit of loading for an athlete and the frequency of exposure of the athlete to that unit.

Extent of training is, therefore, the sum total of hours, kilograms or kilometres of training, calculated from the cumulation of units and their frequency – the whole being expressed over a unit, microcycle, mesocycle, macrocycle, or, indeed, annual cycle (figure 22.1).

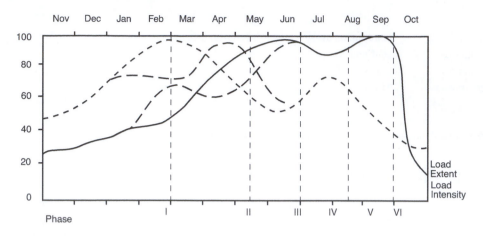

FIGURE 22.1 The suggested relationship between extent and intensity of loading in the annual cycle of single and double periodised years (from Matveyev, 1965)

Progressive loading

'Progression of loading in pursuit of progression of performance improvement' might, in a nutshell, represent the whole purpose of training. From the above discussion of adaptation and loading, 'progression of loading' will be seen as greater extent, higher intensity, longer duration, greater density or increased frequency, or a combination of some or all of these. Loading must always bear a particular relationship to the athlete's present loading capacity. Consequently, no 'absolutes' can be given in terms of loading progression. However, the following general principles do operate to guide the coach when increasing loading:

1. In technical and tactical training, loading is increased by imposing greater demands on the coordination required of a technique. This can be achieved by:

   - demanding greater speed in execution and/or selecting correct technical solution;
   - requiring technical exactness in an endurance situation;
   - combining various elements of practice;
   - changing external conditions;
   - learning more complex technical variations;
   - offering competition pressure.

   Not only do such practices develop technical efficiency, but they also develop specific physical capacities such as mobility and the ability to make rapid and correct adjustment when a loss of balance threatens technical precision.

2. For endurance, strength, speed, elastic strength, etc., the structure of loading must be altered. The main problem here is to decide exactly the alteration of ratio of intensity to extent from mesocycle to mesocycle, or, for that matter, from athlete to athlete, in the whole range from the beginner to the elite. The problem does not end there, however, because great thought must be given to the question

of which components (endurance, strength, etc.) should be stressed in the increase of loading. To say simply that this varies according to athlete and event, and that herein lies the art and mastery of coaching, is quite an indictment of coaches' progress in establishing firm training principles. It is true that to date the state of knowledge in this field is most unsatisfactory, yet it is equally true that the roots of such knowledge lie with coaches and athletes. However, until knowledge in this area becomes more specialised, it is clear that, in general, when the athlete's degree of adaptation has been raised, loading must then become more comprehensive and more intensive. This means that the athlete must be exposed to raised loadings specific to all facets of his sport and, that such an increase is not one of extent, but of intensity. This generalisation must be applied to specific sports. Consequently the coach must evaluate both sport and athlete and be able to apply this information to improve the athlete's status of adaptation.

3. For the beginner in sport, another general principle is: 'Fit the sport to the athlete – then fit the athlete to the sport'. Once this introductory stage is past, these athletes will achieve more stable adaptation and, ultimately, a greater improvement in performance if intensity is raised cautiously and loading progression is primarily via more extensive training. According to Harre (1973), the progression is:

- raise the frequency of training (e.g. number of consecutive units, say, from twice weekly to daily training);
- raise the extent of loading per training unit, while keeping frequency constant;
- raise the density of loading within the training unit.

This progression can only be applied given stable technical quality. As a rule, it is not acceptable to the athlete to bring about these three stages simultaneously. At first an optimal frequency is sought and only when time is limited should the coach consider increasing the load.

4. Analysis of individual athletes' training has shown that a linear gradual increase of loading is not as effective as increases by 'jumps' spaced at given intervals. It would appear that increasing loading in such jumps suddenly taxes the status of the athlete's capacities and 'disturbs the physical–psychological balance' (Harre, 1973).

   This then forces the athlete's total organism to establish new physical–psychological processes of regulation and adaptation. The most obvious examples of this are seen at the start of mesocycle 1 where extent is advanced by jumps (compared with mesocycles 4 and 6 of the previous cycle), thus affecting rapid strength endurance and aerobic status, and at the start of mesocycle 3 where intensity is advanced due to severe competition specific loadings and is accompanied by rapid improvements in performance. The time interval between such jumps is, again, arrived at individually, but several coaches now tie these in with 4–6 week mesocycles. Chronobiology will almost certainly offer a great contribution to understanding such time intervals. Obviously, the athlete will require some time to adapt to the sudden increase in loading and stabilise his training level, but adaptation of processes and stability do not necessarily advance together.

5. The 'jumps' of increased loading may be formalised by maintaining a six-weekly programme review where progress follows a 'sigmoid' shape (figure 22.2).

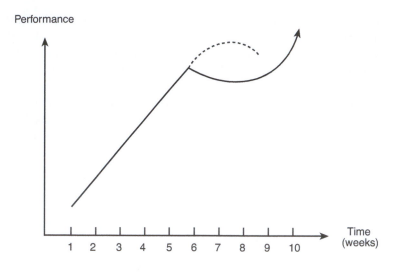

FIGURE 22.2 Although the athlete continues to adapt to the aggregated stressors of a training mesocycle up to around eight weeks, it ensures optimal cumulative training effect when a new mesocycle is introduced at six-weekly (max) intervals

6. The next question is how much to increase loading with each jump, or from year to year. Again, there is little to use as a basis for absolutes, but Matveyev (1965) determined an increase of 20–50 per cent in extent from one year to the next through the developing years. With elite, older athletes there is less increase and sometimes even a reduction. This of course, will vary from sport to sport and will depend on conditions and time available for training. The progressions then will grow from an educated appraisal by the coach of conditions and time, using a logical progression based upon the foregoing general principles. The hardest area of judgement for the coach is when to maintain rather than increase extent or intensity.

On the subject of increasing intensity, personal observation suggests a maximum increment of 2.5–5 per cent per mesocycle where a particular unit or its derivative runs throughout a year. This policy is only altered for testing sessions, or when the very high intensity demanded of mesocycles 3_1, 3, or 3_2 implies work to maximum (see below).

Repetition runs over 300m – female long jumper (100% taken as previous best):
Mesocycle 1: 3 × 75% (4 mins) → 5 × 75% (4 mins)
Test to establish new 100%
4 × 80% (4 mins) → 5 × 80% (4 mins)
Test to establish new 100%
Mesocycle 2: 4 × 85% (7.5 mins) → 5 × 85% (7.5 mins)
Test to establish new 100%
3 × 90% (10 mins)
Test to establish new 100%
Mesocycle 3: 2 × 90% (15 mins)
1–2 × 100% with full recovery
(figures in brackets are recovery times)

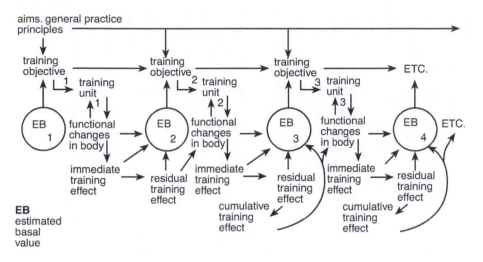

FIGURE 22.3 Summary of the effects of training

7. Within training units, at the exercise level, there can be considerable confusion over the available avenues for progression. There are only three:

- perform the exercise more often (or for greater duration) (endurance factor);
- perform the exercise against increased resistance (strength factor);
- perform the exercise faster (speed factor).

Progression may only be considered when the athlete's performance of the exercise is technically sound. If the performance breaks down to a comfortable compromise, then clearly there is no basis for progression.

8. It is important that the coach fully understands that the athlete experiences three separate effects of training. They are: the immediate effect; the residual effect; the cumulative effect. Each contributes to the pattern of events which have been represented in figures 21.2 and 21.3 (page 333).

- The immediate effect is a breaking down or depleting of the adaptation energy reserve – so it is the catabolic effect of training (figure 21.2a).
- The residual effect is the regenerating and overcompensating process – so it is anabolic (figure 21.2b and c).
- The cumulative effect is the continuing process of capitalising on the advantage which the overcompensation phase (figure 21.2d) affords and is represented by figure 21.3.

The overall picture is summarised in figure 22.3.

This is all very straightforward when the training objective is singular, for example in progressing leg strength through a weight training programme. The situation becomes more complex when several training objectives are being pursued. Figure 22.4 represents the weekly microcycle of a decathlete, and shows how pursuit

TRAINING PHASE PLAN Name (Athlete/Team). _____

Phase No: 2

Commencing: 18 . X . 87

Ending: 28 . XI . 87

No. of Weeks: 6

Objectives: 1. SPECIFIC RUNNING ENDURANCE

2. SPECIAL STRENGTH - THROWS

- JUMPS

3. TECHNIQUE

Progression by Weeks or Sessions

Unit Detail (left block)

Day	Unit 1	Unit 2	Unit 3	Unit 4	Unit 5	Unit 6
1.	T4	HURDLES DRILLS	JAVELIN	GENERAL JUMPS	DRILLS	STRENGTH B
2.	T3(4)	HURDLES DRILLS	JAVELIN	DISCUS	HIGH	STRENGTH A
3.	T1(4)		SHOT DRILLS	DISCUS	POLE	STRENGTH B
4.	T2	HURDLES ENDURANCE	JAVELIN DRILLS		LONG	STRENGTH A
5.	T4		SHOT	DISCUS DRILLS	POLE	STRENGTH B
6.	T1(6)	HURDLES DRILLS	JAVELIN DRILLS		HIGH	STRENGTH C
7.	T3(6)		GENERAL THROWS	DRILLS		
8.						
9.						
10.						
11.						
12.						
13.						
14.						

Cycle of 7 Days Registered 6 Times

Right-hand unit detail / progression columns (1–10):

T 4:30 MINS FARTLEK HILLS — 6X 200m HILLS

3X3 X 60m HILLS

T3(4) 2X (300 250 200) — 48 37.5 28

(6) X 200m

3 X 4(4) (300 500m 200) — S1 30

450 300 150 — 75 42 21

T2 SPRINT : HOLD : SPRINT : HOLD : SPRINT (30m : 30m : 30m : 30m : 30m)

3 X 3 X 3

T4 4 X 3 X 3 — 100m BUILD UP (2)

2 X 3 X (6) 40m STANDING START

2 X 3 X 30m ROLLING START (6)

HURDLES DRILLS

LEAD LEG & TRAIL LEG ISOLATION PLUS FULL TECHNIQUE

HURDLES ENDURANCE -

2 X 4 X 12 HURDLES

TECHNIQUE AND SPECIAL STRENGTH DRILLS ARE BLENDED

INTO TRAINING UNITS OF 90 MINUTE DURATION FOR ALL FIELD EVENTS

Progression recovery notes:
- RECOVERY: JOG 200m REST 4 mins
- RECOVERY: 3m - 2m - 3m - 2m - 3m
- RECOVERY: 6 min
- 150 (3 min) 300 (4 min) / 450 (5 min) 300 (4 min)
- RECOVERY: WALK BACK REST 10 mins
- RECOVERY: WALK BACK REST 5 mins
- RECOVERY: WALK BACK REST 5 mins
- REST 15 mins
- 1 STEP : 3 STEP : 5 STEP : 7 STEP
- RECOVERY: 3 mins 40mins

Unit Detail (strength/running progression table, columns 1–10):

Unit Detail	1	2	3	4	5	6	7	8	9	10
STRENGTH B										
HARNESS RUNNING	4X 75m	4X 75m	5X 75m	5X 75m	6X 75m	6X 75m				
HIGH KNEE RUNNING	4X 60m	4X 60m								
HURDLE REBOUNDS	6 HURDLES	6 HURDLES	8 HURDLES	8 HURDLES	10 HURDLES	10 HURDLES		HURDLES 3' HEIGHT		
TWO-FOOT JUMPS	4X 30m	4X 30m	5X 30m	5X 30m	6X 30m	6X 30m				
DOUBLE HOPPING R.L LR LL	4X 30m	4X 30m	5X 30m	5X 30m	6X 30m	6X 30m				
STANDING 5 BOUNDS	4X	4X	5X	5X	6X	6X				
POWER RUNNING	4 X 100m					→				
	RECOVERY: WALK BACK BETWEEN EACH									
	REPETITION : 3 mins BETWEEN EACH NEW EXERCISE									
STRENGTH A										
POWER CLEAN	3 - 5 X 5 X 85% MAX									
BENT ARM PULL-OVER	3 - 5 X 10 X 30 KG									
BENT ARM FLIES	3 - 5 X 10 X 15 KG									
DUMBELL RAISE	3 - 5 X 10 X 10 KG									
INCLINED DUMBELL PRESS	3 - 5 X 10 X 35 KG									
HANGING BACK EXTENSION	3 - 5 X 8 X 10 KG									
STRENGTH C										
1/2 SQUAT WITH JUMP	8 X 25	8 X 25	8 X 30	8 X 30						
PRESS-UP WITH JUMP	8 X 20	8 X 23	8 X 25							
SIT-UP WITH JUMP	8 X 40	8 X 45	8 X 50	8 X 50						
TREADMILLS	8 X 30	8 X 33	8 X 35	8 X 35						

FIGURE 22.4 Example of a microcycle for a decathlete, and progression through a mesocycle

of the stated objectives will proceed over a six week mesocycle. The proposed progressions for individual units are sound as they stand – but they may not be if the aggregate cumulative effect of all training units is such that the aggregate residual effect cannot reach the level of overcompensation. At this point the overall training load will damage rather than benefit the athlete. The importance of responsible interpretation by the coach and the athlete of the athlete's subjective evaluation of training effect is clearly highlighted here, and there must be a flexibility built into the programme for adjustment to progressions within the meso-cycle. Clearly, progressions in pursuit of all objectives cannot proceed at the same rate.

SUMMARY

To conclude this discussion of adaptation to loading, the basic guiding principle should be:

- Step 1 – preparation for training
- Step 2 – training for competition.

Without doubt, the most rapid development of performance will come from high intensity specific loadings, but where these are used to too great an extent, they quickly wear out the physical and psychological potential of the athlete. The more thorough and extensive step 1, the longer will be the amount of time before such 'wearing out'. Nevertheless, there are occasions when the athlete appears to have gone 'stale' for reasons that are not always apparent. This phenomenon has critical implications for coach and athlete and will be examined in the following chapter.

The defining of optimal loading for an athlete is critical to progression of his fitness and maintenance of his health. It demands fine judgements on the part of the coach. The cycle of adaptation, application and regeneration must be followed at all levels. This emphasises the importance of a thorough and extensive preparation part of the cycle and of viewing stimulus plus recovery as a total process.

REFLECTIVE QUESTIONS

1. Probably the most difficult area of judgement for the coach is the balance between increasing intensity (quality) and decreasing extent (quantity) of loading. What factors do you consider most influential in making that judgement call?

2. Give arguments for and against mixing a) intensity of loading, and b) recovery level within a training unit and between training units in the first mesocycle (core training) for a triathlete.

3. An athlete has just completed her university course and returned to her home town to start her professional career as a landscape gardener. She is moving into her own flat and is now engaged to the father of her baby. Unfortunately her father has been ill for some time. She nevertheless returned a performance in her final year that meets a standard which given normal improvement, will challenge for

Olympic selection two years away. Three months into preparation mesocycles, training performance is falling short of target. Outline a strategy to help the athlete return to training target in terms of lifestyle and mesocycle design.

4. Prepare a basic weight training unit for a shot-put athlete (your gender choice). The athlete will complete this twice per week over six weeks. Explain (see figure 22.3):
   a. Possible functional changes and immediate effect in week 1
   b. Possible functional changes and residual effect in week 3
   c. Possible functional changes and cumulative effect in week 6

5. In the course of preparation for a major championships, an adaptation programme must accommodate, in addition to the year plan, dry heat adaptation, altitude acclimatisation (venue is 1,750m), time change (8 hours ahead, i.e. east) and there is an air pollution (particulate) possibility. Outline the factors you must consider and your strategy for addressing the collective adaptation issues.

23 TRAINING V STRAINING

Our capacity to adapt protects us from threats to our wellbeing and also enables us to realise our performance potential. At the one extreme it equips us to survive when our very existence is in peril; at the other, it may be applied to enable us to go beyond our present performance limits when challenged to do so. Adaptation is as essential to the effectiveness of our immune system as it is in preparing to raise our game to perform better in progressively tougher arenas. It is an inbuilt auto-regulative feature of our physiology which operates without us realising it, yet can be constructively manipulated and managed in pursuit of performance objectives.

Training programmes based on the performance-related sciences, training theory and coaching methods aim to bring about the adaptations necessary to improve the athlete's performance advantage. However, training is only one of several stressors that persistently and cumulatively bombard the athlete each day (see figure 13.4, p. 220). They include studying, domestic and social life, relationships, health, general lifestyle, cultural demands and so on. Where the total load of these stressors is in keeping with the athlete's ability to deal with them, training will progress normally and performance will improve. This demands that the athlete is at the overcompensation phase as illustrated in figure 21.2, p. 333. It is important then to understand fatigue.

FATIGUE

Fatigue is a natural occurrence in physical activity. Its cause may be physical or mental.

- **Physical:** Muscles, ligaments, joints, nerve cells, bones, etc., are all subject to the process of fatigue, which is a temporary, reversible reduction of function, linked with the disinclination for further loading.
- **Mental:** This is the temporary reduction in capacity to maintain focus and optimal cognitive competence.

Mental fatigue may also bring physical fatigue. This connection has introduced the argument that fatigue is a psycho-physiological phenomenon. Noakes (2012) suggests fatigue is a brain-derived emotion, proposing that it is the brain which controls the process.

> 'The brain regulates exercise performance by continuously modifying the number of motor units that are recruited in the exercising limbs. This occurs in response to conscious and subconscious factors that are present before and during exercise, and those which act purely during exercise. The goal of this control is to ensure that humans always exercise with reserve and terminate the exercise bout before there is a catastrophic failure of homeostasis. The brain uses the unpleasant (but illusory) sensations of fatigue to ensure that the exercise intensity and duration are always within the exerciser's physiological capacity.'
>
> (Noakes 2012)

Noakes proposes 'The Central Governor Model of Exercise Regulation' where the brain is the central governor. 'This model therefore predicts that the ultimate performances are achieved by athletes who best control the progression of these illusory symptoms during exercise.' (Noakes 2012). Sport psychology affords techniques for learning such control.

The fatigue following exposure to the stimulus of exercise load is an essential feature for adaptation of the organism to increasing demands (figure 21.2). Such fatigue should be overcome relatively quickly, depending on the nature of loading; even after very heavy loadings, the athlete should be at the overcompensation phase within 24–48 hours. This sort of fatigue is normal. The athlete will be ready to tackle normal physical, mental and emotional challenges after the training loads and should feel well rested and fully recovered the morning after.

On the other hand, the cumulative stressors may be too much for the athlete and this will be referred to as overstressing the athlete. Short of complete and regular bioprofiles on athletes, which demands access to physiological testing laboratories, the coach has very little with which to assess the contribution of training to the sum total of stressors. This said, in some countries it has become an accepted feature of the National Performance Programme that athletes will undergo periodic 'stress' monitoring to reduce the risks of overstressing the athlete. In Finland, at Vierumakki, athletes present themselves for such monitoring on the following basis:

Stress level	Chronic long-term training stress-disturbances at hormonal level.	Acute short-term training stress-disturbances in muscle membranes and in energy production.
Relevant measurement	Measuring the ratio of testosterone:cortisol levels in blood serum.	Measuring urea/creatinine/ creatinekinase concentration in blood serum.
Timing of measurement	Four times per year; twice during the main preparation phase, once during the competition preparation phase, once one month before the main competition.	During hard training micro cycles (e.g. training camps) samples taken each morning. Also 2–3 hours post-unit. (Grosser 1986: overstressing if serum urea >8 mmol/ litre.)

Clues which the coach might pick up on are shown in table 23.1.

A low white cell count is also an indicator of the onset of chronic stress – specifically a low quantity of natural killer cells (NK cells), which are the leukocytes that assist in the destruction of foreign substances in the body. More recently, S-IgA (secretory immunoglobin A) levels and the ratio of anti-ageing hormone, DHEA (dehydroepiandrosterone) to cortisol are considered key indicators of physiological stress.

Clearly, the failure to ensure adequate recovery and regeneration should not be dismissed as being 'a little more tired than usual' as it can lead to the weakening of the immune system.

It is critical, then, that coaches ensure that the recovery or regeneration component in training is designed and delivered as carefully as the stimulus. If not, intended adaptation will not occur. The adaptation process occurs because the athlete's physiology recovers into overcompensation. This will happen when, on the one hand, the training load is consistent with the athlete's capacity to accept its challenge against the background of his total stressor profile, and on the other, if the recovery is effectively managed through appropriate timescales.

	Optimal loading	Excessive loading	Recovery after excessive loading
Skin colour	flushed	very flushed	paleness for several days
Sweating	heavy sweat in upper body	sweating throughout body	night sweats
Co-ordination	slight loss of precision as unit proceeds	loss of precision, distressing confusion, increased reaction time	reduced precision beyond 48 hrs or in extreme cases beyond 72 hrs
Concentration	reducing span of attention; reducing capacity to solve technical problems; reducing power of identifying irrelevant cues	inability to concentrate for even relatively short periods; forgets instructions	unable to correct technical errors for more than 48 or even 72 hrs; unable to concentrate on academic work
General health	progressive muscular weakness, reduced efficiency	possible muscle and joint pain, light-headedness and stomach upset. General feeling of malaise, even headaches	difficulty in sleeping; pulse remains higher than normal for up to 24 hrs. continued physical inefficiency and discomfort
Approach to training	desire for longer recoveries but eager to train	desire for complete rest; doubts on value of training; fear of further loading	disinclined to train next day; negative attitude to coach perhaps even inventing excuses for avoiding training

TABLE 23.1 Symptoms of tiring after optimal and excessive loading of training

Because training affects, and will focus on, different levels of the athlete's physiology, it should be borne in mind that the adaptation cycle is operating across different timescales. Figure 23.1 is a schematic of recovery of various aspects of physiology following a training stimulus.

It is here where the importance of the relationship between structure of loading (intensity and extent) and training ratio (loading and recovery) are underlined. More than that, is the need to appreciate the importance of recovery and regeneration.

The most fundamental medium affording rest, recovery or regeneration, is sleep. If the right quality and quantity of sleep is not routinely in place, it is hard to imagine how any training programme can be effective or how performance potential can be realised.

Sleep is an important component in the preparation for and recovery from strenuous activity, whether physical, emotional or mental or a combination of these. Sufficient sleep on the one hand aids functional efficiency and on the other, facilitates repair and regeneration of muscle and tissues.

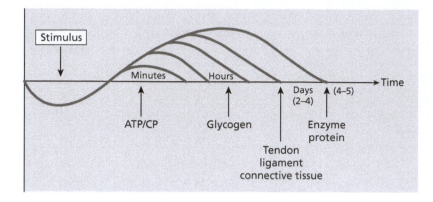

FIGURE 23.1 Variations in post stimulus recovery and adaption timescale in selected system function

Generally speaking, we need seven to eight hours quality sleep each day. For high performance athletes there is an argument for at least eight hours. A comfortable mattress and pillows, a quiet and dark room, and 21°C temperature are the best environment.

Establishing a sleep preparation routine helps ensure quality sleep. The following is adapted from Clyde Rathbone, Australian Institute of Sport:

1. 30 minutes before bedtime, turn off radio/computer/TV and excess lights.
2. Check diary for next day and write down related actions and thoughts.
3. Shower, go to the toilet, brush teeth.
4. Set alarm.
5. Get into bed.
6. Either read easy-reading book for 10–15 minutes and/or listen to relaxing music which switches itself off after 15–20 minutes – or go immediately to step 7!
7. Switch lights off.
8. Relax and reflect on calmness (think about places and situations that are calm and peaceful)
9. Normally sleep commences any time up to 20–30 minutes.

Eating habits can help with falling to sleep and getting enough quality sleep:

- No eating after two hours before bed time.
- No caffeine after four hours before bed time.
- Avoid spicy foods for final meal of the day.
- Avoid hard-to-digest foods in final meal of the day (e.g. cheese can cause problems for some people).
- Drink a calming hot drink such as Horlicks or Ovaltine.

For high performance athletes, it is sensible to monitor sleep hours, sleep efficiency and sleep quality. There are several smartphone apps and other technologies designed for this purpose.

The idea of 'power naps' has gained popularity with high performance athletes especially where there is more than one period of training per day. An hour of sleep between training sessions enhances recovery from the previous and readiness for the subsequent period. At least 30 minutes should be allowed after the nap before resuming training.

Once again, attention to ensuring recovery and regeneration is essential. Athletes must return to the over-compensation phase of the adaptation cycle. If not, the athlete is being exposed to the risk of failure to meet training and competition targets and, if continued over an extended period, to breakdown and burnout.

Overstressing causes progressive fatigue. Capacity is not restored after training in this situation and will continue to deteriorate until the causes of overstressing are removed. If they are not, the athlete may become ill.

Israel (1963) points out that overstressing can produce either of two extremes of response: over-excitement of the system (over-stimulation), or over-depression (over-inhibition). He refers to the former as basedovoid overstressing and suggests that, within the training context, this occurs chiefly as a result of suddenly increasing the density of sub-maximum intensity loadings in the training programme, or of making excessive demands on the power of concentration. He refers to the latter as addisonoid overstressing, and this is brought about by very comprehensive endurance programmes with persistent over-emphasis in the extent of loading.

While there is general agreement among coaches and training theorists with Israel's observations, these broad causes of overstressing are seldom exclusively so. In fact they should be viewed more as major contributors to the syndrome. The fact is that the phenomenon of overstressing arises from the cumulative effect of many stressors – which leaves the individual exposed to a reduced threshold of stress tolerance; reduced capacity to adapt to stressors or cope with stress; and, in extreme cases, may contribute to chronic fatigue syndrome and other clear warning signs that the immune system is under threat. Other stressors include the following:

1. Principal faults in the training process: recovery is neglected (mistakes in the build-up of micro and mesocycles, and inadequate use of general exercise sessions for recovery); demands increased too quickly so that adaptation cannot be consolidated; too rapid an increase of loading after forced breaks (injuries, illness); too great an extent of loadings of maximum and sub-maximum intensity; too high an intensity of duration loadings in endurance training; excessive and forced technical schooling in complicated courses of movement without adequate recovery; excess of competitions with maximum demands, combined with frequent disturbance of the daily routine and insufficient training; excessive bias of training methods and units; lack of trust in the coach; repeated setbacks as a result of the coach setting sights too high; inability of athlete or coach to maintain adaptation: application: regeneration balance.

2. Factors reducing performance:

   - Lifestyle – inadequate sleep; irregular daily routine; dissolute behaviour; use of alcohol and tobacco; excess of caffeine; distracting company; lack of free time or inability to relax; nutritional deficiencies ('empty calorie' foods, lack of vitamins or antioxidants, low water intake, etc.); frequent necessity to adjust bodyweight; accepting more stressors when already at capacity.
   - Environment – poor living conditions (overcrowding, etc.); excessive family duties and tensions; difficulties in personal relationships; dissatisfaction with career, studies, school; poor marks in school, studies, etc; conflict with attitudes hostile to sports (family, superiors); excess of stimuli (TV, cinema); temporary upsurge of anxiety (e.g. exams).
   - Health upsets – feverish colds; stomach or intestinal upsets; glandular fever; chronic infections (e.g. of tonsils, teeth, ovaries, sinuses); after-effects of infectious illnesses (e.g. sore throats, lingering cough, etc.); injury; neglected infections (e.g. athlete's foot, rashes, etc.).

Management of the athlete's lifestyle outside the sporting context, while finally resting with the athlete, requires knowledge and skill in areas including time management; personal health and hygiene; control of interpersonal communication and relationships with people in social and business situations; and direction in pursuit of career. There is no single 'educator' here. Learning resources include parents, family, teachers, friends and coaches. Because of this, it is often wrongly assumed that 'someone else' is taking care of such matters. The truth is that all of the athlete's potential 'educators' must accept responsibility for relevant input. Ideally they all should work in partnership as a support team. Before anyone loads the athlete with yet another stressor, the existing stressor profile should be known, and help afforded in ensuring that the athlete's tolerance to stress is not overloaded.

It is the coach who must coordinate such input and lead the team of 'educators'. This role will be discussed further in chapter 24.

Within the sporting context, there is much the coach can do in the area of preventing overstressing. With careful planning, means and methods to encourage recovery or regeneration can be included in the training programme. This will ensure that the aggregate effect of the training programme does not constitute a stressor which will tip the athlete into the overstress situation.

The means and methods may be considered at three levels: intra-unit, inter-unit and inter-micro/mesocycle.

Intra-unit (between repetitions and/or sets)

The period of time involved here is measured in seconds or minutes. During this period the athlete must recover to a level which permits the objective of the training unit to be met. For example, if the unit is interval training, the degree of recovery, monitored by noting heart rate, must allow the athlete's heart rate to fall to around the midpoint of the total range. If resting heart rate is 60 and maximum is 180, then the athlete's heart rate should be around 120–130 before he performs the next repetition.

If maximum quality of performance is required over a number of repetitions, say for speed, recovery must be complete between runs. A unit of 3 × 60m then, will require at least 10 minutes between repetitions.

If incomplete recovery is required to guarantee cumulative fatigue for development of anaerobic tolerance, time periods are chosen to ensure that the athlete can perform sufficient repetitions to guarantee a training effect. This effect may or may not require that the athlete maintains a minimum quality of performance in each repetition. If it does, then clearly the time periods are larger and the quality of performance is submaximum.

Recovery activities include:

- lying down
- walking
- jogging
- doing a related activity
- doing an unrelated activity
- massage
- changing footwear
- warming up
- sipping water or glucose/mineral replacement drinks.

Intra-unit recovery is, by definition, part of the training load. However, it may also be considered part of the stimulus in certain types of training. For example, in some special strength work, where the objective is to accelerate strength levels, instead of load = stimulus + recovery, it becomes load = stimulus 1 + stimulus 2.

So, in leg work, the training unit might become:

stimulus 1–5 × 85% max ½ squat
stimulus 2–5 × rebounds over 8 hurdles at 90 cm.

Immediately on completing stimulus 2, the athlete starts again with stimulus 1. The total unit is 3–5 × (stimulus 1 + stimulus 2).

Inter-unit (between units on a given day or from day to day)

The period of time involved here is measured in hours or days. Few athletes outside the endurance group pursue the same training objectives in successive units. Having said this, many endurance athletes follow a pattern of 'hard unit'–'easy unit' alternation. In-built to most training programmes then, is a form of recovery from the stressor of specific training loads.

Coaches must learn to feel comfortable not only at including rest days and rest units in the microcycle, but also at introducing periods of up to several days recovery when necessary. The flexibility of programme design, as suggested in chapter 22 in connection with the aggregate cumulative effect of training, should allow for this.

Recovery activities include:

- Special diets, lying down, sleeping, massage, jacuzzi, sauna, change of venue, work/study, going out to a show, watching TV, listening to music, etc.
- Doing another event/sport at recreational level, e.g. swimming, golf, cycling, etc.
- Variety – in the training objective; the level of athlete involvement in decision-making; routine; between training and competition.
- General activity units.
- Warm-up units.
- 'Feel good' sessions.
- 'Finding space' sessions.
- Relaxation units – dynamic/passive.
- Dance, aesthetic expression.

Although it seems common sense to include such activities, both athletes and coaches can occasionally abandon common sense under pressure. For example, it is not unknown for programmes to be made harder rather than easier when performance in training does not come up to expectation. For athletes who are achievement-orientated, lack of commitment or hard work is not an acceptable explanation for performance problems. Motivation is not the problem but avoiding demotivation can be. It is more likely that the athlete has been over-committing and over-working, or that the work has been inappropriate. Whatever the explanation may be, the coach must ensure that units for recovery or regeneration not only appear in the programme, but are also carried through.

Inter-micro/mesocycle (normally at transition or regeneration macrocycle)

The period of time involved here is measured in days or weeks, and suggests that such training cycles should be considered and introduced to the programme at the same time as the year plan itself is set out. This is not to say, of course, that given certain circumstances, such a training cycle may not be introduced in pursuit of a specific regenerative objective, at any time in the year.

The 'early planned' regeneration mesocycle is normally between conclusion of the competition macrocycle and commencement of the introductory mesocycle of the year plan. It should be planned in such a way that the athlete returns to training highly motivated and fully prepared to commit himself to the rigours and discipline of training. This is best achieved quite simply by taking a vacation. This suggests:

- a different climate
- different surroundings
- different routine
- different social environment
- different physical activities
- different diet
- different emotional and mental demands.

The 'introduced' regeneration mesocycle is normally associated with recovery from crises. Unexpected and critical defeat; selection for a major championship; serious injury/illness; all represent possible crises which may require a regeneration mesocycle to help bring things back into focus. However, it should be said that the crisis situation seldom arrives out of the blue. It can often be spotted early. Timely regeneration will help avoid the situation becoming virtually irretrievable.

We have established that coaches have, over time and through experience, created a reasonable reference framework for the design and delivery of effective recovery. But can we expand this?

A mixture of Eastern and Western influences have now opened our minds to a host of possibilities that focus on a holistic approach to regeneration – often with the sense of sanctuary offered by spas. Such measures are variously described as treatments or therapies which enhance or restore wellbeing. They focus for the most part on rest, recovery, recuperation, relaxation, recreation, rehabilitation and regeneration; some are rooted in oriental and alternative medicine, others in the cosmetic industry.

Within this world, it is certain there are areas of practice which, if understood and founded on sound principle, must surely enrich the training process when thoughtfully applied.

It is beyond the scope of this book to list all such therapies and treatments. But it may be worth outlining the general bases of some, to encourage further thought and study of effective recovery and regeneration management. For example:

The exteroceptors
Electromagnetic waves

The eyes are sensitive to light, dark and colour. We may respond to how we see or interpret what we see in movies, pictures, what we witness etc. with a range of emotions.

The skin is sensitive to touch, pressure, light, heat, cold and pain. (We use the effect of electromagnetic waves via the skin in magnetic resonance, electrical stimulation of muscle, light therapies including ultraviolet and infrared etc.)

Mechanical vibration

The skin again. (We use such in massage, jacuzzis, ice therapies, bathing in salts or essences, soothing the skin with various substances, and so on.)

The outer, middle and inner ear are sensitive to sound waves. These set up a series of mechanical stimuli translated by the cochlea, the essential organ of hearing, into perceptions of loudness, pitch and timbre. The non auditory part of the inner ear, the labyrinth, accommodates the vestibular apparatus. It is stimulated by movement of the head enabling balance to be maintained.

We use music and sounds to stimulate or relax, emotionally, intellectually and physically.

Chemical changes

The nose is sensitive to smell and we have a most sophisticated memory bank for aromas. Once experienced, a smell, even years later, will conjure up the original experience. Aromatherapy uses this sense to advantage.

The tongue is sensitive to taste. We use this sense in food and drink flavourings and via digestion to stimulate, soothe etc.

The propriocetors

Propriocetors respond to stretch, tension or pressure in the locomotor system.

They provide information about movement, position, balance and coordination.

They are located in muscles, tendons, joints and the labyrinth apparatus in the ear. We use this knowledge in a range of therapies including reflexology, and in the work of chiropractors, osteopaths, manipulation masseurs and so on.

The interoceptors

The interoceptors are located in the viscera and monitor the internal environment; they are sensitive to distension in the hollow organs. Most therapies here involve preventing situations which lead to distension.

The senses are also involved in creating emotional, physical and intellectual changes as a consequence of how we personally interpret the conduits referred to above. That said, there is much we don't know or understand of why certain treatments or therapies are effective. For example, acupuncture has eluded satisfactory scientific explanation, yet, clearly, it works for some. Some medical practices now offer both conventional and alternative medicines, including acupuncture, and alternative therapies have been included in athlete's performance services resources. Coaches must work closely with the research areas of sports science in making responsible decisions in the interest of an athlete's wellbeing, development and performance. This is now even more important in the context of regeneration strategies.

Stress

But what if the athlete becomes overstressed? The coach should be aware of the following.

1. Psychological symptoms: increased irritability; obstinacy; increased argumentativeness; 'flying off the handle'; complaining about trivial things; defiance; anxiety; melancholy; avoidance of contact with coach and colleagues; oversensitivity to criticism; blaming everyone else for problems; laziness; fullness; 'imagining things'; depression; insecurity.

2. Performance symptoms:

- Techniques – increased incidence of disturbance in the basic technical model, e.g. reappearance of old faults; cramps; inhibitions; loss of confidence; disturbance in the rhythm and flow of the movement; reduced ability to differentiate between right and wrong movement.
- Condition – diminishing endurance, strength, speed; longer recovery times needed; loss of 'bounce' in training – becoming almost a 'slog'; loss of personal effervescence on and off track.
- Competitive qualities – reduced readiness for competition 'action'; fear of competition (or rather of losing); giving up under pressure; confusion in competition such as departure from competition plan or inability to respond correctly to the strategy of the opposition; easily demoralised; loss of belief in self and abilities; talks about lack of point in continuing the struggle; wants out!

3. Somatic functional symptoms: sleeping difficulties; lack of appetite; loss of weight; 'addictive' eating; increase in weight; disturbance in digestive function; longer recovery of pulse to resting rate, increased resting heart rate; dizzy spells; night sweating; increased susceptibility to injury/infection; loss of vitality. Should such symptoms arise, especially if there are several symptoms, the coach should:

- have the athlete check with his doctor;
- put the athlete immediately on a regeneration programme.

Selection of components to be included in the regenerative programme vary according to whether the athlete's reaction is basedovoid or addisonoid. Israel (1963) identified examples of such variance and these have been divided into three sections.

Basedovoid

- **Diet:** encourage the athlete to eat more; choose basic foods such as milk, vegetables, fruit, and organic foods; eliminate foods with preservatives and/or artificial colourings; avoid spicy or greasy sauces/dressings; avoid coffee, tea, chocolate and soft drinks containing caffeine; reduce protein consumption, especially red meat; take a concentrated course of vitamins, especially B complex plus the antioxidants; take small quantity of alcohol e.g. a glass of sherry prior to sleeping; take tonics and nutritional drinks which are approved by anti-doping bodies.
- **Physical therapy:** swim outdoors; bathe in the evening for 15–20 minutes (at water temperature 33–37°C) with additives such as Radox, Badedas, extract of pine needles, etc; take jacuzzis; in the morning, take a cold shower followed by a brisk towelling; take soothing massage and relevant aromatherapy; do soothing slow pace aerobics/exercises to music with emphasis on slow stretching.
- **Climate:** move to a quiet area, e.g. forest or mountains; avoid intense ultraviolet radiation; live in moderate temperature of 18–24°C.

Addisonoid

- **Diet:** encourage maintaining a strict three meals a day routine; increase protein intake, e.g. meat, cheese, eggs, cereals; prioritise organic foods and eliminate foods with preservatives and artificial colourings; take a concentrated course of vitamins, especially B12 plus the antioxidants; avoid alcohol; take occasional caffeine-based drinks with meals.

- **Physical therapy:** take alternate hot/cold showers in the morning and in the evening; take saunas in the middle or high range of temperatures; take vigorous massage using approved rubbing lotions; do vigorous fast pace aerobics/exercises to music, with emphasis on elasticity.
- **Climate:** move to a bracing climate – windy seaside location is ideal; look for moderate ultraviolet radiation; seaside in a warm climate allows the benefits of hot sun and high temperatures to be alternated with plunges in the sea; live in moderate to high temperatures of 22–28°C.

Because several people may be involved in an athlete's development and lifestyle, they should all understand the complex business of overstressing. Consequently, there should be regular communication through the 'support team', to help establish that balance of stressors which will not harm the athlete.

SUMMARY

The effect of training may become negative if the athlete's lifestyle outside sport is poorly managed, so the total content of that lifestyle must be known. The coach must accept a responsibility to help ensure sound management in this direction, and also to develop an understanding of the unique aggregate of stressors represented by the athlete's lifestyle.

Both the structure of loading and the training ratio must be carefully planned if negative training effects are to be avoided. More specifically, the coach must ensure adequate recovery before the athlete is exposed to subsequent loadings. Means of accelerating recovery in normal training and in the event of possible overstressing, should be understood and applied. Quality and quantity of sleep are important.

Close observation of the athlete for early identification of symptoms of over-stressing may help eliminate any serious damage to the athlete's fitness status in the long term.

REFLECTIVE QUESTIONS

1. Prepare a fifteen minute presentation for 16–18-year-old professional tennis players about to embark on the International Tennis Federation (ITF) circuit, which may take them all over the world. Success at this level is a stepping stone to the Association of Tennis Professionals (ATP) circuits. The topic is: 'Quality Sleep is the Key to Quality Performance'.

2. Design a strategy for monitoring stress levels including preparing athletes for their role in doing so. The athletes should be in the sport of your choice.

3. Design an attractive email for coaches to download on what helps or hinders in ensuring that the beginner and early developer athletes they work with get the positive value of training and not the negative of straining from their programmes.

4. Parents are critical partners in the development of young athletes. What would you include in a fifteen minute webinar introduction for parents on fatigue to better equip them for their role in the process? Suggest some questions they may wish to ask you following your 15 minute piece.

5. Following a search of studies on regeneration, relaxation and recovery, prepare a chart for athletes, scoring out of 10 the value you would give to those practices and processes you have sourced under the headings indicated.

Conduct	Practices/processes	Physical	Emotional	Intellectual
Electromagnetic waves	e.g. light therapy			
Mechanical vibration	e.g. massage			
Chemical changes	e.g. aromatherapy			
Proprioceptors	e.g. reflexology			
Interoceptors	e.g. bioneurofeedback			
Psychology related	e.g. meditation			

24 COMPETITION PERIOD

COMPETITION

The purpose of a competitive athlete's training programme is to produce optimal performance in competition. After all, there are no awards offered for world records in training! This point must be emphasised. The coach is preparing the athlete to improve his competition performance and to deliver intended performance 'on the day', and therefore all training is in pursuit of this end. The concept of periodisation implies producing or reproducing the high point of performance in a particular competition.

Training competitions

Bridging mesocycles 2 and 3 is a 'grey area' where specific training is mainly composed of competitions themselves. These competitions have immense importance in the development of the athlete's training status and his competition performance. Moreover, they are a means of evaluating status and stability of performance. These competitions are seldom used to evaluate status relative to other athletes. Instead, they may evaluate the athlete's status relative to his own previous competition performance, or those at the same time last year, etc. It seems reasonable to refer to all such competitions as 'training competitions'. These may be simple competitions to assess training status, or progressively sophisticated in terms of objective (and frequently referred to as 'build-up competitions'). It is worth pointing out that these competitions may well include events other than the athlete's own. For example, a 400m hurdler may run 500m to assess speed endurance, or a breaststroke swimmer may swim medleys to assess strength endurance, and so on.

Principal competitions

Apart from these training competitions, one should also distinguish principal competitions. These competitions dictate the patterns of mesocycles in the competition macrocycle, just as the pattern of the complete annual cycle is dictated by the climax of the competition macrocycle. The mesocycles must be so arranged that the best possible performance can be produced in each principal competition. The principal competitions should be seen as including the 'main' and the 'major' competitions. These main competitions are the final preparations for the major competition or the 'competition climax'. According to the nature of the sport, Matveyev (1965) believes two or more peaks (including the competition climax) are possible. However, from practical experience, it is most unusual for an athlete to produce more than four peaks even in the explosive sports where the technical component is high.

By way of summary of these points, the competition programme for a long jump athlete is set out in table 24.1.

Date	Level event	Mesocycle	Mesocycle content	Mesocycle objective
April 5		2	Progression into optimal	Rapid increase in
12	(a) 200m: 110H: 4 x 100		competition frequency: loading	competition performance.
19	(a) LONG: TRIPLE: HIGH		extent reducing: training itself	Training competition
26	(a) LONG: 100m: 4 x 400		reduced but loading not yet	hardness. Evaluation of
			at optimal intensity. Probably	technical performance and
May 3			one mesocycle only.	training status. Stabilising
10	(b) LONG: 100m			competition performance:
17	(a) 200H: 200m		Emphasis on training:	putting together competition
	(b) 100m: LONG		correction of technical faults	experience.
24	(a) 100m		found in previous mesocycle:	Correction of technical
31	(c) LONG: 4 x 100		intensity progressing steadily.	faults: preparation for 3/3½
June 7		3 or 3½		based on above evaluations:
14	(a) LONG: 100m: 4 x 100	4		commencement of main
21	(d) LONG: 4 x 100	5		competitions.
28	(a) 100m		Main competitions with	
July 5	(c) LONG: 200m		gradual reduction of extent as	Stabilising optimal
12	(d) LONG: 4 x 100		loading now moves to optimal	competition performances.
	(a) 4 x 100: 4 x 400		intensity, but structure of	Recording these in main
19	(b) 100m: 200m		loading is still in keeping with	competitions. Collection of all
26	(b) LONG		event requirements. There will	relevant data on behaviour in
Aug 2	(d) LONG		be several mesocycles here.	all competition situations.
9			Period of special preparation.	
16			Extent of loading rises for	
23			3 wks then decreases as	
30			intensity reaches opitmal –	Special preparation for major
			and highest in the annual	competitions based on
			cycle. The whole of this phase	analysis of 3/3½.
			is a complete mesocycle.	

TABLE 24.1 Possible distribution of competitions for an athlete whose main discipline is long jump. Note that from approximately April 12 to May 21 there is almost a 'grey area' where mesocycles 2 and 3 are bridged.

Competition v training

But why should competitions have anything more to offer training than, say, a trial in a training session? In training, one can only simulate competition situations. In competition, the athlete, due to the experience of competition and its emotional demands, emerges more completely exhausted than in training. Consequently the stimulus for adaptation to high or maximum loading is more effective than that which can be reproduced in training. Just as important, however, is that competition is the most specific training that exists to master emotional excitement, and in such a way that it helps the athlete surpass present limits of performance. It is not unusual to hear of an athlete producing superb achievements in training, yet experiencing disasters in competition. He has failed to master himself in competition, reacting negatively to the threat of insecurity of living life on the edge of challenge. Once back in the quietness and security of the training situation, all is well again. Competition is the only means of adapting to the stressor of competition and to avoid its particular stress simply increases the stress potential of the next one.

It is essential that the level of competition is perceived by the athlete as a challenge relevant to the stage of preparation. So preceding a major competition with 'soft' competition is pointless. There is no adrenaline and, consequently, there is no rehearsal of competition intensity sharpness – intellectually, physically or emotionally.

In addition to this factor which validates competition as a training means, exposing the athlete to a wide variety of competition situations lessens the likelihood of him being confronted with the unfamiliar. Every competition has a character of its own, determined not only by the physical environment of stadium, wind, humidity, and so on, but also by the group of athletes involved. Athletes must be encouraged to seek out opposition, especially if the opposition is known to be better. By competing with the same opponents, a system of stereotyped, albeit efficient, reactions will evolve. Varied opposition and environment develops the capacity to adapt more readily to varying competition conditions.

Competition frequency

Frequency of competition is determined by athlete preference and relevant competition availability at one extreme, and the structure of sports competitions at the other. Weather conditions also play a part in the UK!

Time is needed for recovery from the physical and emotional stress of a main or build-up competition, and also to correct training deficiencies. Consequently, the 'build-up' and principal competitions should be 7–10 in number. Any additional competitions should be low key, at the level of 'simple training' status. Against this background, speed and elastic strength events in track and field can amount to one or two per week, while strength endurance and the longer track events can be separated by up to 14 days.

Occasionally there are instances where athletes saturate part of the competition season with a concentration of quality performances. In 1965, Ron Clarke raced 21 times in 56 days, lowering the 5000m record twice, and the 10 mile record once. Moreover, in the month preceding this period, he set a world record for three miles; and three months after this period, in the space of 40 days he set world marks on three occasions: 3 miles/5000m, 3 miles, and 6 miles/10,000m. In 1980, Sebastian Coe also established three world records over a very brief timescale:

July 3	Oslo – 800m	1 min 42.33 sec
July 17	Oslo – 1 mile	3 min 48.95 sec
August 15	Zurich – 1500m	3 min 32.03 sec

Only after several years preparation can such a programme be contemplated – and it certainly cannot be repeated over two or three successive years. At this level, the concept of using a year to regenerate is not uncommon. On the other hand, at the lower end of the scale, it has already been suggested that the young and developing athlete seems to be quite uninhibited in his appetite for competition. In fact, according to Thiess (1967), improvement in performance is directly proportional to competition frequency. He recommended, following the 1966 Spartakiad, taking part in 20–30 competitions in the period cycle leading up to the major competition.

Before moving on to competition preparation, and by way of summary, the following points should be noted:

- The athlete must compete as often as is necessary to achieve and stabilise a good competition performance.
- The better opponent must not be avoided without good reason.
- The athlete should only compete when he is physically and emotionally prepared for it.
- Too many competitions (especially when they are close together or involve considerable travel) not only interfere with training progression, but cause cumulative psychological fatigue.
- Competitions should be in ascending order of difficulty, building up towards a major competition with all other competitions subordinate to it.

Long season sports

A team at the top of the FA Premier League may, due to the success of the club, have roughly 60 competitions in the course of approximately 270 days. Some of the players will also have international duties, and no allowance is made here for any replays. It still means, however, that for 75 per cent of the year, players are potentially in line for one competition every 3½–4½ days!

In such cases, competition frequently becomes a central factor in maintaining a player's level of conditioning. It also, of course, saps the player's physical and emotional energies establishing a climate for the negative effects of stress.

Managers and coaches must, then, create a rotating cycle of development for each player, where regeneration is ensured and conditioning status is updated to give consistent high performance and motivation. It should not be injury or illness which determine when a player is rested, but value judgements related to an individual player's conditioning and motivational status. A system of player rotation must be understood by players and coaches, and fitted into the year phase in a way which allows the club to meet team and player development objectives. For the non-competitive 25 per cent of the year it becomes essential that all players build the greatest possible conditioning base and regenerate fully from the competition season, so that the 'player rotation' approach can be effected with minimal difference to team performance.

Competition preparation

Specific competition preparation assumes a given status of training in the athlete for a given sport. This understood, the coach must carefully prepare units, etc., leading up to the competition itself. The following points should then be taken into account:

1. The specific objective of the competition must be known by, and discussed with, the athlete. If it is not known, there is no means of evaluating success or failure, nor is there any distinct purpose to training. The objective may fall into one of two categories, or be a combination of both:

   - Competition with the athlete himself. These contests are to advance training status, improve performance, etc. Here, the opposition is used to aid pursuit of the objective. This is about performance.
   - Competition with an opponent. These contests are to win a point for the club/country, qualify for the next round, eliminate opposition, win a title, etc. Here the opposition is to be defeated. This is about results.

2. An athlete's or team's game plan for a given competition must be constructed to his or its strengths. The opposition should be obliged to address that game plan. There may be a plan A and B, but it is negative thinking to enter the arena with the primary objective of countering the opponents' game plan. The opposition are always better at their game plan than yours; and less equipped to play yours! So a high ranked athlete must not play down to a lower ranked athlete. That said, the opposition must be clearly identified and known to the athlete, as not all athletes in a contest may be opponents. Information on each opponent should include previous best performance, recent history of competition, and behaviour in competition (e.g. how effective they are in aspects of play which may challenge your game plan).

3. It is difficult to adapt quickly to unfamiliar conditions (a strange surface, humidity, altitude, temperature, etc.). Where possible, training should involve similar conditions to those at the competition venue.

4. The chronobiologist encourages the coach to understand the peak and trough of human performance in terms of body rhythms of daily and longer cycles. The athlete must be able to compete at specific times and the coach should make allowances for adjustments in body rhythms. For instance, if travel has meant an east/west time shift, the athlete should arrive at his destination with enough time to spare to 'reset' his body clock. If this is impossible, the athlete's normal day must be 'shifted' in training.

5. The athlete should be educated towards complete independence and the capacity to act 'executively' in the competition situation, and must take his opposition seriously yet concentrate upon the task in hand. The athlete must never be afraid of the opposition and certainly never be encouraged to avoid opponents equal, or superior, to himself. In fact, the athlete should be hungry for such opposition, looking forward to these encounters with a positive anticipation. After all, this level of opponent represents the highest stimulus to increased adaptation levels and higher performance (see also chapter 10).

6. Despite the athlete's physical and emotional concentration on the forthcoming competition, any anxiety must be managed. The contest must not be seen as some kind of threatening monster. In the last few days, the coach should stimulate the athlete's belief in success (see pp. 171–2), aid relaxation via recreation and reading, avoid boredom between training units by organising interesting but relaxing outings, and so on. Autogenic training, as formulated by Schultz (1956), or by the variation advanced by Machak (1964) may have something to offer in the control of 'pre-start reaction'. The athletes are originally 'trained' to relax by the coach, but eventually may induce the same state of relaxation themselves. Hypnotherapy is also very effective in affording a deeper state of relaxation. Hypnosis, of course, does not allow an athlete to adjust his behaviour to an unexpected situation that might occur in competition (see also chapter 10).

7. Athletes naturally vary in their behaviour immediately prior to competition. Puni (1961) refers to this as 'pre-start reaction' and tabulated variations of this are shown in table 24.2. If the athlete shows start-fever, warm-up should be relaxed, while for those with start-apathy, the warm-up should be vigorous and lively. According to Vanek and Cratty (1970), both extremes should benefit from autogenic training. Athletes also vary in their degree of sociability during warm-up, and over the last few days before a competition. A stronger feeling of security can sometimes come from being in a group, but this is not always the case. Many athletes seek to isolate themselves in order to concentrate a tighter focus on the forthcoming challenge (see also chapter 10).

8. The younger athlete will especially benefit from observing other events prior to his own. The more mature athlete may learn something of the atmosphere of the stadium, the temperature, variations in wind, and so on. There is always the morale boost, of course, when witnessing a successful performance by a colleague. On the other hand, morale can slide with an early defeat. While this can be turned to advantage as a spur to other team members, the athletes who are yet to compete should not be exposed to the demoralising effect of discussing the defeat with the unfortunate athlete. There will be time for this after the day's competitions are over. The coach should ensure that there is careful management of the pre-competition environment to the athlete's advantage.

9. It is the athlete's responsibility to check his personal equipment, but it is the coach's responsibility to ensure that the athlete knows what is the specific equipment required.

10. In the construction of the special competition preparation cycle, the following should be noted:

- A decision must be made by the coach whether to programme for improved performance or stabilisation of the existing performance level. There are times when to demand increased levels of intensity will 'burst the bubble'.
- The athlete's own status, that of his opposition, and the competition environment must be evaluated.
- Microcycles must allow complete recovery between units.
- Any additional competition must not itself be a peak but rather a build-up. Errors here will deplete reserves of emotional and physical energy. At least one such competition should be at, or near, the venue of the major competition, especially if the athlete must travel east/west, to altitude, to extreme humidity, and so on.
- The coach must develop the athlete's emotional focus and his appreciation of the need for complete preparation for the forthcoming contest. Too often an Olympic qualifying mark is reached, an athlete selected, and apathy follows. Or, again, a player who has gained international selection may lose his edge in the next game for his club – as if gaining selection was the major objective.

Once targets have been reached, new targets must be set or qualifying targets should be higher than is necessary:

- The first week of the special mesocycle leading up to the major contest should emphasise general development, relaxation and the recharging of batteries before the concentrated four weeks of build-up are started. This will be interpreted variously according to the patterns of performance in the previous mesocycle.
- No technical variations should be attempted.
- A thorough check by a physiotherapist or sports medicine specialist should be sought in the first week of this five-week mesocycle.
- Rules and regulations specific to the forthcoming competition should be clearly understood by the athlete. Moreover, commands and instructions in a foreign language should be rehearsed, where applicable.

11. While the content and composition of units, microcycles and mesocycles vary between individual athletes, all are focused on ensuring that the athlete is intellectually, emotionally and physically prepared to compete with distinction in pursuit of the agreed goal.

State of readiness for competition	Start-fever (nervous anticipation)	start-apathy (listlessness/inhibition)
All physiological processes proceed normally.	The athlete radiates great excitement; acute physiological changes (considerable increase in pulse rate, trembling in the limbs, feeling of weakness in lower extremities, etc.).	Listless, completely inhibited movements, yawning.
Slight excitement, enjoyable and rather impatient anticipation of the coming challenge, optimal power of concentration in complete control of own behaviour, radiating energy.	Great nervousness, uncontrolled movements, forgetfulness, absent mindedness, uncertainty of action, haste, unnecessary activity.	Limp, lazy, apathetic, anxious; low spirits; desire to 'cry off' from competition, tired, 'sour', unable to get going.
The athlete enters into competition in a highly organised way and exactly according to plan, sees the way ahead clearly, masters the situation, all forces at his disposal are brought into use in a tactically correct way; the anticipated result is achieved or surpassed.	Athlete's activity is disturbed, partially disorganised, he competes rashly, departs from his usual tactical line, loses the feeling for tempo, exhausts himself prematurely; movements are uncontrolled, accumulation of mistakes in face of high technical demands; very cramped.	He does not compete energetically, will-power soon abates, the athlete is incapable of mobilising the strength he possesses, action does not flow; after competition he is not exhausted because all reactions were on a low level.

TABLE 24.2 Principal forms of pre-start reaction from Harre (1973) according to Puni (1961)

On the day, only one person can bring the hours of work to a successful conclusion. The athlete's own will to coordinate all that has been learned and worked on, and to bring character, through his personality, to fruition within the opportunity represented by the challenge of the arena, are the most vital qualities of the successful athlete. He takes the risk of winning.

When the competition is over, the athlete will have a post-event reaction. This will be coloured by whether or not the acknowledged objectives of the competition have been met. Those who have not met the objective need not be reminded of it! Those who have been successful need little encouragement to be aware of this! The coach should encourage a state of normality and relaxation for the rest of the day of competition. Certainly there must be no criticism unless the athlete has for some reason misinterpreted the result relative to the objective. Review of the competition, evaluation of performance and clarification of lessons learned, should be pursued in the hours immediately after competition, or at the latest the next day. Such evaluation and modification is part of the athlete's preparation for the next competition and must not be neglected, whether the competition outcome was excellent or fell short of excellent.

One final point: a major tournament such as an international games, world cup/championships, tennis grand slam, etc, requires a mindset that sees each round, even the earliest, as if it is a final. Such intensity and the limited time between rounds demands highest levels of skill as the coach addresses focus, performance under pressure and recovery. Each round becomes not only the gateway to the next, but is preparation for it.

SUMMARY

It is in the competition period that the objectives of the periodised year are met. Each competition should be seen as fulfilling several roles. It serves as training for future competition, is a test situation for evaluation status, and is the raison d'être of training. The athlete's objectives in competition will vary and they must be identified prior to a given competition. The coach, in planning and distribution and frequency of competitions, and in identifying competition objectives, must have detailed knowledge of the competition programme available and the level of each competition. Only then can he bring the athlete to each competition prepared to meet the identified objectives.

REFLECTIVE QUESTIONS

1. 'Results are things over which you do not have total control, you only have total control over your performance.' Defend or attack this statement and outline your approach to delivering your argument in practice to athletes.

2. Coaching effectiveness in high performance sport may be defined by the coach's athletes or team delivering on the day. Discuss how you would use training competition to achieve this.

3. In a sport of your choice, select two athletes or teams who compete in the same annual competition. Record performances/results through at least two competition seasons. Examine data for trends and inconsistencies and then discuss factors which may influence such. You may need to do extra homework in this!

4. In preparation for a major tournament, a national team often has a match against quite weak opposition. Discuss the pros and cons of this.

5. There are five weeks between selection and your athlete's Olympic discipline. Prepare a personal checklist of points you must have covered and been fully satisfied with the outcome in the run up to the competition.

25 FITTING THINGS TOGETHER

To create a context for the content of *Sports Training Principles*, it may help to consider the process of preparation for a major international championships or games. There are two aspects to this: preparation of the athlete or team, and preparation for the athlete or team.

PREPARATION OF THE ATHLETE/TEAM

Preparation of the athlete of course began with the earliest days of the athlete's long term development and performance pathway. Given responsible application of relevant sports sciences and training theory, as the athlete has progressed in that pathway, and given high performance potential, the athlete will challenge for major competition selection.

Preparation for major international championships is the responsibility of the athlete's/team's coach, or the national coaching 'team' supported by the sports sciences and medical professionals (SSMP) or high performance director (HPD). In professional sports where clubs are involved in international competition (e.g. UEFA Champions League; Super Rugby in southern hemisphere Rugby Union), the responsibility also rests with personal coaches and club coaching teams.

Where the coaching team is led by a head coach (HC), he works with or through the personal coach (PC) to ensure the level of coaching and performance-related support meets the athlete's preparation needs and the overall team preparation strategy.

The objective here is to prepare the athlete and team to produce peak performance in the games/championships tournament or cup competition. The cumulative effect of annual training plans combined with what is learned through experience at the one-off competitions, championships and major tournament levels are the major factors in this preparation. They are, of course, tempered by interpretation of team preparation information.

Each competition serves as preparation for the next. Preparation for the target competition (TC), however, commences normally at least four years before. This means learning through experience of:

0–4 yrs	Previous TC experience (competing to establish performance platform)
0–3 yrs	Other high level competitions, international matches/team meets, other major championships (competing to raise performance)
0–2 yrs	Other high level competitions, international matches/team meets, other major championships (competing to prepare/learn)
0–1 yr	Other high level competitions, international matches/team meets, other major championships and selection process for the TC (competing to win)

Each experience might be considered as a 'dry run' or cumulative 'dry runs'. They afford critical insight into how the athlete handles the tournament situation, athlete's village, etc. and the coach's competence in preparing the athlete/team. Coaches can adapt the preparation models used here in shaping the 'end game' of the TC preparation. Coaches may also use the year's run-in to the 'dry run' as an essential source of reference for fine-tuning the one to two year TC run-in. This may require a very specific use of out of season competition.

This said, the four-year preparation cycle as a whole, and each annual cycle within it, will take the general shape of alternating emphases:

- General/related/specific.
- Development/stability of conditioning and technique.
- Adaptation; application; regeneration.
- Goal setting; planning; executing; reviewing.
- Performance monitoring/coaching adjustments.
- Throughout there will be a growing value to the athlete and coach of network interdependence.

Coaches must, then, be able to differentiate between the annual or lesser frequency training emphases and be able to prepare the overall annual plans for them in fine detail. More than this, they must be able to draw the athlete back from the urgency of competition in what may be a more 'regeneration' type year, macrocycle, mesocycle or microcycle, and set the right motivational environment in the more 'testing' type of year, macrocycle, etc.

This approach is consistent with the argument that performance progression is not linear; rather, it progresses in 'jumps'. It has an ebbing and flowing rhythm.

Before embarking on the TC final year programme, athletes must be fully recovered from the previous season via a carefully constructed regeneration programme and indicated rehab following a thorough post season medical check. It is also worth considering a programme of flu jabs for athletes and staff to help avoid loss of preparation days.

Any experiment in terms of mesocycle and microcycle length, unit detail and so on has no place in a TC year. This must be done in a testing year, two years previously or in 'regeneration' years. By the start of the TC preparation year, details must have been sorted out, right down to the choice of exercises, repetitions, sets, recoveries, progressions – and the precise length of mesocycles and microcycles. This is about fine tuning and understanding the 'end game'.

Of course, we are in the considered risk business by this time, but considered risks do not include taking chances in the structures of loading, training ratios etc. Rather, the risks lie in the area of taking energy and defence systems to the limit and exposing structures to new levels of stress. Rapid access to expert medical support and accurately interpreted biochemistry is of the utmost importance. Methods of monitoring cumulative training effect and acute chronic stress indicators must be built into the training system lest ambition and motivation threaten the athlete's well being.

Without doubt, the single greatest attributes for coach and athlete are persistence and patience in the year leading through to the TC. It is most certainly not a year for cutting corners in getting back to training after injury or illness; nor is it a year for making the intensity gradient steeper than in previous years. The extent of loading may be less than in the preceding year – and the intensity peak higher. The trick is knowing how far to go in interpreting the concept of overload. It is the dilemma facing every parent when they are blowing up a party balloon! When do you stop putting in more air? This underlines the need for a 'dry run' – and for careful evaluation of that experience.

Coaches must appreciate that athletes learn to listen to their bodies. Feedback from athletes – and a certain freedom to interpret units according to mood – are vital components of decision making on preparation plan adjustment. Neither coach nor athlete should be a slave of a system. Inbuilt flexibility is essential.

Where there is the need to review or develop coaching skills in delivering the above, the HC must work together with the PC to address that need. The samples of debriefing forms referred to in chapter 10 (see appendices A and B) are valuable in this.

To draw together performance-related data for ease of synthesis in decision making, the coach may use some form of athlete preparation plan pro forma. Appendix C is an example and a growing number of electronic versions are emerging to facilitate athlete tracking.

Preparation for the venue as much as the TC occasion must be accommodated within the programme. The particular stressors, which the venue represents, such as variable conditions, should be a feature of selected competitions athletes experience in advance of the TC. This can be used to reinforce the athlete's motivational climate. Looking ahead, it should be borne in mind that heat adaptation can be started at home and commences from first exposure to the stress. Nevertheless, experience of high temperature/humidity living and pressure competition should be pursued abroad and well before the TC (see chapter 7).

It should go without saying that the coach will stay ahead of the game in terms of training theory interpretation, new coaching methods and so on. He must retain the capacity of overview through multi-year and annual plans while being able to adjust detail to meet needs and mood of athlete(s) and current development in performance related matters. All coaches should design and deliver their own continuous professional development (CDP) plan.

What may require stating, however, is the need for 'management' of the athlete's lifestyle. This goes beyond factors which are directly performance related. It concerns the setting of objectives relating to entourage (see below), occupation, athletic ambition and commercial commitments; deciding on means of meeting these objectives; and the management of time in their pursuit. If a coach does not actually afford direction in this area, he is at the very least part of the counselling team involved (see overleaf).

Once objectives, means and time management are in place, the scene is set for creating the right motivational climate for success. The coach is central to this, generating a 'winner attitude'. Winner attitudes' start by believing in oneself. Such belief is borne of self-knowledge, pursuit of knowledge and successful application of knowledge. The positivity this creates is most infectious. The athlete believes in the coach and in the programme – and feels part of a *winning team*. For a growing number of athletes, that team includes family, agent and performance support personnel (the athlete entourage). More than that, because the athlete is encouraged to be involved in the decisions which affect his athletics – and lifestyle – bringing order and achievement, he believes more and more in himself. Coach and athlete share and welcome responsibility for achievement *and* hiccups! In this climate, winners grow – and TC preparation is accepted as an exciting and realistic challenge.

Finally, the outcome of the preparation process must find the athlete individually and/or collectively, competent to take ownership of each moment in his arena, to make the right decision and judgement calls and to deliver personal and/or collective excellence. The coach and performance support team have done their job; only the athlete and team can deliver in their arena.

PREPARATION FOR THE ATHLETE/TEAM

This is the work of the sports management team and ultimately the team manager.

The objective here is to create an environment where the athlete and team can fully express their talents in pursuit of competitive achievement. The idea is to spare the athlete unnecessary expenditure of energy in dealing with situations which break concentration on the task in hand. The athlete is preparing for the highly specific demands of producing his best possible result in a given championship discipline on the day (and through each stage of the tournament, if applicable).

Preparation for the team must evaluate what is required to create that environment – then take the necessary steps to establish it. In doing so, success becomes more probable – failure less possible.

It should be said that planning for a major championship (e.g. world, area, Commonwealth, Olympics) begins with evaluating the experience of the previous one; and the cumulative experience of equivalent competitions. However, it must also be recognised that each major championship or cup competition adds to the pool of resource to which we can refer.

The experience of the previous given championships would have been reviewed in the 6–8 weeks following it. This would have been made possible by preparing for such evaluation before those championships. Each member of the management, coaching and performance support team would have been delegated to certain review duties. This technical input, plus an account of preparation prior to the championships, affords a high quality report, which will prove of immense value in putting together a preparation plan for the next competition; and to those coaches who will be involved in athlete or team preparation.

It should be understood, then, that review of and learning from the forthcoming experience must be planned in advance.

The first two steps in preparation for the team are, therefore:

- Learn from review of preparation for and experience of previous championships (specific and other).
- Ensure that there is review of the next games/championships for the following ones.

The third step is to afford athlete and team coaches experience of good practice in major competitions. Associated with this should be a policy of sending information to those who need it as soon as it is available. Pre-championships preparation reports must be sent to athletes, personal coaches, team coaches, management, administration, SSMP and press liaison at commencement of the annual preparation cycle. This allows personal coaches and athletes to adjust their programmes in tune with recommendations made by the HC. It is suggested that a press and media briefing regarding the preparation report helps a broader sense of teamship.

In preparing the pre-championships preparation reports, counsel from athletes is fundamental to eventual recommendations. This will be part of coach-athlete debrief (appendices A and B) and campaign debrief. This ensures that a tighter focus on operational realities is brought to input from personal and team coaches; managers and SSMP; and an intelligence trawl by the HC.

TIMESCALE IN BUILDING TOWARDS TC PREPARATION REPORT

The process of setting out a preparation report for a given target competition (TC) will be followed for each TC so it is possible that this process is being pursued at different stages for different TCs. A 4-year cycle of events is clear for Olympics, rugby and cricket World Cups, etc. Where the TC is every other year (e.g., in football, European Cup and World Cup) the 4-year cycle for the venue specifics still applies, but there is an additional progress monitoring and learning experience two years out. Where the TC is annual, (e.g. European Athletics – World Championships; European Championships; World Championships; Olympic Games) again the 4-year cycle should be applied to each where possible and sensible, with annual progress monitoring and learning.

For Olympic sports, the priority TC for athlete and federation is the Olympic Games. For non-Olympic sports it is normally the World Cup/Championships.

0–4 yrs   After digesting reviews of the previous games, championships, cup etc., early notes are made regarding some of the general aspects of venue evaluation for the TC, planning process and team support service. These constitute the framework for building a cumulative briefing programme that will culminate with the TC preparation report for the final preparation year.

0–3 yrs   Recommendations would have been made in these notes/reviews and decisions taken on major expenditure items (e.g. holding camp – need for special adaptation training etc.). Co-ordination of resources are pursued, and links with key partners (e.g. National Olympic Committee) forged to prepare the ground for team support up to and at the TC; partnerships with businesses and sponsors wishing to offer support are established.

0–2 yrs   Lessons learned from Olympics, World Championships and Cups, Area Championships and Cups, Commonwealth Games, Age Group Championships, Internationals, etc. are constantly fed into the growing report. The reference framework in this is 'what can we do to make it work better for the athlete/team?'

0–1 yr   The TC preparation report is prepared and is operational. All reviews and reports will, in the first instance, go to the TC team management group (HC, team manager, team doctor, team administrator, HPD) if applicable and possibly also other national performance staff. The group will consider recommendations and make decisions based on these. Published reports will subsequently go to the athletes, personal coaches, team coaches, management, administration, performance support staff and press liaison.

The HC will go to the TC venue with the team administrator three to four days before the first wave of the team arrives. Athletes' entry to the village should be consistent both with what they are comfortable with and what the team management (and e.g. the National Olympic Committee general manager) considers acceptable within their rules and regulations.

EVALUATION OF THE VENUE AND PREVIEW FINAL YEAR

It is this that becomes the meat of the preparation report.

A simple checklist is worth following in evaluating a new venue and the specifics of a final run in to TC. Athletes must feel comfortable and not strange in the competition environment.

1. **Conditions**. Analysis of the conditions where competition is to take place is essential to inform management, coaching and support. Whereas conditions for indoor sports are clearly more readily controlled than outdoor, all conditions must find the athletes and teams equipped to cope with them.
   - Time change (1 day per hour plus 1)
   - Altitude (if significant – plan adaptation programme)
   - Temperature max–min each day and during competition times (if significant – plan adaptation programme)
   - Humidity (if significant – plan adaptation programme)
   - Intensity of sunlight (medical advice regarding protection factors and ensure applied in training or whenever exposed to sun)
   - Wind direction – in stadium and for roads and courses (where appropriate)
   - Sun's angle and shadow spread in stadium and for roads and courses (where appropriate) (sunglasses provided if necessary)
   - Rain patterns (possible kit implications)
   - Competition surfaces
   - Competition equipment
   - Indoor competition climate control
   - Unique competition area features

2. **Accommodation**. Athletes must have optimal conditions for rest and sleep.
   - Room-mates – ensure athletes are comfortable with the person they are sharing room with
   - Numbers per room (preferably two per room to be managed against programme)
   - Toilet/shower facilities
   - Length of beds – order 2m + as necessary and well in advance, also, mattress hardness/pillow filling and dimensions should be checked
   - Temperature in rooms/ventilation/air conditioning
   - Storage amenities (for safety as much as comfort)
   - Noise insulation
   - Opportunities to move athletes out of village/hotel when their competition is over

3. **Food** (in village)
   - Counsel athletes regarding overuse of 24-hour restaurant service
   - Athletes to check weight daily on team scales
   - Water (bottled) – hydration charts in all toilets
   - Variety/nature of meals – discourage experimentation – glycaemic index notes
   - Approved supplements – only those cleared by team doctor
   - Note: Athletes should not eat outside the village, nor take drinks with ice outside the village. If drinking outside the village – known brands only, or bottled water from the village.

4. **Training facilities.** Training facilities must be of such form and quality that permit athlete/team to effectively perform final rehearsal for the competition or to fine tune their fitness/conditioning/strength.
   - Conditioning – gymnasium range of machines and free weights and other equipment, etc.
   - Technique – surfaces/equipment same as competition?
   - Roads, courses, etc. – access, safety, competition routes?

- Learning/review – video material and statistical data from competition at accommodation area for post competition analysis every day for that day
- General, e.g. toilets, changing facilities, transport, security, communication, etc.

5. **Recreation and regeneration.** In the final days pre-competition or between rounds, the athlete must have the opportunity to maintain the right balance between the   physical, mental and emotional stimulus of the competition and recharging batteries in recovery.
   - In village – quiet rooms, etc.
   - Outside village – sanctuary – calming options – stimulating options
   - Programming – activities, music, movies, etc.

6. **Transport.** Travel carries its own set of stressors from comfort, mobility and dehydration to time adjustment and meeting timetable demands. All logistics must be understood and managed.
   - Travel from home country to venue – (logistics/times/duration)
   - Public – at venue as emergency fall back
   - Team – organisation buses and team car access
   - Transfer to airport – accreditation/village (duration, logistics)
   - Village – training (duration/logistics)
   - Village – stadium (duration/logistics)
   - Timetables for all transport as part of information pack for all team – and posted on team noticeboard

7. **Local Support Staff/Resources.** Team support often requires a greater number of persons than in official staff.
   - Families – facilitate family support, e.g. club venue, link to travel/accommodation/ticketing organisations
   - Supporters – cooperate with supporters' association club, e.g. 'Meet the team evening'
   - 'Aunties' – friends of the sport and local known persons who can afford personal support
   - 'Rest Houses'/sanctuary – havens for regeneration/recovery
   - Support committees – local organisations to provide team support programme
   - Relationship management – build and maintain strong partnerships across greater team population
   - When abroad embassies or consular offices can be a most valuable resource. They often will offer an evening reception.

8. **The TC headquarters support services.** In Olympics, Commonwealth Games, other multi-sport games, and major international championships/cups it is necessary for management to work closely with general national and/or international management. A sense of partnership is required.
   - Administration and relationship to team management
   - Pre TC training and orientation regarding games/championships organisation
   - National/international management relationship to team management
   - Central medical relationship to team medical staff and ease of access when required
   - Meetings in situ – daily as briefing to all team management, coaching and support staff

9. **Village amenities.**
   - Geography – walk through with athletes and staff on arrival
   - Services – establish a complement for those not provided as required

- Medical – to be identified as emergency back-up – this includes dentist, optician etc.
- Restaurant(s) – (see previous caution regarding use)
- Shops (and local shopping)
- Distractions – village life itself can be a distraction – establish guidelines
- Information – where is the technical information accessed daily and, information centre? Know them well (keep personnel sweet!)

10. **Communication.** Keep all who must be in the loop informed as planning and operations progress ensuring all intelligence is clear, transparent, open and consistent with national federation policy and practice.
    - Routine:
        - Years 0–4, 0–3 quarterly team and preparation news update
        - Year 0–2 monthly team and preparation news update
        - Year 0–1 fortnightly team and preparation news update
        - News flashes/breaking news as appropriate
    - Staff briefings – following team management group meetings (all staff)
    - Preparation report – produced at commencement of annual preparation cycle
    - TC team meeting – purpose and frequency and protocols
    - TC staff briefings/debriefings – daily pre breakfast
    - In competition – staff mobile/radio contact
    - Trouble shooting strategy – regarding appeals, injuries, accidents, anti-doping, discipline issues, etc.
    - Daily team programme – produced and distributed each night
    - Team policy reference:
        - i. communication conduits – e-form, printed form, phone
        - ii. social media policy, e.g. team confidentialities and at TC
    - Strategy regarding athlete entourage
    - Press and media briefings – routine, pre TC and during TC
    - Post competition – immediate athlete/team debrief; post TC observations, analysis, recommendations

11. **Local pests/hazards.** All possible issues regarding health and wellbeing and other performance threats must be understood, analysed and prepared for.
    - Medical – thorough intelligence regarding exposure to health risks and protection
    - Physiological – adaptation/acclimatisation requirements
    - Physical – general safety and security
    - Daily health/wellbeing check to ensure no secrets nor surprises

12. **Camps and courses.** Preparation for the team is a continuous process of learning fast from experience and realigning or revising. So in any year there are camps, courses, clinics, etc. To ensure timely briefing and debriefings, each camp etc. must have an agreed purpose within the process. In the final year each is focussed on fine tuning preparation for the TC wherever possible, procedures protocols, etc. should be rehearsal for how things will be at the TC. This 'familiarisation' reduces probability of distraction when all energies must be channelled on performance.
    - Specific focus in camps, courses, clinics:
        - i. athlete/team preparation/orientation

       ii. team management training/orientation
       iii. coach CPD/orientation
       iv. SSMP CPD/orientation
       v. regeneration and recovery
       vi. adaptation and acclimatisation (where relevant)
- Potential holding camp (where applicable)
       i. location (distance from competition venue)
       ii. relevant 1–11 (above)
       iii. economics
       iv. transfer from holding camp to venue and timing

13. **Competitions.** Each competition in the athlete/team calendar is on the one hand an end in itself in terms of agreed specific objectives, but on the other a stepping stone of learning experience in preparation for the TC. So the competition opportunity must be there, ordered within a season, then season on season to accommodate each level of athlete/team development needs. There must be a sense of relating each competition to the rhythm and cycle which will prepare the athlete/team to deliver 'on the day' – whatever that day brings in the shape of conditions and circumstances.

14. **Selection policy.** The purpose of selection policy is to ensure that the athletes/team most competent to effectively address the challenge of the TC or other international competition on behalf of the nation, are/is selected. Ideally, selection commences with a selection matrix, based on performance structure, for a progressive squad system.
- No compromise – this principle must not be compromised by inflexible rules. There must be margin for discretion and professional judgement.
- Focus
       i. Athlete/team challenging for gold
       ii. Athlete/team challenging for silver
       iii. Athlete/team challenging for bronze
       iv. Athlete/team challenging for top eight
       v. Athlete/team competing with distinction in delivering season's or lifetime best on the day whether i–iv or missing out on final eight
       vi. Young potential high achiever athlete who will learn from the experience
- Squads matrix – different matrices for regional – national – TC
       i. Build in reflection of performance structure
       ii. Apply judgement to high potential performers outside matrices
- Team staff
       i. all team staff are appointed by team management group
       ii. team managers and administrators are trained for these roles
       iii. team SSMP are trained for these roles
       iv. team coaching staff are selected by HC on basis of delivering the performance end game and competence to draw intelligence from experience for benefit of review and planning for next TC.

15. **Team kit and personal equipment.** The importance of kit, from competition clothing and footwear to weatherproof clothing, cannot be overstated. Consultation with athletes and thorough researching of

manufacturers against the specific environmental demands is part of the preparation programme. This also applies to technical equipment for the discipline. It is management's responsibility to arrange safe and timely passage of technical equipment from home to venue and return.

EVALUATION OF THE COMPETITION

The TC in a given year must be viewed as representing for athletes and team the highest priority competition – the primary focus of all preparation and competition. As such the TC will represent high pressure, yet the quality of preparation for the team should have each athlete comfortably seeing it as 'just another competition'. There is a balancing act here between harnessing the excitement of the occasion and remaining focused.

A SIMPLE CHECKLIST:

- Dates
- Venue
- Time frame
- Timetable – including technical meeting
- Official TC qualifying standards
- Prognosis of performances for gold, silver, bronze, final 8 (if quantifiable)
- Principle opposition intelligence
- Warm-up arrangements
- Reporting arrangements
- Technical equipment (where relevant)
- Language critical terms used
- Course maps (where relevant)
- TC – specific rules

The preparation report: The preparation report is produced annually for the TCs of a given season. It is the final outcome of a four year process. Its content sets out essential preparation input for the athlete/team and their coaches and posts intent on preparation for the team. It should also invite input from athletes and coaches to enrich the preparation process.

The contents will include:

1. Introduction and 4-year rolling calendar

2. Fixture/competition list for forthcoming season and selection dates

3. General and TC selection dates

4. TC1 detail – this is the top priority championships for the national federation

5. TC2 detail (there may be more than one major target competition) – this is the next level of priority. If other TCs, they are dealt with in turn and in detail.

6. Junior and/or other TC championship detail for national federation or professional club operating at this level. If no championships, then the key international or national event. Note: each TC detail will include:
   - Competition title
   - Venue
   - Dates
   - Travel
   - Accommodation
   - Timetable
   - Qualifying standards
   - Time change
   - Temperature/humidity
   - Altitude (if applicable)
   - Competition specifics (if applicable)
   - Previous national performance
   - Performance prognosis
   - Accreditation (extra)
     1. General information regarding season
     2. Contact persons and details.

RECOMMENDATIONS AND ACTION

Once all relevant intelligence is gathered and evaluation is in place the HC and the HPD or relevant SSMP should work together (where applicable) to draw up recommendations for action. All recommendations are based on the idea that we should endeavour to have the athletes enjoy a final run-in to competition in an environment, which is as close to 'normal' as possible. This has given birth to the idea of a 'holding camp'. This means that while helping aid recovery, for example, after a very long and tiring air journey; recovery through jet lag; adaptation to time change; and topping up on previous acclimatisation to high temperature and high humidity, the athlete is spared the 'hype' of the village until he is ready for it.

On the one hand the recommendations are aimed at performance related matters, and on the other at organisational and administration matters. Once decisions are made by the team management group, relevant action is taken. All performance related matters are followed through by the HC.

The preparation report is prepared, published and circulated as early as possible so that coaches and athletes can have guidance in that preparation.

PRE-COMPETITION

The holding camp situation permits personal coaches to join team coaches in affording a coaching service through to entry into the village. This helps ensure a stable preparation environment as late as possible. In team sport situations holding camps should only involve team staff.

Delegation of discipline or technical-specific duties ensures that each athlete's final days are overseen. Team coaches share responsibility with management in keeping as close a personal contact with athletes as the situation requires. In team situations this is fundamental; in non-team situations it requires sensitive handling to fit individual needs.

The need to 'escape from' or to 'join with' the main group should be spotted through such contact. Essential team communication must be maintained.

Recreation support and technical feedback can both be via video/TV. PCs, videos, DVDs etc. should be brought in, with TV or PC providing transmitted material for coaches and athletes to examine when occasion permits.

Each athlete will be requested on selection to arrange with their personal coach to bring a personal training programme to the holding camp. This should apply, even if the coach is accompanying the athlete. This will on the one hand help in meeting athletes' training requirements, and on the other afford valuable insight into each coach's concept of the 'end game' of preparation.

Movement from holding camp to the TC athletes village must be decided on the basis of personal preference timetable and transport logistics.

In those locations which are within 2–3 hours travel from home, the concept of a 'holding camp' does not have a strong argument. The 'normal' or 'home' environment is real when at home! On the other hand, if there is immense media and other pressure, it may be sensible to have a remote base should athletes require it.

It is strongly recommended that even in this very commercial age, athletes/team should have no promotional obligations in the six week run in to the TC. The only focus should be on preparation for, and delivery of, performance.

ON THE DAY

This is 'countdown time' from the organisation point of view and 'being available time' from the coaching point of view.

Countdown

- Breakfast/lunch details
- Check onto bus/accompany
- Check into warm-up
- Check out of warm-up
- Report/accompany
- Competition time
- Meet post competition to support and constructively debrief

Be available:

- At breakfast/lunch
- Warm-up
- Coach/advise
- Rest/quiet place
- Shade

- Information
- Back-up
- Inter-round
- After competition – whatever the result

But most important – it is 'be positive time'. 'This is your day' – right through to positive evaluation when it's over. Review and evaluation is not about judgement, it is about learning. Review must take place as soon as possible after the competition for athlete and team. Overall review of the athlete and team preparation from the perspective of the athlete, coach, national performance team coach and plan should be completed within six weeks of TC conclusion.

This whole business of preparation for the team is about giving each athlete the best chance to give his or her best possible shot. It is about snakes (getting rid of the things that prevent best performance on the day) and ladders (ensuring that those things which make the best shot happen are provided).

THE LAST STEP INTO THE ARENA OF THIS CHAMPIONSHIP IS THE FIRST TOWARDS THE NEXT

The consequence of delivering the four-year strategy in preparation of and for the athlete and team for a major target competition campaign is measured in performance and results in the arena. Just as there is learning through review built into the cyclic process of Dream – Plan – Do – Review for athlete and team (see page 164 and figure 10.3) and strategy in general in pursuit of agreed objectives – OPERA (page 223), so also for the four-year strategy. Role and responsibilities of all who have been involved in its design and/or delivery must be evaluated in the review and debrief programme.

The seven review headings are:

- Results – intended and actual
- Performance under pressure of athletes and teams
- Professional competence of all staff – coaching, management, administration and performance support
- Effectiveness of athlete and team staff in preparation planning
- Effectiveness of overall campaign strategy/current year plan/applied game plan
- Leverage of high performance intelligence and resources, e.g. systems and technology
- Quality of chief coach decision making and judgement calls

In addressing these headings, six fundamental points in preparation for the next four-year strategy are:

1. Extrapolated numbers for winning results, performance and components of future performance
2. Perceived successful technical training and tactical trends
3. Effectiveness in preparation and in the arena
4. Strengths and vulnerabilities
5. What could be done differently and what different things can be done to perform better and gain competitive advantage next time
6. Identify the people who will grow a winning dynasty.

In terms of timescale – a full report with action recommendations based on debrief analysis should be completed within six weeks of the major target competition and the next four-year strategy be in place after a further six weeks.

SUMMARY

Sports Training Principles hopefully helps shape quality decision making in a process which takes an athlete from beginner to high performance in major championships.

The performance quality of the athletes in a TC, then in future TCs will be governed by how well they have been prepared to express their talents on the day; and how totally their preparation and competition environment in these competition venues permits such expression. Appendix D will help in this.

Preparation for the team aims to establish, through strong partnerships, the right environment in TCs and informed counsel leading through to selection and final approach. Appendix E will help in this. Preparation of the athlete aims to create the right climate of motivation and a custom-built preparation programme through to the final test in the TC arena. Appendix F will help in this.

Everyone involved has a role to play within the preparation team – not only for the immediate TCs but for all those to follow. That role means a responsibility! One that can only be accepted by those who believe in themselves and in what can be achieved by our athletes when they are afforded the support they deserve. I know we each have a positive self-belief and that we believe in the character and talents of our athletes. The responsibility, then, is ours to accept by living the principle that we are each accountable for what we do and how we do it.

REFLECTIVE QUESTIONS

1. Design a strategy for creating the intelligence you need to prepare the best supportive environment for athletes and staff in your team for the World Junior Championships (U/20) in your chosen sport (or in a sport which has World or Area Junior Championships). Assume that venue and date are known four years in advance.

2. The debrief following an Olympic Games or World Championships comes at the end of a four to six year campaign. So there are many people, positions and parts of the sport and its partners who have been involved. Design a strategy that will deliver the depth and detail of review and debrief necessary to prepare for the next campaign.

3. List the people and positions who will have possible input to the content of appendices D, E and F per item.

4. Following consultation with SSMPs, suggest an appendix G.

5. Prepare recommendation for a social media agreement for all members – athletes and staff at a major championship. What are the advantages and disadvantages of proposing such an agreement throughout the year?

SUMMARY OF PART 5

When planning the athlete's annual training programme, the coach must have access to a considerable volume of information and also have the ability to interpret this in the light of current training theory. The structure of this programme begins to take its final shape during the transition macrocycle at the conclusion of the previous competition season. However, this is not to say that the programme is inflexible. The coach must appreciate the dynamic nature of his work and be prepared, where appropriate, to make any necessary adjustment within the structure. Information required by the coach is as follows:

1. He should know the programme of competition available to the athlete or team and the precise nature of each competition.
2. He should know how to plan the year to accommodate the best competition programme for the athlete's development and/or the team's.
3. He should know the theoretical distribution of general, related and specific training in each mesocycle of the year.
4. He should know the number of training units and the training environment available to the athlete or team.
5. He should know the relevant training practices, structures of loading and training ratios for development of specific fitness each athlete requires to meet his training objectives.
6. He should know the principles of unit, microcycle, mesocycle and macrocycle construction, and their variations according to its position in the annual cycle.
7. He should apply the 11-step approach on pages 368–70.

The final product should reflect the coach's interpretation of training theory and application of experience in a programme designed to meet the unique needs of an athlete to persistently perform better than before.

The athlete's fundamental objective in sport is pursuit of competitive advantage. It represents a serious commitment of time and effort, but is nevertheless undertaken for the pleasure which that commitment brings. To be invited to direct the athlete's growth and development in sport is a great honour; to accept that invitation is to acknowledge an immense responsibility. The coach must know that his work with the athlete will provide a systematic progression towards his fundamental objective, while contributing to his total wellbeing. Such knowledge is born of an understanding of those areas of study which feed into the science of sport as outlined in parts 1, 2 and 3, and of an appreciation of how these relate to the athlete via training theory, as presented in parts 4 and 5. It is my belief that when the coach thoughtfully weaves this knowledge into the fabric of practical experience, the athlete must certainly achieve his fundamental objective. The athlete's life in sport will, then, be a purposeful and enjoyable experience which will add a lasting richness to his life outside sport. Moreover, the visionary coach will not only contribute to the athlete's or team's lifetime achievements, but will learn through the experience to contribute to establishing a dynasty of excellence.

REFERENCES FOR PART 5

Carl, G. *Gewichtheben*. Berlin: Sportverlag. (1967)

Endemann, F. 'Throws conditioning'. *4th Coaches' Convention Report*. (1973)

Gundlach, H. 'Zur Trainierbarkeit der Kraft und Schnelligkeitsfahigkeiten Im Prozess der Korperlichen Vervollkommnung'. *Theorie Und Praxis Der Korperkultur* 17. (1968)

Harre, D. *Trainingslehre*. Berlin: Sportverlag. (1973)

Hettinger, T. *Isometric Muskelkrafttraining*. Stuttgart: Thieme. (1968)

Hollmann, N. and Venrath, H. 'Experimentelle Untersuchungen zur Bedeutung Eines Trainings Unterhalb Und Oberhalb Der Dauerbelastunsgrenze'. In *W.u.a., 'Carl Diem Festschrift'*. Frankfurt. (1962)

Israel, S. 'Das Akute Entlastungssyndrom'. *Theorie Und Praxis Der Korperkultur* 12. (1963)

Matveyev, L. P. *Die Periodisierung, Des Sportlicher Trainings*. Moscow: Fiskultura i Sport. (1965)

Noakes T. D. 'Fatigue is a brain-derived emotion that regulates the exercise behavior to ensure the protection of the whole body homeostasis'. *Frontiers in Physiology* 3: 82. (2012)

Osolin, N. G. and Markov, D. P. *Distribution of Training* (part translation from Russian). Moscow: Lehka Atletika. (1972)

Puni, A. Z. *Abriss Der Sportspsychologie*. Berlin: Sportverlag. (1961)

Schultz, H. H. *Das Autogene Training*. Stuttgart: Konzentrative Selbstentspannung. (1956)

Ter-Ovanesyan, I. 'Ter-Ovanesyan on the long jump'. *Modern Athlete and Coach* 4(4). (1965)

Thiess, G. 'Wettkampfhaufigkeit Im Nachwuchstraining'. *Theorie Und Praxis Der Korperkultur* 16. (1967)

Yakovlev, M. M., *Sport Biomechanic*, Leipzig: J. A. Barth (1977), in vol 14 of Sportmedizinische Schriftenreihe

BIBLIOGRAPHY

Bauersfeld, M. and Voss, G. 'Neue wege im schnelligkeitsteaincing'. *Trainer Bibliotek* 28. (1992)

Bellotti, P. 'A few aspects of the theory and practice of speed development'. *New Studies in Athletics* 6(1). (1991)

Bonov, P. *2nd International Scientific Congress Report: Sport, Stress, Adaptation*. Sofia: National Sports Academy. (2001)

Bosco, C. 'Eine neue methodic zur eimschatzung und programmierung des trainings'. *Leistungssport* 22(5): 21–8. (1992)

Craig, T. 'Analysis of female athletic injury frequency'. *4th Coaches' Convention Report*. (1973)

Dick, F. W. 'Foundation of jumps development and initial conditioning'. *Proceedings of EACA Congress, Berlin*. (1993)

Donati, A. 'The development of stride length frequency in sprinting'. *New Studies in Athletics* 10(1). (1995)

Gladwell, M. *Blink*. London: Penguin. (2006)

Hettinger, T. and Müller, E. A. 'Muskelleistung und Muskeltraining'. *Arbeitsphysiologie* 15: 111–26. (1953)

Karvonen, M. J., Kentala, E. and Mustala, O. 'The effects of training on heart rate'. *Annales Medicinae experimentalis et Biologae Fenniag* 35. (1957)

Kruger, A. 'Periodisation or peaking at the right time'. *Track Technique* December. (1973)

Machak, M. 'Relaxacne–Aktivacni, Autoregulacni Zasah, Metoda Nacviku a Psychologicka Charackteristika'. *Czechoslovakian Psychology* 3. (1964)

Mah, C. D., Mah, K. E., Kezirian, E. J. and Dement, W. C. 'The effects of sleep extension on the athletic performance of collegiate basketball players'. *Sleep* 34(7): 943–50. (2011)

Matveyev, L. P. 'Die Dynamic Der Belastungun Im Sportlichen Training'. *Theorie Und Praxis Der Korperkultur* 11. (1962)

Prindle, D. '5 easy ways to track your sleep habits with technology'. Available at www.digitaltrends.com/home/5-different-ways-track-sleep-get-better-rest (accessed 16 January 2014). (2014)

Reilly, T. and Edwards, B. 'Altered sleep–wake cycles and physical performance in athletes'. *Physiological Behaviour* 90(2–3): 274–84. (2007)

Samuels, C. 'Sleep, recovery and performance: The new frontier in high-performance athletics'. *Neurologic Clinics* 26(1): 169–80. (2008)

Samuels, C. 'Sleep, recovery and human performance: Developing a comprehensive psychometric sleep screening program for Canadian athletes'. *SIRCuit* 2(1). (2011)

Schiffer, J. 'Overtraining'. *New Studies in Athletics* 9(3). (1994)

Schmolinksy, G. *Leichtathletic*. 7th edn. Berlin: Sportverlag. (1974)

Sinkkonen, K. 'The programming of distance running'. Paper presented to ELLV Congress, Budapest. (1975)

Vanek, M. and Cratty, B. J. *Psychology and the Superior Athlete*. Toronto: Macmillan. (1970)

Walton, G. M. *Beyond Winning*. Champaign, IL: Leisure Press. (1992)

Zhelyazkon, T. and Dasheva, D. *Training and Adaption in Sport*. Sofia: Digital. (2001)

APPENDIX A

Please visit bloomsbury.com/9781472905277 and follow the link under online resources to download and print these forms.

POST-RACE DEBRIEF: ATHLETE

Competition: _____   Time/Placing/Splits (if possible)

Event: _____   Heat: _____

Date: _____   Semi: _____

Race Conditions: _____   Final: _____

_____

Overall I am satisfied with my performance for this event.   ☐ Yes   ☐ No   ☐ Partially

Psychological Debrief: *Rate on a scale of 0–6 (0 = not at all and 6 = very much)*

Pre-Race I felt

1. Physically warmed up	0 1 2 3 4 5 6	6. Feelings of anxiety 0 1 2 3 4 5 6
2. Healthy	0 1 2 3 4 5 6	7. Worried about performance 0 1 2 3 4 5 6
3. Mentally prepared	0 1 2 3 4 5 6	8. Distracted 0 1 2 3 4 5 6
4. Eager to race	0 1 2 3 4 5 6	9. Focused 0 1 2 3 4 5 6
5. Confident	0 1 2 3 4 5 6	10. Technically prepared 0 1 2 3 4 5 6

During the Race   **Comments**

1. I found myself thinking of unrelated things   0 1 2 3 4 5 6   _____

2. I was able to focus on my race plan   0 1 2 3 4 5 6   _____

3. I was able to use emotions to my advantage   0 1 2 3 4 5 6   _____

4. I felt overwhelmed and not confident   0   1   2   3   4   5   6   _____

5. I let my focus drift to others around me   0   1   2   3   4   5   6   _____

Technical Debrief: *Rate on a scale of 0–6 (0 = extremely poor and 6 = excellent)*

Start/Transition/First 1/5th of the race   0   1   2   3   4   5   6
Comments:

_____

_____

_____

Middle section (100–400, 200–800)   0   1   2   3   4   5   6
Comments:

_____

_____

_____

Last 100m/200m/Finish   0   1   2   3   4   5   6
Comments:

_____

_____

_____

What parts of my performance went really well? Why?

_____

_____

_____

What parts of my performance can be improved?

_____

_____

_____

_____

_____

Is there anything I would like to improve about the way I approach my preparation or performances (attitude, perspective, focus, consistency, level of intensity, or state of relaxation)?

_____

_____

_____

_____

Actions: Based on the above evaluation, list the necessary steps that you will take in order to improve your performance. What can I do better today to improve my performance and prepare to perform my best in my next performance?

_____

_____

_____

_____

_____

_____

_____

APPENDIX B

POST-RACE DEBRIEF: COACH

Competition: _____

Time/Placing/Splits (if possible)

Event: _____

Heat: _____

Date: _____

Semi: _____

Race Conditions: _____

Final: _____

_____

Overall I am satisfied with my athlete's for this event.　☐ Yes　☐ No　☐ Partially

Psychological Debrief: *Rate on a scale of 0–6 (0 = not at all and 6 = very much)*

Pre-Race I felt　　　　　　　　　　　　　　　　　　**Comments**

1. My athlete was prepared　　　　0　1　2　3　4　5　6　_____

2. My athlete was focused　　　　　0　1　2　3　4　5　6　_____

3. My athlete was calm and ready　0　1　2　3　4　5　6　_____

During the race I felt　　　　　　　　　　　　　　　**Comments**

1. My athlete executed the race plan　0　1　2　3　4　5　6　_____

2. My athlete was focused　　　　　　0　1　2　3　4　5　6　_____

3. My athlete was nervous　　　　　　0　1　2　3　4　5　6　_____

Technical Debrief: *Rate on a scale of 0–6 (0 = extremely poor and 6 = excellent)*

Start/Transition/First 1/5th of the race   0   1   2   3   4   5   6
Comments:

_____

_____

_____

Middle section (100–400, 200–800)   0   1   2   3   4   5   6
Comments:

_____

_____

_____

Last 100m/200m/Finish   0   1   2   3   4   5   6
Comments:

_____

_____

_____

What parts of the performance went really well? Why?

_____

_____

_____

_____

What parts of the performance can be improved?

_____

_____

_____

_____

Actions: Based on the above evaluation, list the steps that you consider essential to take in order to improve performance.

_____

_____

_____

_____

_____

_____

_____

_____

APPENDIX C

ATHLETE PREPARATION PLAN

Athlete: _____   Position/Discipline: _____   DoB: _____

Result Target: _____   Performance Target: _____

Current Status: _____   Current Status: _____

Result Prognoses

	For Target Competition	Challenge(s)	Current Performance Challenge(s)
Gold	_____	_____	_____
Silver	_____	_____	_____
Bronze	_____	_____	_____
8th	_____	_____	_____
Personal Best	_____	_____	_____

Key Performance Determinants (KPDs) and KPD Measures/Scoring (M/S)

KPD	M/S	KPD	M/S
1. _____	_____	5. _____	_____
2. _____	_____	6. _____	_____
3. _____	_____	7. _____	_____
4. _____	_____	8. _____	_____

Month on Month Progress History

Month/Year	Year				Year				Year				Year			
	Perf	KPD1	KPD2	KPD3	Perf	KPD1	KPD2	KPD3	Perf	KPD1	KPD2	KPD3	Perf	KPD1	KPD2	KPD3

Summary (as basis of performance structure)

Best Performance _____   Performance Target _____   Current Performance Status _____

KPD1 KPD2 KPD3   KPD1 KPD2 KPD3   KPD1 KPD2 KPD3

____ ____ ____   ____ ____ ____   ____ ____ ____

Current Annual Cycle Plan
Intended (I) v Action (A)

Month	Performance Progression		KPD1		KPD2		KPD3	
	I	A	I	A	I	A	I	A
_____	_____	_____	_____	_____	_____	_____	_____	_____
_____	_____	_____	_____	_____	_____	_____	_____	_____
_____	_____	_____	_____	_____	_____	_____	_____	_____
_____	_____	_____	_____	_____	_____	_____	_____	_____
_____	_____	_____	_____	_____	_____	_____	_____	_____
_____	_____	_____	_____	_____	_____	_____	_____	_____
_____	_____	_____	_____	_____	_____	_____	_____	_____
_____	_____	_____	_____	_____	_____	_____	_____	_____
_____	_____	_____	_____	_____	_____	_____	_____	_____
_____	_____	_____	_____	_____	_____	_____	_____	_____
_____	_____	_____	_____	_____	_____	_____	_____	_____
_____	_____	_____	_____	_____	_____	_____	_____	_____

Preparation Components

	At Plan Commencement	Retest Date	Retest Date
Technique(s)	**Assessment:** 7 (high) – 1 (low)		
Optimal biomechanical model	_____	_____	_____
Effective execution	_____	_____	_____
Robust under pressure	_____	_____	_____
Analysis frequency	_____	_____	_____
Analysis process	_____	_____	_____

Conditioning

	At Plan		
		Commencement	**Retest Date**	**Retest Date**

Assessment: 7 (high) – 1 (low)

Strength	General (basic)	_____	_____	_____
	General (balance)	_____	_____	_____
	General (max)	_____	_____	_____
	Specific (max)	_____	_____	_____
Endurance	General (aerobic)	_____	_____	_____
	Specific (strength/endurance)	_____	_____	_____
	Specific (speed/endurance)	_____	_____	_____
Speed	General co-ordination (agility)	_____	_____	_____
	General (decisions)	_____	_____	_____
	Specific (max/race/in play)	_____	_____	_____
Mobility	General (all joint)	_____	_____	_____
	Specific (posture/competition)	_____	_____	_____

Tactical

	At Plan		
		Commencement	**Retest Date**	**Retest Date**
Strong in: _____		_____	_____	_____
Vulnerable in: _____		_____	_____	_____
Options: _____		_____	_____	_____

Assessment: 7 (high) – 1 (low)

	At Plan		
		Commencement	**Retest Date**	**Retest Date**
Tactical delivery focus:		_____	_____	_____
Effective response to opposition tactic:		_____	_____	_____

Health and Wellbeing

Height: _____

	At Plan Commencement	Retest Date	Retest Date
	Amber/Red	Amber/Red	Amber/Red
Conditions (e.g. diabetic/allergies)	_____	_____	_____
Illness _____ _____ _____			
Hot spots (musculo/skeletal weaknesses	_____	_____	_____
Injuries	_____	_____	_____
HR (resting)	_____	_____	_____
Bodyweight	_____	_____	_____
Hours/night quality sleep	_____	_____	_____
Hydration	_____	_____	_____
Dental status	_____	_____	_____
Optical status	_____	_____	_____
Aural status	_____	_____	_____
Medications	_____	_____	_____

Physiology

Nutrition analysis	_____	_____	_____
Nutrient status	_____	_____	_____
Nutrient allergies	_____	_____	_____
Full blood biochemistry	_____	_____	_____
Urinalysis	_____	_____	_____
Respiration capacities	_____	_____	_____
Aerobic capacities	_____	_____	_____
Lactate/metabolite tolerance	_____	_____	_____
Testosterone/cortisol	_____	_____	_____
Immunoglobin A (IgA)	_____	_____	_____
Heat adaptation	_____	_____	_____
Day humidity	_____	_____	_____
Pollution/hypoxia adaptation	_____	_____	_____
Time change management	_____	_____	_____
_____ :	_____	_____	_____

Psychology

Attitude/motivation (profiles of resilience, drive, focus etc.)

	At Plan Commencement	**Retest Date**	**Retest Date**
	Amber/Red	*Amber/Red*	*Amber/Red*
General	_____	_____	_____
Training	_____	_____	_____
Pre-competition: In lead (up)	_____	_____	_____
In pursuit (down)	_____	_____	_____
Start	_____	_____	_____
Main body of competition	_____	_____	_____
Finish	_____	_____	_____
Post competition	_____	_____	_____
Crisis management	_____	_____	_____
Lifestyle balance	_____	_____	_____
Personality profile	_____	_____	_____
Coach/athlete relationship debrief	_____	_____	_____
_____	_____	_____	_____

Technology

For discipline or for performance

Support

_____   _____   _____   _____

_____   _____   _____   _____

_____   _____   _____   _____

_____   _____   _____   _____

_____   _____   _____   _____

Analysis   _____   _____   _____

Feedback   _____   _____   _____

Optimal training venue/equipment   _____   _____   _____

Technician support   _____   _____   _____

Opponent Analysis

Technique   _____   _____   _____

Conditioning   _____   _____   _____

Tactics   _____   _____   _____

Health/wellbeing   _____   _____   _____

Physiology   _____   _____   _____

Psychology   _____   _____   _____

Technology   _____   _____   _____

Strong in   _____   _____   _____

Vulnerable in   _____   _____   _____

APPENDIX D

MAJOR CHAMPIONSHIP PREPARATION CHECKLIST

Athlete

	PERSON RESPONSIBLE	TARGET BY	COMMENTS	COMPLETED
TECHNICAL				
Personal training				
Year plan and competitions				
Championships programmes				
Selection – championship programme				
Opposition/challenge intelligence				
Championships performance focus				
Self monitoring discipline				
Injury/illness/wellbeing controls				
TEAM				
Selection agreement				
Team agreement				
Team code of conduct				

	PERSON RESPONSIBLE	TARGET BY	COMMENTS	COMPLETED
Teamship preparation and commitment				
Team priorities				
Buddy system				
VILLAGE				
Eating/hydration discipline				
Daily weigh-in				
Preferred room mate				
Family/friends issues				
Daily routine planning				
Distraction management				
OCCASION				
Pressure/anxiety management				
Media training and discipline				
Social/community responsibilities				
Life balance through championships preparation – no big changes				

APPENDIX E

MAJOR CHAMPIONSHIP PREPARATION CHECKLIST

Manager (and administrator)

	PERSON RESPONSIBLE	TARGET BY	COMMENTS	COMPLETED
TECHNICAL				
Camps and competitions logistics and administration				
Technical equipment collection/ transport/delivery				
Team entry for championships with CEO				
Daily athlete entries per event				
Athlete reporting for event				
Official technical pre-championships paperwork				
Technical meeting preparation				
Crisis management				
Appeals process with CD				
Official kit/equipment check				
Anti-doping process with team doctor				

	PERSON RESPONSIBLE	TARGET BY	COMMENTS	COMPLETED
VILLAGE				
Team maintenance and support services in championships				
Team purpose, policies, roles, responsibilities				
Team communications system				
Liaison and meetings with general team management (if relevant)				
Policy re mobile phones, laptops, social media, etc.				
Manage media pressure/ attention				
Media relations contact person				
Policy re entourage and relationship management				
Manage balance between sponsor commitments & training/preparation				
Manage team v athlete personal network situations				
Ticketing issues process				
Daily routine planning including 'time out'				
Accommodation management				
Weighing scales provision				

	PERSON RESPONSIBLE	TARGET BY	COMMENTS	COMPLETED
Complementary accommodation items				
Village life briefing				
Village recreation/leisure programme (with athlete group)				
Entry dates into village and orientation				
Accreditation procedures – team and personal coaches				
General relationship management and team agreement compliance				
Conflict resolution processes				
Rotation plan in dining with team members				
Role in daily competition schedule				
'Being there' for athletes and all staff				
GENERAL				
Team management training and CPD				
Championships management experience				
Team management group involvement				
Transport and logistics through year and at championships (official and team transport)				

	PERSON RESPONSIBLE	TARGET BY	COMMENTS	COMPLETED
Staff and team meetings, planning and programming				
Policy re media relationships and statements				
Media briefings and 'enlightenment'				
Athletes and staff media training				
Distraction management briefing (over year and in championships)				
Strategy re team member protection from outside threats to focus				
Provisions, expenses, etc.				
Team noticeboard				
OCCASION				
Real/virtual pre experience				
Pressure/anxiety management				
National federation media strategy				
Social/community responsibilities during and post championships				
Official team events – opening/ closing ceremony, embassy visits, photographs.				

APPENDIX F

MAJOR CHAMPIONSHIP PREPARATION CHECKLIST

Coach – national (HC and staff)

	PERSON RESPONSIBLE	TARGET BY	COMMENTS	COMPLETED
TECHNICAL				
CPD plan – personal				
Championships experience				
Comprehensive intelligence of championships				
Camps strategy/planning (including holding camp)				
Selection preparation and selection				
Coach–athlete year plan support/ guidance (training/competition/ recovery)				
Coach–athlete championship briefing				
Coach–athlete in–championship support (coach present)				
Coach–athlete championship debriefing				
Technical meeting preparation				
In championships video/ notational analysis and performance reviews				

	PERSON RESPONSIBLE	TARGET BY	COMMENTS	COMPLETED
Training programmes management/supervision in holding champ and championships				
Conditions adaption/ acclimatisation planning (if appropriate)				
Athlete and coaching staff regeneration/recovery planning and facilitation in championships				
Daily competition schedule for athletes and all support staff				
Inter-round briefings/debriefings with athlete (and coach if present)				
Coaching staff meetings				
Overall technical review of championships, observations and recommendations, etc. and preparation of technical report				
Crisis management				
Appeals process with manager				
TEAM				
Team management				
Team code of conduct				
Management teamship preparation and commitment				
Team training, tactics, tournament strategy				
Team meeting preparation				

	PERSON RESPONSIBLE	TARGET BY	COMMENTS	COMPLETED
VILLAGE				
Eating/hydration discipline				
Daily weigh-in				
Personal coach accreditation				
Personal coach liaison				
Daily routine planning including 'time out'				
Learning on the move				
Professional networking				
'Being there' for athletes and coaches				
Communications plan for rapid contact and intelligence distribution				
Technical information access				
Team management meetings				
Rotation plan in dining with team members				
OCCASION				
Real/virtual pre experience				
Pressure/anxiety management				
National federation media strategy				
Social/community/PR/media responsibilities during and post championships				
Leverage to enrich national coach development programmes				

INDEX

Note: page numbers in *italic* indicate figures and tables.